Conscience and Critic

Conscience and Critic: The Selected Works of Keith Tudor brings together 35 years of Keith Tudor's finest contributions to the field of mental health. Covering a wide range of subjects that encompass psychotherapy, social policy and positive mental health or wellbeing, Keith reflects on practice and theory from his wealth of experience in various fields of practice, including probation, counselling, field, hospital and psychiatric social work, psychotherapy, supervision, and education and training.

Over the span of his professional career, Keith's concerns and contributions have focused on the interface between psyche and society. This is reflected in his writings on the politics of disability, mental health reform, class-conscious therapeutic practice, the application and critique of theory, health and professional regulation and registration.

Conscience and Critic will be of interest to psychotherapists and mental health practitioners, as well as students of psychotherapy.

Keith Tudor is professor of psychotherapy and head of the School of Public Health and Psychosocial Studies at Auckland University of Technology, Aotearoa New Zealand. He is the editor of *Psychotherapy and Politics International*, a fellow of the Critical Institute, an honorary senior research fellow at the University of Roehampton, London, and a visiting associate professor at the University of Primorska, Slovenia.

World Library of Mental Health series

The *World Library of Mental Health* celebrates the important contributions to mental health made by leading experts in their individual fields. Each author has compiled a career-long collection of what they consider to be their finest pieces: extracts from books, journals, articles, major theoretical and practical contributions, and salient research findings.

For the first time ever the work of each contributor is presented in a single volume so readers can follow the themes and progress of their work and identify the contributions made to, and the development of, the fields themselves.

Each book in the series features a specially written introduction by the contributor giving an overview of their career, contextualising their selection within the development of the field, and showing how their own thinking developed over time.

Titles in this series:

Towards a Radical Redefinition of Psychology – The Selected Works of Miller Mair
Edited by David Winter and Nick Reed

Living Archetypes – The Selected Works of Anthony Stevens
By Anthony Stevens

Soul: Treatment and Recovery – The Selected Works of Murray Stein
By Murray Stein

A Developmentalist's Approach to Research, Theory, and Therapy – The Selected Works of Joseph Lichtenberg
By Joseph D. Lichtenberg

Existential Psychotherapy and Counselling after Postmodernism: The Selected Works of Del Loewenthal
By Del Loewenthal

Love the Wild Swan: The Selected Works of Judith Edwards
By Judith Edwards

Conscience and Critic: The Selected Works of Keith Tudor
By Keith Tudor

Conscience and Critic

The Selected Works of Keith Tudor

Keith Tudor

Routledge
Taylor & Francis Group
LONDON AND NEW YORK

First published 2017
by Routledge
2 Park Square, Milton Park, Abingdon, Oxon OX14 4RN

and by Routledge
711 Third Avenue, New York, NY 10017

First issued in paperback 2018

Routledge is an imprint of the Taylor & Francis Group, an informa business

British Library Cataloguing in Publication Data
A catalogue record for this book is available from the British Library

Library of Congress Cataloguing in Publication Data
A catalog record for this book has been requested

ISBN 13: 978-1-138-20785-1 (pbk)
ISBN 13: 978-1-138-68236-8 (hbk)

Typeset in Sabon
by Out of House Publishing

To Louise – with thanks and love

CONTENTS

ACKNOWLEDGEMENTS

First, I wish to acknowledge Joanne Forshaw, my editor at Routledge, who I have known for the best part of 20 years. Over this time, I have appreciated her interest in and encouragement and support of my writing and various publishing projects; our lunches, still lovely, though more occasional, due to the fact that we now live in different hemispheres; and, specifically, her invitation to contribute to this series, which I regard as a great honour. Thank you.

Second, I wish to acknowledge and thank my wife, Louise Embleton Tudor, for her unfailing support for my writing. Over the past 27 years, which encompass all but two of the papers in this volume, she has seen and supported me: moving from someone who was uncertain about and unconfident in my ability to research and write, through the ups of successful publications and good sales (relative to the market), as well as the downs of losing chapters to my own technological shortcomings, rejections, bad reviews, hostile responses and even hate mail, to my current employment and success as an academic. We met (for the second time) in 1988 and soon realised that we wanted to be together. Within 2 years we applied for and were appointed to one position, that of a development and training officer (mental health), which we did on a job-share basis. From that time on, we have spent more of our professional life working together and alongside each other than not: we co-founded and then managed Temenos, Sheffield for some 17 years (eight of which with our colleague and friend Keemar Keemar); we have designed training courses together, and co-facilitated training groups; for 3 years, we worked as co-therapists of an intensive therapy group; and we have co-authored some 18 publications. We have also raised two children – and homes – and have been actively involved in wider relationships in what we referred to as "chosen family" before we came to live in Aotearoa New Zealand where the Māori word "whanau" refers to a concept of family that is more extensive and inclusive than the given and nuclear family. For as long as Louise and I have known each other, we have exchanged ideas, and debated them – and each other! We have been partners in our intellectual as well as our emotional lives, and I have learned enormously from her. It is to her that I dedicate this volume with profound appreciation and love.

Third, I want to acknowledge the Auckland University of Technology, for which I have worked for the past 6 years, for its welcome and support of me and my work. I still regard it as a priviledge to be employed as an academic and to be able to access resources to support my reading, writing, and publications. With regard to this specific project, I have very much appreciated its support for a research assistant, Jyoti Smith, who as well as being an astute editor is a valued colleague. Thank you.

Finally, as no man – or writer – is an island, my writing would not exist without mentors, friends, comrades, colleagues, and supervisors. In reviewing my work in order to select what appears here, I have been struck by and enormously appreciative of just how many people are in and/or behind these pages. Rather than naming them all here, which, in any case, would be an impossible task, I have retained the original acknowledgements and, in some instances, made additional specific dedications to people in my retrospective introductions to each chapter.

PERMISSIONS

The context of this book is such that all but two of the chapters have been published before. I am, therefore, grateful to the following publishers for permisison to reproduce the original articles or chapters.

Critical Social Policy for permisison to publish "The politics of disability in Italy: La Lega per il Diritto al Lavoro degli Handicappati" (Chapter 3), and "One step back, two steps forward: Community care and mental health" (Chapter 4).

Changes for permission to publish "Being at dis-ease with ourselves: Alienation and psychotherapy" (Chapter 5).

Person-Centred Practice for permission to publish "The personal is political – and the political is personal: A person-centred approach to the political sphere" (Chapter 6).

Sage Publications for permission to publish "Mental health promotion" (Chapter 7).

The International Transactional Analysis Association for permission to publish "'Take it': A sixth driver" (Chapter 8), and "There ain't no license that protects: Bowen theory and the regulation of psychotherapy" (Chapter 11).

Neopsiche for permission to publish "Transactional analysis is radical or it is not transactional analysis" (original title "L'analisi transazionale o è radicale o non è analisi transazionale" (Chapter 9).

Psychotherapy and Politics International for permission to publish "Southern psychotherapies" (Chapter 12).

Person [The International Journal for Person-Centered and Experiential Psychotherapy and Counselling] for permission to publish "The relational, the vertical, and the horizontal: A critique of 'relational depth'" (original title "Das Relationale, das Vertikale und das Horizontale: Eine Kritik von 'Relational Depth'" (Chapter 13).

INTRODUCTION

When I was invited to submit a proposal for a book in this series, I was both honoured and humbled. It is an honour to be thought of as someone who has made a significant and international contribution to mental health (in the broadest sense of the term), and, with such honour comes a certain elevation. It is also profoundly humbling in that I think of myself as a simple man who, in many ways, is close to the ground, whence humble (from the Latin *humus* meaning ground, and *humilis* meaning low or lowly) and not a "name". I remember, some years ago, after I'd introduced myself and had been talking with someone for a while, they suddenly said "You're not *the* Keith Tudor are you?" I had quite a strong, physical reaction to this, which included spontaneously looking back over my shoulder, as if they were talking about somebody else. In my view, between honour and humility lies responsibility, that is, my responsibility for my words and actions, and for ensuring that the latter match the former, a matching that I and Mike Worrall referred to as "philosophical congruence" (Tudor & Worrall, 2006).

I am most grateful to Routledge, and, as I have acknowledged, Joanne Forshaw, for the invitation to contribute to the series and, thereby, for the opportunity to present my work in this way. The brief of the series (www.routledge.com/series/WLMH) is to compile:

> a career-long collection of what [the author] consider[s] to be their finest pieces … so readers can follow the themes and progress of their work and identify the contributions made to, and the development of, the fields themselves … [including] an overview of his career, contextualising his selection within the development of the field, and showing how his own thinking developed over time.

In addition to this brief, I had the benefit of some excellent peer reviews of my original proposal, which encouraged me to offer more critique of my own ideas, some illustration of how I have changed over the years; and some detail as regards the ethical basis of my therapeutic and political positions.

I have tried to meet these expectations and encouragement both in this introduction as well as the retrospective introductions to each chapter. I have divided the book into four parts, representing my writing during four decades: the 1980s, the 1990s, the 2000s, and the 2010s (to date). At the beginning of each part, I have outlined what I was doing in the particular decade in terms of employment and/or voluntary work and have included my membership of relevant professional and political organisations, as well as some significant personal events. I have always had a strong association with the number 13: I was born in a house (no. 13) and, for 17 years lived in another house with the same number; this is my thirteenth book, and so there just had to be 13 chapters!

A career-long collection

This collection – or selection – represents my career as a practitioner and theoretician. My practice has encompassed social work, including probation (1976–1977), mental health/psychiatry (1987–1990), and training (1990–1992); counselling, including research (1981–1985); teaching English as a foreign language (1985–1987); psychotherapy (from 1987), including supervision and training (from 1992); and academia (from 2009). This work has included being employed in the public sector (1976–1977, 1987–1992 and from 2009), and in the voluntary/independent sector (1981–1985); being unemployed (1979–1981), and self-employed (from 1987), including, with my partner, Louise Embleton Tudor, establishing and running Temenos (www.temenos.ac.uk) (1993–2010), and managing the Sheffield Natural Health Centre (2000–2006). I have been a member of three different trade unions (1981–1985, the Association of Clerical, Technical and Supervisory Staff; 1987–1992, the National Association of Local Government Officers; and, from 2009, the Tertiary Employees Union), including serving as a shop steward (1988–1990). I have been a manager for brief periods (1988–1990), managed a business, including staff (1993–2010), and (from 2013) have been in different managerial roles at Auckland University of Technology. I have worked and done voluntary work in three different countries, i.e. the United Kingdom (1976–1985, and 1987–2009), Italy (1985–1987), and Aotearoa New Zealand (from 2009). I have presented my work in a number of countries in addition to the UK and Aotearoa New Zealand, i.e. Canada, Lithuania, Australia, The Netherlands, India, Italy, Spain, the United States of America, Japan and Slovenia; and have had my work translated into six different languages, i.e. French, Portuguese, Italian, German, Japanese and Serbian. As far as writing and publishing is concerned, I have had an unusual career in that I have been an independent academic for many years, but only employed as an academic since 2009, completing my PhD in 2010.

In making this selection, I have been concerned to represent both the variety of my work in a career that has spanned a number of fields, and also a certain coherence over time. In terms of variety, the papers represent three specific, 'though related fields:

1 Influenced by my social work background, the social world, including *social policy*, i.e. Chapters 1, 2, 3, 4, 7, and 10;
2 *Positive mental health or wellbeing and its promotion*, the subject of my first book (Tudor, 1996b) and my doctoral thesis (Tudor, 2010e), i.e. Chapters 7 and 10; and
3 *Psychotherapy*, i.e. Chapters 5, 6, 8, 9, 11, 12, and 13.

In terms of coherence, these papers all represent a critical perspective. When, in 2009, I emigrated/immigrated to Aotearoa New Zealand to take up the position I had been offered at Auckland University of Technology, I was delighted to learn that the New Zealand Education Amendment Act 1990 (§4), which outlined the characteristics of universities, included the statements that: "They are primarily concerned with more advanced learning, the principal aim being to develop intellectual independence" (§4(i)), and that: "They accept a role as critic and conscience of society" (§4(v)). I was delighted to read this as these statements represent values that inform my practice as an educator, academic, practitioner and activist – and hence the title of this volume. The phrase "critic and conscience" also has a personal resonance for me as, during the second world war, my father, who was a teacher, had been a conscientious objector. From him I derive both a love of teaching – or, rather, education – and a commitment to embody conscience in my work, as well as a willingness and an ability, when necessary, to object! (see especially Tudor, 1999c, 2000, 2007e, 2008b, 2008d, 2008f, 2010c, 2011b, 2011e, 2012a, 2013d).

As far as this collection being "career-long", the grammarphile will note the definite articleinthesubtitleofthebook;however,whilethesearenamedas"*The*SelectedWorks…" they might, more accurately be "*These* Selected Works …", as my career is not over yet and that there is more to come!

"Finest pieces" from various sources

The various sources of this selection encompass: a newspaper article of limited circulation (Chapter 1), some unpublished pieces (Chapter 2, and half of Chapter 5), peer-reviewed journal articles (Chapters 3, 4, 5, 8, 9, 12, and 13), other articles (Chapters 6 and 11), a book chapter (Chapter 7), and extracts from my PhD (Chapter 10). Some chapters began life as conference presentations (Chapters 9 and 12), and some were invited contributions (Chapters 7, 9, and 13).

Notwithstanding the fact that I am not an island or, arguably, an individual (see Tudor, 2016b), one of the selection criteria for this volume was that it is all my own work. As I have co-authored and co-edited quite a lot over the years – contributions that represent some 26 percent of my total outputs (and I am glad to say that this has not diminished since I have become an employed academic) – this set some significant limit. Also, the format of the series is that the authors make their own selection, which I have done, although this task benefitted from the peer reviews of the original proposal as well as my own editing of the manuscript, as a result of which I made several changes to the final "play list".

In terms of whether this selction represents my "finest pieces", I would say that they – and perhaps I – have matured with age. Thus, I have included some early writing – "early Tudor", as one of my colleagues referred to them, perhaps evoking images of half-timbered English medieval houses! – in order to fulfil the aspect of the brief that the reader might see the development of my thinking during my career to date. The selected contributions comprise three papers from each of the 1980s, 1990s and 2000s, and four from the current decade, three of which have been written since I emigrated to my new adopted homeland, and one of which was written in both hemispheres. Although I do think that some of this is my finest writing, as I am continually refining my writing, I hope my finest is yet to come!

In order to maintain historical accuracy and to account for the development not only of my thinking but also of my style, I have largely retained the language and style of the original papers, editing only for an overall consistency for the presentation of this as a whole book, to which end I have collated all references into one list (and, therefore, altered the citations accordingly). In editing the book as a whole, I have used the house style of the American Psychological Association (6th edition) throughout, and thus removed footnotes from one contribution (Chapter 3), whilst retaining or (in the case of articles originally published in American journals) reverting to the original British English spelling. The few substantial or significant additions or alterations are marked by square brackets, thus: [...]. At certain points I have inserted the word "then" in order to clarify the different timeframes, i.e. the there-and-then of the original publication and the here-and-now of 2016. I have made two other alterations. The first concerns lists of citations, which I put in chronological rather than alphabetical order, as I think this better represents the development of the history of ideas: thus, for instance, Winnicott precedes Tudor. The second concerns dates, mainly in the list of references in which I use British and New Zealand English regarding the order, thus "2016, 1 December" and not "2016, December 1". Call me old fashioned, but there you go! I enjoy embracing the pluralism and sometimes the contradictions of being radical in my thinking and conservative (some might say archaic) in my language. Other delights in store for the grammarphilic reader include the use of archaic forms of words, for example, "whilst" rather than "while"; extensive use of the Oxford comma; and, of course, a zone free from split infinitives!

I began to edit this book at a residential writing retreat, funded by the School of Public Health and Psychosocial Studies of the Auckland University of Technology – to which I am grateful – during which some colleagues were playing and discussing music. At one point during the residential the music being played was that of the era (in that case, the 1980s) of one of the articles I was editing. This was not only synchronous and nostaglic, it also helped me to "get back", to paraphrase the words of Paul McCartney (1970), to where I once belonged. Since that retreat, as I have gone through the chapters in chronological order, and have been thinking about where and when I have belonged, lived, worked, loved, contributed, and lost, I have played the music I was listening to at those times, a conceit that has helped me relocate and remember the original work and, therefore, my retrospective introductions.

An overview of my career

I have begun this in this introduction, and develop this in the introductory pages to the four parts. In common, I am sure, with that of many others, my career has unfolded more than it has been particularly planned, and has been more cirtuitous than linear; moreover, whilst I am ambitious (and I don't think that's a bad thing), I have not been particularly career-minded. For instance, I became interested in probation as a result of having an inpsiring and creative tutor, Dr Roger Hood, who, as part of a paper/course on the philosophy of punishment, took a group of students to the local prison to meet some long-term prisoners. For the cost of some packets of cigarettes we listened to their stories – and I have to state that, as far as arguing about different philosophies of punishment, they ran rings around us! Something about their stories and demeanour fascinated me, and that experience eventually led me to applying for and obtaining a 1 year position as a temporary probation officer, which, in turn, led to training as a social worker, and so on.

Also, in common with others, my life and career has reflected certain values, some of which I have inherited, others of which I have adopted. Here I note certain themes which reflect the ethical basis of my therapeutic and political positions and have informed my career, and, specifically, the contributions reproduced in this book.

Social – and political – service

I come from a long line of social service: my maternal grandfather was a Unitarian minister, my mother was a social worker (as was my Godmother, and my eldest brother), and my father was a teacher and a lay preacher. I was told that my grandfather, Ralph Philipson, who christened me, thought that our task in life was to leave the world a better place than when we found it, whence and hence the importance of being of service and making a contribution. This perspective reflects the ethical principle of beneficence, which goes back to the Hippocratic Oath (5th century Before Common Era). Some years ago, I came across the writing of Jessie Taft, who was influenced by Otto Rank and who, in turn, influenced Carl Rogers, and, amongst many other contributions, coined the term "relationship therapy" (Taft, 1933). She commented that: "The word 'therapy' has no verb in English" (p. 3), going on to reflect that the Greek noun from which the word "therapy" is derived means "a servant" and its associated verb is "to wait". She continued:

> I wish to use the English word "therapy" with the full force of its derivation, to cover a process which we recognize as somehow and somewhat curative but which, if we are honest enough and brave enough, we must admit to be beyond our control.

I like this connection between therapy and service, waiting, and humility, and would make a further connection between this approach to therapy and the concept of "clinical hospitality" (see Orange, 2012). More recently, I came across a more political perspective on this, from Alice Walker: "Activism is my rent for living on this planet" (from a poster advertising the film *Alice Walker: Beauty in Truth* (Parmar, 2013)).

My own expression of my grandfather's view on life has been my involvement – and activism – voluntarily in various projects (political, social, educative, and therapeutic), and professionally by doing pro bono work and offering reduced fees. As I am passionate about writing, I am equally passionate about encouraging others to write and, to that end, have done a lot of editing (largely on a voluntary basis) and co-authoring. As far as this book is concerned, I suggest that this value and theme both informs and is reflected specifically in Chapters 2, 3, and 12.

Free thinking and conscience

I was brought up by parents who were Unitarians. Influenced by the Enlightenment, Unitarianism is based on "faith, freedom, and reason", and a critique of Trinitariansim. From this background I inherited an appreciation of faith and faiths; of freedom, liberty and more generally, of liberal values; and of rational argument: perspectives which were enhanced by my study of and first degree in philosophy and theology. This theology and philosophy supports and is expressed in ethical principles of fidelity, intellectual responsibility, and human rights. Apart from the obvious connection between having a conscience and the example of my father's conscientious objection, there is a more general ethic that conscience informs practice. This is expressed well by the characters Robin Oakapple and

Richard Dauntless in *Ruddigore* (I was also brought up with Gilbert and Sullivan) when they sing about obeying the dictates of their hearts and conscience:

> Richard. Hold, my conscience made me!
> Withhold your wrath!
>
> SOLO – Richard
> Within this breast there beats a heart
> Whose voice can't be gainsaid.
> It made me thy tru rank impart,
> And I at once obeyed.
> I knew 'twould blight thy budding fate –
> I knew 'twould cause thee anguish great –
> But did I therefore hesitate?
> No! I at once obeyed!
>
> (Gilbert & Sullivan, 1886/1961, *Ruddigore*, Act I, pp. 521–522)

Broadly, this free-thinking and liberal background, supported by a liberal education (at primary, secondary, and tertiary levels) has led me to be independent minded, and idealistic, both of which have given me a strong sense of being able to embody values, including, as the Quakers put it, of speaking "truth to power" – and have got me into conflict (see introduction to Chapters 8, 11, and 13). Specifically, with regard to the education (and training) of therapists, I have been very influenced by Rogers' work *Freedom to Practice* (1969, 1983), which theory and title has guided my approach to the education and training of therapists (see Embleton Tudor, Keemar, Tudor, Valentine, & Worrall, 2004; Tudor, 2007g, 2009c), influenced my work with Mike Worrall on person-centred supervision (Tudor & Worrall, 2004, 2007), and informed my perspective on regulation and registration (Tudor, 2011e), and recognition (Tudor, 2013b). Clearly, this theme is part of the thesis of the book and is particularly reflected in Chapters 8, 9, and 11.

Internationalism and locality

As a child, I remember my parents welcoming foreign students, especially those from Germany – my father was a German teacher, and loved both the German language and literature. In the 1960s my parents also took us (my two brothers and me) on holidays in continental Europe, which my father planned meticulously (and, in those days, this was all done by correspondence and post). This, together with my parents' liberal values, led me to being interested in other cultures, being open to different experiences, being curious, and learning the social and cultural courtesies of being a host and a guest. My involvement in politics, and in two therapeutic approaches (transactional analysis and the person-centred approach), each of which have strong international communities and organisations, and, more recently, with *Psychotherapy & Politics International* (http://onlinelibrary.wiley.com/journal/10.1002/(ISSN)1556–9195) (which I edit) have all fostered my internationalism. In my early 30s, I lived in Italy (where the word "ospite" encompasses both the roles of host and guest), and learned how it was to be the Other, the "straniero": the foreigner, the stranger. This experiential learning about culture (see Rogers, 1951), together with the discipline and the challenge of learning another language, was not always easy, and, indeed, was sometimes painful; nonetheless, it was transformative. Following on from learning about being "othered", I discovered my Englishness and became more aware of my own culture and of being "intentional" about culture (see Shweder, 1990) and other aspects of (my) human experience such as being white (Naughton & Tudor, 2006). This led me to a greater appreciation for the local as well as the international, a perspective which has been further inspired by Totton's (1999) work (which, in turn, was informed by van der Ploeg's (1993) work); and, following my move to Aotearoa New Zealand, by a greater appreciation of "local" indigenous knowledge.

With regard to ethical principles, this theme and value is reflected in those of charity (love), peace, reciprocity, and respect, and, I suggest, in Chapters 3, 4, 9, 11, and 12.

Radical and critical

During the year I was a temporary probation officer, I had a number of experiences by which I was radicalised. It was as if I woke up – or was woken up – from a certain comfort and complacency that liberalism affords. I knew I was missing something and made a very clear decision to enrol on a social work course that would educate me in radical theory and practice. As part of my training I read feminist theory, did a placement at a women's prison, and wrote my social work thesis on women and crime (Tudor, 1979). I also became interested in theories of education and training about which I wrote and in 1981 had my first article published (Brown & Tudor, 1981). Shortly after finishing the course in 1979, I moved to London and quickly became involved in housing politics – I was part of establishing a housing association in west London and lived in its first custom-designed collective house; in community politics – I joined a local collective that produced a community newspaper, *Bush News* (see Chapter 1); and in national politics – I joined a libertarian socialist organisation called *Big Flame* (see http://bigflameuk.wordpress.com/). *Big Flame* was influenced by the politics of movement (as distinct from party); by feminism and the politics of *autonomia* (autonomy) in Italy (see Lotringer & Marazzi, 1980), and by race politics; and by a libertarian socialism (see Howell, 1981), by which it – we – aspired to reflect a "prefigurative politics", i.e. ways of being, relating, and organising that articulated and reflected personal and social liberation before the revolution. Since arriving in Aotearoa New Zealand, I have been very influenced by the politics of biculturalism, and am grateful to have the political education I had with regard to autonomy as this has helped me to begin to understand my new context: a bicultural nation with a multi-ethnic society.

Thus my intellectual journey has been one from liberal to radical; from one which focused on unity to one that acknowledges and understands disunity, including the significance of difference and diversity; and one on the basis of which I did things for "the good" to one on the basis of which I am more concerned to do things to put something right, in other words, from supporting equality to promoting equity. My politics are (still) broadly Marxist; the ethical principle by which that is expressed is that of justice, themes and values which are reflected specifically in Chapters 4, 5, 8, 9, 11, 12, and 13.

Collectivity and community

From the mid 1970s to 1990, I lived in shared houses, including, for 7 years in the 1980s, in two different collective houses, one of which was very political, the other of which was more psychologically-minded, including having the support of a group therapist, with whom the adults in the house met monthly. During my training as a therapist, I was a member of a therapy group. As a therapist I have run therapy groups, at one point, three groups; and, for a number of years, worked more in and with groups than with individuals, experience on which I drew to write a book on *Group Counselling* (Tudor, 1999a). As a trainer, all my work has been in groups, and, for most of my working life, I have run and facilitated supervision groups. All my political work has been in groups. Although I have lived for more of my life in the context of the nuclear family, I remain very group- and, indeed, organisation-minded.

Interestingly, western – and, in effect, northern – psychology and psychotherapy places a high value on autonomy and less value on its corollary, homonomy (see Angyal, 1941), a concept I have been promoting for a number of years (Tudor, 2006, 2007a, 2007b, 2008e, 2010e; Tudor & Worrall, 2006). As autonomy represents and promotes self-determination and self-organisation, homonomy acknowledges the human urge and desire to belong to and be in groups: family, tribe, community, organisation, and so on. Indeed, in his closing comment in a workshop we ran together (Steiner & Tudor, 2014), Claude Steiner, a transactional analyst and a proponent of radical psychiatry, suggested that working in groups was perhaps the most radical contribution that transactional analysis had made – and that we, as practitioners, could make. Although there isn't a chapter in this volume which specifically focuses on groups, the ethical values and principles of homonomy, reciprocity, and partnership inform much of my work, in theory, in my practice, politically, and organisationally.

The context of my selection within the development of the field(s)

When I was an independent academic (i.e. when I was not employed as such), I wasn't particularly concerned about the development of the fields in which I was writing, or, specifically, measuring the impact of my contribution to the particular field. When I undertook my doctoral study, and especially given the particular pathway, i.e. that of a PhD by public (published) works, I was challenged to assess the impact of my writing on the field – and did so, a process and a task that I have subsequently taken forward (see, for instance, Tudor, 2014a). In this volume, which has also been a heuristic process, I do address the specific context of my selection within the development of the field in the retrospective introductions to each chapter. In terms of developing the field, I would suggest the following:

- That my work on alienation and psychotherapy (Chapter 5) is part of developing the field with regard to class-conscious practice.
- That my use and advocacy of the feminist slogan "The Personal is Political" (Chapter 6), whilst not new, is nevertheless still useful and supportive of others who promote a similar analysis.
- That my work in promoting positive mental health (represented here in Chapter 7), has advanced the field and has had a certain impact – albeit that it has largely failed in changing people's use of the term; and, for some time, I have thought that the term mental wellbeing or, simply, wellbeing, will outlast that of (positive) mental health.

- That my elaboration of a transactional analysis informed by radical psychiatry (Chapter 8) represents a significant contribution to revitalising this tradition within transactional analysis and, indeed, the original radicalism of transactional analysis itself (Chapter 9).
- That my use of heurism and Moustakas' (1990) heuristic method was an appropriate methodology for my doctoral work and, specifically, my context statement in support of linking three public (published) works, which, to my knowledge, was pioneering in this particular pathway to a doctorate (see Chapter 10).
- That my work on the regulation of psychotherapy and the registration of the title psychotherapist (represented here in Chapter 11) has helped to advance a pluralistic approach to this area of the field, especially in the relatively few countries in the world in which psychotherapists are registered and/or regulated by legal statute. In a review of my book, *Mental Health Promotion*, McNulty (1997) commented on this aspect of my work, which, he wrote, "offers the opportunity for informed pluralism to replace both interprofessional and interdisciplinary defensiveness and the well-intentioned naive eclecticism that characterises much of mental health work" (p. 121). However, whilst I am pursuaded by and optimistic about pluralism, I fear that the debate about statutory regulation and state registration, at least within the psychotherapy profession in Aotearoa New Zealand, has, in effect, simply outed those colleagues who are, it transpires, unilateralists, with the result that opinions, when aired, are possibly more polarised than ever. My contribution to the same debate in the field of counselling (see Tudor, 2013b) has been more welcomed and influential.
- That my application of "Southern Theory" to the field of psychotherapy (Chapter 12) offers (to date) a unique analysis, and is one which has the potential to contribute to the development of a specific, local, radical, and critical praxis.
- That my contribution to person-centred theory (represented here in Chapter 13) honours a specific aspect of its history, i.e. its roots in organismic psychology, argues that it has a specific and important reading of the relational (which predates the more recent "relational turn"); and advances it as a critical theory and practice (see Tudor, 2015), a contribution that, interestingly enough, has been both rejected (see Chapter 13) and invited (Tudor, 2016a).

This work represents both continuity and progression, in both transactional analysis (Chapters 8 and 9) and the person-centred approach and its psychology (Chapters 6 and 13), and, within each of those approaches, a specific development of the "relational turn".

Whilst these points focus on my own contribution, I am nevertheless both appreciative and proud of my collaborations in a number of fields:

- Social work education (Brown & Tudor, 1981);
- Therapy (Embleton Tudor & Tudor, 1994; Tudor & Hargaden, 2002; Smith & Tudor, 2003);
- Therapy and culture (Singh & Tudor, 1997; Naughton & Tudor, 2006; Komiya & Tudor, 2016; Ioane & Tudor, 2016);
- Person-centred therapy (Tudor & Worrall, 1994, 2004, 2006, 2007; Sanders & Tudor, 2001; Tudor & Merry, 2002; Embleton Tudor, Keemar, Tudor, Valentine,

& Worrall, 2004; Embleton Tudor & Tudor, 2009; Rogers, Tudor, Embleton Tudor, & Keemar, 2012).

- Transactional analysis (Summers & Tudor, 2000; Tudor & Widdowson, 2008; Tudor & Summers, 2014; Minikin & Tudor, 2016);
- Biculturalism (Green & Tudor *et al.*, 2014; Tudor & Grinter, 2014; Came & Tudor, 2016);
- Professional regulation (Smith & Tudor, 2015; Tudor & Shaw, 2016).

How my thinking has developed over time

For a long time, I have been interested in the idea that all theory is autobiographical or, more precisely, that the theory in which we are interested is strongly informed by our autobiography. In the home in which I was born and grew up, my parents had a little alabaster statue of a seated boy, which they referred to as "the little philosopher", with which I had an ambivalent relationship but also identified. Fifteen years later, I studied philosophy (and theology) at university; and later still wrote a book about therapy as "clinical philosophy" (Tudor & Worrall, 2006). I am a doctor of philosophy, and now supervise others studying to gain this degree. Given my family's religious background, I am also interested in the fact that, whilst I myself am not religious, I have been approached by a number of students and have agreed to supervise dissertations and theses which explore aspects of religion and spirituality in psychotherapy. I think that living in Aotearoa New Zealand, and working in the public sector, in which many of us observe aspects of Māori protocol, such as karakia (blessings) and waiata (singing), has led to me being more open to the spiritual and to the unknown.

In terms of my politics, I don't think I have changed that much. If anything, I think they – and I – have simply become more so, which, as people point out, is a feature of growing old, 'though on this, I am with Rogers (1977/1980) in reframing this as "older and growing" (p. 70)! As my son, Saul, put it recently: "You're not petering out; you're just finding new things to get upset and incensed about" – and I think he's right! Two years ago, as part of my 60th birthday present, I attended the Marxism 2015 Conference in Melbourne, Australia, and thoroughly enjoyed it, including getting annoyed at and with the Party hacks who, at the end of each presentation each gave a 3-minute speech about why it was important to join The Party, orchestrated interventions which, of course, left no time for discussion or disagreement. I still favour autonomous organisation(s) over Leninist party, and consider that my main political work in the context in which I live and work is supporting and promoting biculturalism. I am still an idealist.

In terms of my psychology, I have changed in that I have become more aware of myself, my patterns and proclivities, as well as my shortcomings; in this my doctoral work (see Chapter 10) was invaluable in helping me to reflect on and process the dynamics of polarisation and fight(ing). Whilst, in some ways, I have become psychologically and psychotherapeutically sophisticated, I also enjoy a certain freshness, even naivite, that derives from my idealism, which also fuels my interest in and commitment to action alongside reflection, and I continue to be critical of psychotherapists who priviledge and reify reflection at the expense of action, whether it be personal and/or social/political. As Marx (1888/1975b) put it: "The philosophers have only interpreted the world … the point is to change it" (p. 423).

Over the 35 years represented in and by this book, I have learnt much (and forgotten much) and, now in my seventh decade, am still learning. I have very much enjoyed putting this volume together, a process which has included inhabiting for some time quite a retrospective space – and, whilst I have enjoyed the task, I also want to acknowledge some attendant sadness and grief as I have remembered colleagues and comrades lost through disagreements, drifting apart, and dislocation, as well as death.

To those who have gone and to those still present, including, you, the reader, warm Pacific greetings: kia ora, talofa lava, kia orana, malo e lelei, fakaloha lahi atu, bula vinaka, tēna koutou, tēna koutou, tēna koutou katoa!

PART I

THE 1980s

Employment, other work, professional qualifications, and memberships

1979–April 1981	Living in west London; unemployed; community and political activist
1979–1985	London W12 Housing Co-operative, member, and, 1981–1983 living in its first, custom-designed collective house-Big Flame, member
1981–1985	Upstairs Project (Hammersmith Crisis Intervention Centre), counsellor/researcher
1982	Meets Christine (Louise) Embleton
1983	Moves to live in second collective house
1984	Pellin Diploma in Gestalt Therapy and Contribution Training (Pellin Institute, London)
1985–1987	Living in Italy
	Freelance teacher of English as a foreign language, and translator
1987	Scuola Media 150 Ore (Italian school leaving certificate) (Scuola Media Statale "E. De Marchi", Ministero Della Pubblica Istruzione, Milan, Italy)
	Moves back to west London
1987–1990	Hammersmith Social Services, 1988–1990 senior social worker (mental health), and approved social worker, also National Association of Local Government Officers' shop steward
From 1987	Self-employed vounsellor, and, 1987–1994 psychotherapist in training
1987–1994	Institute for Transactional Analysis, UK, member; European Association for Transactional Analysis, member; International Association for Transactional Analysis, associate member
1988	Meets Christine (Louise) Embleton (for the second time), begins relationship
1989–1991	Guild of Psychiatric Social Workers, member

CHAPTER 1

GAZETTE UNSTUCK

"Glue sniffing" (1980)

Retrospective introduction

In 1979 I completed my social work training at the University of Kent in Canterbury, where I had been very influenced by radical social work theory and practice and specifically by my contact with Mike Brake (and, specifically, with regard to sociology), Janet Sayers (psychology), and Vic George (social policy). At the end of the course I moved to London where I quickly became involved in Left politics both locally, as a part of which I joined a collective of activists who produced *Bush News*, a local socialist community newspaper, and nationally, through my membership (1979–1985) of Big Flame, a revolutionary socialist organisation (see https://bigflameuk.wordpress.com/). My involvement in *Bush News* was a great training, not only in politics and collective action, but also in how to write to a specific word length, to edit, to layout, to print, and, of course, to sell a newspaper.

During my social work training, I had come across the work of Michael Schofield and, specifically, *The Strange Case of Pot* (Schofield, 1971), in which he challenged common myths about cannabis, including the supposed escalation from smoking pot to using heroin; and, more broadly, the work of Stanley Cohen (1972) on *Folk Devils and Moral Panics*, in which he suggested that such a panic occurs when "[a] condition, episode, person or group of persons emerges to become defined as a threat to prevailing social or cultural values and interests" (p. 9). The article reproduced here was provoked by two articles published in the *Shepherds' Bush Gazette*, which, in my view, had precisely represented such a panic: "Parents are worried that young children could be coaxed into joining a teenage gang of glue sniffers". (Editorial, 1980: 3). A brief textual analysis of this editorial would suggest that the use of the word "parents" is intended to imply all parents; and that it is significant that the potential childen are named as *young* children, and that they will be "coaxed", thereby implying coercion, and that the glue sniffers are made into a gang. The Editorial went on to quote a local Tory councillor, who had said that: "a lot of parents are worried … Glue sniffing can kill … there has been an increase … We want the police to get the situation under control". (Editorial, 1980: 3). A week later, the situation – or, rather, the response – had, with no reference to any facts or evidence, escalated: now a senior police officer was calling for a change in the law! This was supported by two articles, reporting "A nightmare in the park for Robert, 13", and a cafe owner getting rid of some kids whom he *suspected* of glue-sniffing (Penn & Langton, 1980). At the time, I was doing voluntary work in the community with young people; worked with colleagues from Release, the west London drug agency (http://www.release.org.uk/, now the oldest such agency in the world); and knew some of the young people involved. I thought this moral panic needed a response, and so wrote the article which was published in *Bush News*. The article provoked quite a response, with letters published in both the *Gazette* and *Post* and *Bush News*, which, of course, came under attack in part because it was a socialist newspaper, letters to which both individuals and the collective also responded.

I have included this short article in this collection for a number of reasons. First, it is one of my earliest published pieces, written just over 35 years ago, and thus gives a starting point for this volume. Secondy, it reflects my long interest in advocacy and commitment to social justice, especially for people who and issues which are misunderstood, misrepresented, and marginalised. Third, in terms of development as a thinker and a writer, it represents and prefigures my interest in and concern about the way in which the social – and the political – impacts on the personal, as well as reflecting a voice that has sometimes evoked or even provoked a strong response (see also Chapter 10). My own critique of this piece is that it is somewhat polemical. Whilst, in part, this was due to the nature of the publication, I think it detracts somewhat from the argument. On reflection, I would include statistics about deaths from tobacco and alcohol (which would have made the argument stronger), and would not end with the comment about leaving them kids alone (as that was not what I was suggesting). Whilst I stand by the argument about moral panic(s), with the benefit of further experience, knowledge, and training, I would also want to talk about the depressant effect of solvents on the central nervous system (by activating the brain's dopamine system), the dangers of inhalation (e.g. irregular and rapid heart rhythms), and the risk of death from toxic shock. I would also want to talk more about the causes of solvent abuse and the psychosociological dimensions and impact of poverty, alienation (see Chapter 5), isolation, and lack of resources, especially in poorer communities.

The *Shepherds Bush Gazette* has done it again! Its article "Parents warn of young glue sniffers" (5 June) is the latest example in a long tradition of irresponsible and inaccurate coverage of activities among youth. This kind of "moral panic" became most obvious in the '60s when reports about cannabis smoking talked in terms of "addiction", of "leading to" heroin dependence, and causing sex orgies, violence and – with usually a heavy racist twist – mugging.

So a few facts for Tory councillor Tony Hennessy, his three children and the 40 parents who signed the petition.

1 "Glue-sniffing" should properly be termed "solvent-sniffing", as it is the volatile agents (such as toluene, acetone, and certain carbon and benzene compounds, etc.), i.e. the solvents in various substances which are inhaled and not the substances themselves (glues, fluids, adhesives, etc.).
2 There is very little evidence to suggest permanent physical deterioration, and physical addiction is extremely rare. A leading Scottish researcher stated at one conference that she had only come across one case of addiction in the several hundreds she had dealt with. Solvent-sniffing is almost totally confimed to the 14–16/17 age group.
3 Since 1975, when the death of an 11-year-old boy was attributed to suffocation resulting from the inhalation of toluene (a constituent of Evo-Stick), there have been about 40 deaths which can be said to have been caused by this activity. During the same period how many people have died as a result of smoking tobacco? During the same period how many people have died due to socially "acceptable" use of alcohol?

4 Most of the accidents or injuries that have occured through solvent-sniffing have been as a result of the activity taking place in isolated and dangerous places such as canal banks and waste land. Some of the responsibility for such accidents must rest with a society which labels and isolates such activities through ignorance.

So, no scaremongering, no crocodile rears and no double standards. The answer is certainly *not* for the police to "get the situation under control" as suggested in the Gazette's article. Most police still haven't read the facts about existing classified drugs, so goodness knows what they think they know about solvent-sniffing. Any police involvement would only criminalise an activity which at present is not illegal.

What we need is more widespread and accessible information for both genuinely anxious parents and kids. We should also have more health education so that we can become more aware of the effects that various substances have on our bodies. In this way the potential dangers and accidents associated with solvent-sniffing will be minimised. Unless they are prepared to become better informed, Tony Hennessy and the like would do well to just "leave them kids alone".

CHAPTER 2

UNEMPLOYMENT AND MENTAL HEALTH (1983)

Retrospective introduction

I wrote this paper when I was working as a counsellor and researcher for a voluntary sector organisation, the Upstairs Project (Hammersmith Crisis Centre Ltd.). The Project was a small street agency in west London, which was aimed at and attracted young people (which the Project defined as aged between 18 and 25, although we did work with some clients either side of this age range). We had opened in 1981, committed to providing a youth counselling service and to evaluating the service. However, first we had to deal with the fall-out from a research design, a randomised controlled trial, by which it was planned that we would randomly accept or turn away young people from the Project. Another aspect of the proposed design was that we would then follow up the young people who we had turned away in order to compare their subsequent lives with those that we had seen for counselling! A local psychiatrist (who, we subsequently discovered, had control over the Project's finances) attempted to impose this research protocol on us; we refused, and, as a result, were promptly sacked. We picked ourselves up, dusted ourselves down, raised money, and, within a few months, had reopened the centre with an independent management committee, with both staff and management still committed to *practice-based* research.

I have included this paper in this collection as my first sole-authored paper and thus, as another starting point for reviewing the development of my ideas and writing. Its – and my – Marxist leanings are revealed in its reference to the analysis that mass unemployment was a strategy for economic problems, which, in turn, was informed by my study of Marx and Marxist praxis during my social work training (1977–1979), and my membership of Big Flame (1979–1985). Whilst the paper itself is undeveloped (and it is no accident that I did not seek to publish it), and the style of the paper is somewhat youthful, it does capture a sense I had – and have retained – of the importance of the social world. As Marx (1894/1962) himself put it: "It is not the consciousness of men that determines their existence, but on the contrary, it is their social existence that determines their consciousness" (p. 4).

In the paper, I refer to productive work being in short supply. At that time the annual unemployment statistics in the UK had risen from 5.7 percent in 1979 to 7.4 percent in 1980, 11.4 percent in 1981, and 13.0 percent in 1982, a percentage that remained above 10 percent until 1987 (Denman & McDonald, 1996). In the paper I adopted the convention of using "we", partly as an assumed academic style, and partly in the hope that other colleagues in the Project would adopt the thesis of the paper, which, broadly, they did.

> Henceforth the quality of a society and its culture will depend on the status of its unemployed: will they be the most representative productive citizens or will they be dependents?
>
> (Illich, 1978: 84–85).

We have examined some of the literature and research relating to mental health and unemployment. Some studies emphasise the state of unemployment from social/political perspectives; others concentrate on the psychological implications of unemployment; few attempt to come to integrated conclusions for practice, particularly in relation to young people. In this paper, with reference to some of the literature, we explore current thinking on unemployment as it affects young people, ways in which the Upstairs Project approaches the problem of unemployment, and our recommendations and tentative conclusions.

Jahoda (1979) suggested that, apart from having the manifest (economic) function for people of earning and living, employment also has several latent (psychological) functions: it provides time structure, regular shared contacts and experiences, and personal status and identity; it links people to specific goals and purposes; and it enforces activity. The underlying implication is, as Hartley (1980) pointed out, that these functions are positive: they reinforce legitimate relationships between the individual and society, and our cultural values give "employment" (as a concept) moral overtones which derive from the Protestant work ethic. By the same token, as a state in which such functions are not provided, unemployment has negative psychological implications including low(er) and/or loss of self-esteem.

There are two main comments to make about this view of employment as having functional effects. The first is that employment is not always a positive experience. Job dissatisfaction is not a subject that concerns us here, suffice it to say that many people would consider a number of essential jobs to be tedious and unattractive. As a result, interest and concern has been shown in the effects of work motivation, involvement, commitment, alienation and effectiveness. At the same time there is political pressure towards a rationalisation of labour resources in streamlining, speed-up, etc. However, as Warr (1982) has pointed out, research over many decades indicates that people want and need to work even if they cannot afford to do so. The psychological benefits seem to outweigh general occupational stress and the negative aspects of employment. Evidence has shown repeatedly that the majority of people prefer to have jobs even if they bring in less than social security levels.

Second, there is an important distinction to be made, as Hartley (1980) has done, between work as an activity and employment as an economic reward for such activity. This is particularly significant for young people as the positive psychological returns gained from employment are not the same as those experienced on job schemes. Stafford's (1982) study, using Goldberg's General Health Questionnaire (Goldberg & Hillier, 1979), which has also been used in a pilot study at the Upstairs Project, found that participation in a youth opportunities programme (YOP) "acts as a buffer alleviating the detrimental psychological effects of unemployment" (Stafford, 1982: 12). This effect is temporary, however, found only during participation in a YOP, and the detrimental psychological effects of unemployment return for those ex-trainees who are unemployed after the YOP. An additional benefit of YOP schemes is that they provide a longer term improvement in employment prospects. This suggests that, although YOP schemes do not have the same status as a "proper job" and the pay is low, they nonetheless are better than nothing and provide meaningful activity.

We are raised and educated in preparation for work, 'though society as a whole values "productive" work rather than other work such as childcare, housework, and nursing (traditionally women's work) which, while considered important in some respects, is also devalued and generally low or unpaid. Productive work is in short supply, particularly at the moment, yet society still expects people to be employed and values them accordingly. This economic and psychological contradiction is explained in two ways: first, on an economic level, in that mass unemployment has been developed as a strategy for coping with world economic problems; and, second, on an individual level, in that unemployment is still seen as a personal problem, which people are exhorted to solve on a personal level.

It is on this personal level of trying to cope with unemployment that many projects, including our own, come into contact with young people. In working with young people there is a temptation to view unemployment as "job loss" and there have been studies (more with reference to the implications of redundancy and early retirement for those who have been employed for some time), which couch the "onset of unemployment" in similar terms as discussion of bereavement: shock, adaptation and deterioration. For the majority of young people the experience of never having had a job and the (rare) onset of *employment* are much more important issues.

Amongst the young people we see [at the Project] is a large number of school leavers. Bachman and O'Malley (1977) have shown that a school leaver's failure to find work has a direct causal effect in lowering self-esteem. This in turn has repercussions in other areas of their lives such as the establishment of relationships (Erikson, 1956). More recent studies have shown that unemployed school leavers, particularly those from social classes four [which refers to partly skilled workers], and five [unskilled workers] and young women are more depressed, are more anxious, and show a higher incidence of minor psychiatric morbidity than those who find jobs (Gurney, 1980; Stafford, Jackson, & Banks, 1980; Donovan & Oddy, 1982). In addition, it has been found that those with an unemployed father, and West Indians were at greater risk of being unemployed.

Current research findings about young people therefore give great cause for concern. Also of interest to those working with young people are questions about how motivated they are to find jobs and to work, the suggestion sometimes being made that young people are unwilling to do so. In fact, studies have shown that young people show a stronger desire to be involved in work than older people (Warr, Cook, & Wall, 1979) and that those with the strongest work involvement are at greatest risk of poor mental health if unable to find work.

Table 2.1 illustrates those problems which are important to the young people who come to us. They are not mutually exclusive, as young people who come to the Project have multiple problems or needs and they often present their worries in an inter-related way [– in this report with an average of three problems each].

It may be seen from Table 2.1 that problems related to unemployment and work are high on the list after those related to housing and homelessness, but even higher are those related to mental health.

In discussing those areas relating to their mental health and unemployment, the young people we see are in no doubt about how being unemployed makes them feel. A 21-year-old young women described it as "being discarded by society, it makes you feel you are no use to anyone, it's really depressing. I want to work and

Table 2.1 The range of problems of clients presenting to the Upstairs Project (Hammersmith Crisis Centre Ltd.) n = 178 (Upstairs Project, 1982)

Housing/homelessness	99
Drugs/alcohol/gambling	84
Mental health	48
Finance/social security	46
Unemployment/work	41
Family	40
Sexual relationships	38
Identity/sexual	28
Police/legal	23
Health	19
Isolation	16
Violence	13
Childcare	9
Boredom	6
Pregnancy	5
Other	17
Total (identified problems)	**532**

it feels terrible that I'm rejected like this". These feelings of being devalued and worthless come from being brought up with the idea of employment as a natural part of life, yet in practice experiencing enormous competition for jobs and consequent feelings of failure when unable to get one.

Underlying these feelings is the symbolic meaning of employment; that is being defined by society in terms of the job which you do. Society also defines people in terms of how they look and self-presentation, which is especially important to young people; advertising for clothes, make-up, and consumer goods is specifically aimed at them for this reason. Lack of money also results in a more serious lack of control over resources (whether housing, books, telephone calls, dressing for interviews, transport or insurance of property) and, therefore, one's life in general. Living on supplementary benefit restricts one's choice in many areas and is barely enough to cover essentials, let alone money for any form of entertainment. One young 21-year-old man who came to us said he would "just like to have enough money not to worry about what I'm going to eat tomorrow". He has just got a job but it is a casual one with no security of any kind which is an example of how people get forced into taking jobs of lower status, satisfaction, pay and security in times of high unemployment. For hard physical labour he will receive little more each week than he received from supplementary benefit, i.e. "the dole".

Another 22-year-old young man who comes to us described collecting his dole money as

> the one spot of freedom in the whole week. I have my own money on a Thursday which I look forward to all week but if I spend any of it on clothes or going out anywhere I know I'll be short of money for food or the rent. I end up spending it on going to the pub which I don't really enjoy but it's the only time you can spend with other people and feel like them.

He spends the rest of the week depressed.

Boredom is a problem for unemployed young people; it is boring and socially isolating to stay at home and going out is expensive unless you just hang around street corners. Some people we see describe going to King's Road in Chelsea for a change of scenery, and sometimes sniffing glue to break the monotony. After a while, this, in turn, becomes boring and, in any case, can result in being taken into a police station for questioning. More serious results of boredom and unemployment can be getting involved in various types of offending to break the monotony and/ or obtain desired possessions.

We estimate that only a small minority of those who come to us are currently offending, however, and of more concern is the lethargy and apathy which is a result of the lack of stimulation in their lives. One can watch people deteriorate for lack of interesting things to do and they will describe the enormous effort of will it can take even to get up out of a chair. In this state it is very difficult for someone to galvanise themselves into action and create a fulfilling life not based on employment or buying enjoyment.

If money is very important to young people so too are friends. Maintaining friendships with those of a peer group who are in employment if you are not is very difficult and demoralising. Even if friends who are working wish to keep in touch, it can be humiliating and embarrassing to accept money for any entertainment you go to together and many will therefore choose to let the friendships lapse. This results in further isolation with an increased risk of depression. Those friendships that are made tend to be with other unemployed young people and "there appears to be a danger that a social network of 'second class citizens' will develop among youngsters who will progressively have less and less in common with their working peers" (Donovan & Oddy, 1982: 25).

The Upstairs Project counsels young people aged 18–25, some of whom are employed, while others would not be able to cope with employment at the moment because of their problems. For those young people for whom obtaining work is a desirable and realistic goal the Project offers support and aims to rebuild confidence. We try to counteract the feelings of worthlessness and failure, which in some instances may have been reinforced by the young people's families.

We are also able to help in practical ways: providing a telephone for calls about jobs, lending or giving clothes or money for transport for an interview and giving references when appropriate. The Project premises themselves can act as an incentive for people to make the effort to get out of bed. Rather than having nowhere to go, young people can come to the Project, meet each other and take part in any activities that occur within and outside the Project, and have individual sessions with a counsellor. We encourage people to undertake individual and group projects. These can relieve boredom and some involve the young people in servicing the Project, which in turn has a positive effect on their self-esteem. The accent therefore is on self-help without unemployment being seen as an individual's problem and helping people to set realistic goals for themselves, the attainment of which can then encourage more ambitious goal setting. We are also interested in non-occupational bases of self-esteem as the prospects for decreasing the numbers of unemployed seem poor (Friend & Metcalf, 1981). Where it is possible we will put young people in touch with other agencies, which may offer more specific services to the unemployed and with educational courses which offer a meaningful use of young people's time. We also subsidise visits to a local exercise class, which has proved very popular and is a good way of giving the young people more energy for other things.

Researchers and practitioners in the field find that young people want jobs, more so in fact than older people. Unemployment is having a serious effect on the mental health of young people with implications beyond this generation. Although youth training schemes and employment initiatives do have a beneficial effect, their short-term nature results in the deleterious effects of unemployment recurring. One definition of mental health in personal and societal terms is the setting and attaining of realistic goals, and counselling agencies have a part to play in helping young people do this without identifying the lack of a job as an individual failure. Instead, emphasis is put on valuing young people in other ways while helping them make the most of the opportunities that are available to them.

We recommend continuing research into the impact of unemployment so that findings can be used to influence policy. The Upstairs Project is engaged in research into the effects of the work that we do. Particularly relevant will be our findings about the young people's expectations and how far these are achieved.

We would also like to see more local initiatives and self-help schemes. However, one of the problems of working in the voluntary sector is the uncertain nature of funding and shortage of staff, which results in ideas not being developed. One example of a practical scheme would be a small workshop which undertakes electrical repairs on household equipment (irons, radios, etc.) as such services are in short supply. The scheme has been tried elsewhere with little financial outlay and great success, incorporating recycling of old equipment which is donated and then sold to finance the scheme. The benefits to the young people who build up a level of skill and see a tangible product for their efforts have been immense.

One way in which we could be released to develop initiatives like these would be to have more secure funding, on a 2- or 3-year basis with an annual review. At present, voluntary organisations are in the position of obtaining funding from a variety of sources on an annual basis, with applications for renewal often falling at different times of the year. The time involved in the preparation of applications and supporting documentation and meetings can seriously curtail the actual services provided, as well as sapping energy to put into new projects. A full-time development officer for the voluntary sector who could act as a resource for advice and information (perhaps computerised) on funding that is available could cut down the work each individual project puts in to finding out where to go for funds for or donations of office equipment for example. S/he would also report on ideas as they occur so that initiatives are not lost through lack of time and energy.

Longer term solutions to the meaningful use of peoples' time if full employment is to be a thing of the past are outside the scope of this paper, [nevertheless] voluntary organisations have an important part to play in feeding their information and ideas to those in a position to influence policy, that is council members. The good relationships that exist locally between the officers of statutory authorities and staff of voluntary organisations should be built on. A co-ordinated and coherent mental health service to the community is more likely if funding bodies, politicians, planners and practitioners collaborate both at local and national level. Ramon (1982) has analysed the links between policy since the 1959 Mental Health Act and practice in the 1980s, focusing particularly on the development of community mental health. She has argued strongly for practitioner input into policy. We find it encouraging therefore that recent circulars from the Department of Health and Social Security (1983a, 1983b) referred both to representations from and to funding for voluntary organisations directly and through joint finance.

CHAPTER 3

THE POLITICS OF DISABILITY (1989)

Retrospective introduction

This chapter is based on an article, published in the journal *Critical Social Policy*, which examines the politics of disability in Italy by means of an analysis of social policy and a case study of a specific organisation: La Lega per il Diritto al Lavoro degli Handicappati (The League for the Right to Work of the Handicapped). The article was based on my experiences working with members of La Lega as an able-bodied ally for 2 years (1985–1987) when I lived in Italy, mainly in Milan. In the early 1980s, in the UK, I had met and become friends with Dick Leaman of the Union of Physically Impaired Against Segregation (UPIAS) (see Union of Physically Impaired Against Segregation, 1981), and had been the instigator of a rehabilitation study tour to Cuba, which included Dick, Vic Finklestein, and others: allies, activists, family members, and translators. We planned the tour in order to meet disabled Cuban activists and their allies, which we did, and combined some study (see Hunt, Leaman, Tudor, & White, 1988) with a lot of fun. During the first half of the 1980s, I learned a lot from Dick and other members of UPIAS about the politics of disability and so, when in 1985 I went to live in Italy, I made contact with Italian activists who had a similar analysis of disability, handicap, and impairment. I did voluntary work with members of La Lega, attended meetings, and studied the history of the organisation. I also researched the relevant background material for the article, which was published a couple of years after I had returned to the UK.

I have included this article in this selection as it reflects not only my interest in and application of a social model and analysis of disability, but also represents a politics of support for autonomous social movements, which was informed by my membership of Big Flame, and which has influenced my praxis ever since. The article, which shows a qualitative development in my writing from the previous paper (Chapter 2), also marks my decision to study, write, and publish, and, thereby, my career as an independent academic, which lasted over 20 years from 1987 (when I returned from Italy) to 2009 (when I was first employed as a full-time academic). My critique is that the original article was a little long and, whilst thorough, could have done with some editing to sharpen the points made, or to make it into two articles.

The original article acknowledged Gloria Stea Carboni who and whose family I thanked not only for their help and information with this article but also for their welcome, patience, comradeship – and for many enjoyable, long Italian lunches! An Italian version of an earlier draft of this article was available from La Lega. Gloria has remained an activist and, as recently as 2013, presented a paper on architectural barriers to access with the challenging subtitle: "Old and New Excuses". Dick, who also remained an activist, which included getting a job with Lambeth Accord (now We are 336), sadly died in 1999. In the days (most of the 1980s and early 1990s) when the social environment was much less accessible than it is now, I used to carry a tape measure with me in order to be able to measure the width of the doors of toilets in pubs. If I found one that was, I think, from memory, at least 33" wide, then I knew it was a pub where Dick and I could have a drink! I remember Dick and those times with great fondness, and it is to him that I dedicate this chapter with much love and appreciation.

La Lega per il Diritto al Lavoro degli Handicappati and the politics of disability in Italy

This chapter focuses on the work and politics of La Lega per il Diritto al Lavoro degli Handicappati – The League for the Right to Work of the Handicapped ("the League"). The League represents a new politics of disability in Italy and indeed one which, particularly in respect of its insistence on an equal alliance with professionals, is lacking within the international movement of disabled people. This [chapter], based on the author's experiences of working closely with the League while he lived in Italy, looks first at the associations and organisations of disabled people and their relation to the Italian welfare state, including reference to some of the more important legislation affecting disabled people. The centrality of the League's politics of the right to work, looking particularly at the law concerning the allocation of work to disabled people is considered, as is its other work on the abolition of architectural barriers, its theory and practice, its position on professionals ("technicians") and on international work.

The Italian state and "voluntary" associations

The "liberal State" formed at the unification of Italy in 1861 was, until 1912 and a significant widening of the suffrage, increasingly governed by centrist compromises (rather than the alternation of parties and power). It was in this context that the first welfare law, the Crispi Act 1890 n. 6972, brought together existing institutions for assistance and charity (IPABs) under a legislative umbrella and recognised the existence of the private sector in the form of the Catholic Church.

An *ad hoc* state of charitable welfare to the poor and needy continued with some decentralisation after 1937 when, under fascism, local welfare authorities (ECAs) were established, theoretically, in every town (comune). This took place during a 20-year period from 1922 to 1943 ("ventennio") in which there was increased intervention in and regulation of the family by the state. It was under fascism, for instance, that rudimentary forms of welfare legislation, such as family allowances, were introduced. For a discussion of the impact of the policies of the Italian state on women in this period see Caldwell (1986). With the foundation of the Italian Republic (1946) the old IPABs continued as public institutions.

As in other countries, including, similarly, Germany after unification, such welfare legislation had the political purpose of tying the worker to the state through defining welfare in terms of work. In translating English Poor Law into the modern welfare state, German social insurance legislation of the late nineteenth century was of crucial importance. In a social insurance bill of 1887 invalidity – a term borrowed from its French origins describing men unfit to be soldiers – was defined as the total incapacity to work, regardless of age. A disabled person was defined as someone who, because of her or his physical or mental condition, is neither in a position to perform her or his previous work regularly, nor to earn the minimum invalidity pension through other work corresponding to his or her strength and capabilities and existing job opportunities. Such definitions of disability as inability to work, togeher with the need to measure this inability in order to define and control access to welfare and services, have underpinned most European welfare legislation and American insurance programmes. The primary distribution system then is one based on work.

After the phase of post-war reconstruction (1945–1950), capital accumulation in Italy proceeded at an increasingly rapid rate. The conversion from an agricultural to an industrial society, which mainly occurred in the 1950s, resulted in large scale migration of labour from rural to urban areas and the growth of the cities. The basis for economic development was production for export, a highly controlled labour market and the lowest salaries and longest working day in Europe. In short, the so-called Italian "economic miracle" was based on the larqely uncontrolled exploitation of the labour force (Marcelloni, 1979). It was in the context of a new political entity – "a democratic Republic, founded on work" (Article 1 of the Italian Constitution) – and rapid industrialisation that the organisation of the relation between capital and labour and the systems of distribution in Italy required the consolidation of the welfare state and the need for definitions of welfare, health, ill-health and disability.

Thus, in the 1950s a series of sectoral associations were created, such as the National Association for the Crippled and Civilian Disabled (ANMIC), the National Association of Invalids and the Injured at Work (ANMIL) and the National Relief for the Civilian Blind (ONCC) (which was later disbanded in 1970). As can be surmised from the titles of these organisations, they were both sectoral, that is in dealing only with one sector of disabled people, and corporative, that is in organising their particular sector exclusively and "from the top". These public authorities concerned themselves with disabled people and at the same time sought to represent them: each authority representing a different category of disability: the blind, war disabled, civilian invalids, etc.

In 1977 with the devolution of responsibility and organisation of assistance and benefit to the Italian regions, the local ECAs were abolished, as were many of these public authorities, although a few retained their representative status. The prime example of such an organisation is the ANMIC, which has representation on: the local social health centres (USSL) commission for establishing the criteria of "invalidity"; the provincial commissions for public assistance and benefits; and the provincial commissions of the employment exchange.

The criteria of "invalidity" used by the medical/legal commission of the USSL are nothing more than a detailed list of "pathologies", each carrying a percentage of invalidity, which corresponds to the percentage of invalidity benefit an individual receives. Thus, for instance, the anatomical or functional loss of both hands is worth from 91 to 100 percent of the invalidity benefit, while, under the heading "Cardiovascular Apparatus", hypertension with minor increase in the lower pressure (diastolic value) rates as between 0 and 10 percent invalidity.

The extent of the ANMICs influence and power would be advantageous if it were used to promote the interests of disabled people. However, despite the fact that since 1977 it has become a private association with its own membership, it continues to claim to "represent" all disabled people. Such representation is one way. The fact that it does not explain the workings of the various commissions on which it sits, the criteria by which they make assessments and decisions, or the unclear statistics they produce, makes its position on these worse than ambiguous; it colludes with the "buying off" of disabled people, that is, in giving up their right to work in exchange for a lump sum payment (see pp. 31 below).

These associations – ANMIC, ANMIL and ONCC – epitomise and characterise the way in which the welfare state functions in Italy. It is worth considering two aspects of this: politics and financing. The associations themselves reflect the party political state at central and local government levels. Thus the president of ANMIC is a Christian Democrat, while in the "red" region of Emilia Romagna the regional president is a Communist. The role of the ANMIC as an organisation is not so much to provide services for its members as to consolidate the current electoral consensus. The ANMIC provides an information and advice service to its members about benefits and pension rights. It also argues that it is only due to its presence on the various commissions that disabled people can obtain benefits, something which in reality is open to all on the basis of their eligibility, not their membership of a particular organisation.

The history of welfare services in Italy, and their relation to the state since the Crispi Act, is that they have been partly organised by the state, through its regional, provincial and local structures; and partly through its private associations and institutions, which nevertheless derive their funds predominantly from the state. The funds which the Italian state designates for its welfare budget can be categorised thus:

1 Social security – distributed both through the Ministry of Labour and the National Social Security Institute on the basis of contributions from workers and employers, in the form of old age pensions, invalidity pensions, and supplementary old age and invalidity pensions.
2 Health funds – managed by the Ministry of Health on the same contributory basis to cover hospital stays and other medical expenses. Since 1983 a "ticket" system has been introduced as a direct charge for prescriptions and tests.
3 Welfare relief – organised through the Ministry of the Interior since 1977 on the basis of a quota to each region for old age, child and invalidity benefits, payments for hospital costs, and attendance allowances. The Ministry of the Interior is also responsible for the state police, thus defining and regulating those people – the "bad" and the "ill" – as "public order" problems.

In terms of politics and in defining the terms of the distribution of resources, the ANMIC and other such associations have played an important and collusive role in relation to the state. Within the ANMIC it is only in those regions which do not share the national political consensus that a more conflictual position is taken.

It was partly in response to the role the traditional associations had taken and following the political flowering in the late 1960s that since the 1970s other associations came into being, generally organised by the families of disabled people. These organisations, with few rare exceptions, have evolved with a strictly assistential or charitable vision and are rehabilitative only as far as this concerns themselves and their relatives; they are highly sectoral and protective, both in organisational terms and in how they regard disability: they negate the capacity of the disabled person and refuse to support or encourage personal autonomy.

In response to the corporativist approach on the one hand and sectoral associations on the other, local groups of disabled people and their supporters, again since

1968 and particularly since 1977, have been organising at a grassroots level. These autonomous "base groups" have developed a more explicitly political analysis of disability and handicap, as well as a practice which has resulted in many living and work communities being established. The work of this "third estate", as it were, has been made more difficult by the existence of the older organisations, which had already established and consolidated their presence in relation to other public institutions. One example of this monopolistic approach is that the ANMIC, which is the "official representative" of Mobility International (MI) in Italy, refuses to disseminate information about MI.

This then is the context in which the new generation of organisations, of which the League for the Right to Work of the Handicapped is a prime and radical example, has to work. Before looking at the work of the League and particularly in relation to one specific law, it is important to note that some important and progressive legislation which affects the lives of disabled people has been passed.

Following the workers' movements of the 1960s and 1970s, law 1977 n. 517 opened up the schools to disabled people: that is, disabled children gained the right to integrated education in "normal" schools up to the minimum school leaving age – which is usually 13/14, after the third year of Scuola Media (middle school). Law 1977 n. 517 and the subsequent ministerial circular established that disabled pupils must have access to ordinary schools, that classes in which there are disabled people must not have more than 20 pupils, and that for every four disabled pupils in the same school and type of class there must be one specialist support teacher. The main difficulty in implementing this has been the lack of funds for adaptations and helpers, as well as the lack of policy and goodwill on the part of some head teachers. A recent example of this was a court case in which a disabled boy was refused entry to a Scuola Superiore (high school) by a headmaster who argued that the student did not have the right to further education. The judge ruled in favour of the student, saying that the headmaster did not have the right to refuse the student access to higher education. These kinds of issues, however, remain largely unresolved and at the level of individual rights.

The second, and more famous legislation was law 1978 n. 180, passed largely as a result of Franco Basaglia's innovatory work in Trieste, and which "opened" mental hospitals. This has been the subject of much debate, both in Italy and in other countries, and has in Italy certainly changed the face of psychiatric treatment as well as people's attitudes towards psychiatric illness and patients; and, on a practical level, allowed many people with mental illness, learning difficulties and/or physical disabilities to live and work in their communities rather than behind bars [see Chapter 4]. Again, a principal difficulty in many areas has been the lack of planning money and political will; and indeed there is now a reaction to this reform. It is partly following from this law and the movement associated with it that the League integrates disabled people with learning difficulties in all aspects of its theory, practice and membership.

The league and the politics of the right to work

It was in this context that various individuals who had been involved in disability struggles as well as other political movements came together in 1979 to form local "base groups" as well as the national secretariat of a federated National League for the Right to Work of the Handicapped.

In pursuing its activities and policies, the League draws on various articles of the Italian Constitution (1947), which state, amongst other things, that all citizens have an equal right to social "dignity" and that the Republic has a duty to remove social and economic obstacles which impede either a person's full development or the effective participation of all workers (Art. 3); that every citizen has the right to work according to their abilities and choice (Art. 4); that every citizen who is unable to work has the right to social security; and that disabled people have a right to education and professional openings (Art. 38). Inspired by the 1975 United Nations' Charter of Rights of Disabled People (United Nations, 1975), the League began its work with a proposal for a national law of "popular reform" (a mechanism by which a Bill can be presented to parliament by the people if supported by at least 50,000 signatures), to reform the existing law concerning the allocation of work. It is worth looking at this law and the League's criticism of it in some depth as it reflects both the state of legislation as regards handicapped people and the politics of the League in terms of the centrality of the right to work.

Law 1968 n. 482

This law governs the way in which disabled people are "called" to work. First, the degree of a person's disabaility is established by a commission composed of three doctors, which operates from the local social health centre. A person whose disability is ascertained to be greater than one-third can benefit from this law. Those with a two-thirds disability also have the right to receive a monthly invalidity benefit cheque from the prefecture. This is suspended, however, if and/or when the disabled person receives a certificate, the nullaosta (literally, "no obstacle"), which indicates that there is no bar to her or his employability, which thus allows that person to take up employment. Those who are assessed as being 100 percent disabled do not have the right to work and receive instead an invalidity pension and a fixed "accompaniment indemnity" (attendance allowance), which is fixed according to another law, 1980 n. 18, in which the indemnity is clearly related to potential work capacity.

These degrees of disability are not based on any medical/social criteria but on a crude and bargained assessment. Bearing in mind that people who are assessed as 100 percent disabled do not have the right to work it is arguably in the state's interest to establish this maximum degree of disability. The League has therefore proposed the adoption of the World Health Organization's (WHO) classification of disability, which, it argues, gives a more accurate indication of a disabled person's work potential rather than an "assessment" of the type and degee of disability.

Under Law 1968 n. 482 every company which has 35 or more employees must employ, as 15 percent of its workforce, disabled people registered with the Provincial Employment Office for Full Employment (UPLMO). As such, this law has some parallel to the Disabled Persons (Employment) Act 1944 in Britain, which introduced a quota system of 3 percent registered disabled people to be employed in firms with over 20 employees. It also introduced the disability resettlement officer (DRO), whose business it is, amongst other things, and like its Italian counterpart in the Ministry of Employment, to issue exemption vouchers. However, disabled people identified and registered as "civilian invalids" are not the only category of disabled people which benefits from this Italian law; indeed there are seven categories each with its "quota" percentage of the overall 15 percent quota. They are: war invalids (25 percent); civilian war disabled (10 percent); disabled as a result of working for the state (15 percent); disabled as a result of accidents at work (15 percent); civilian invalids (15 percent), war orphans, war widows and refugees (15 percent); and the deaf and dumb (5 percent). This means that a firm of 35 employees is obliged to take on, for example, a disabled person in the "civilian invalids" category: if they are between one-third and two-thirds disabled, if they do not constitute a work safety danger, if they have managed to overcome all the bureaucratic barriers, and then only to the extent of 15 percent ("civilian invalids" category) of 15 percent (percentage of disabled people in the workforce). This works out at 2.25 percent of the total workforce, which in effect means that a company must have at least 45 employees before it is obliged to employ, say, one wheelchair-dependent person.

These two aspects – the classification of the disabled person and the obligation to employ disabled people – are fundamental to this law (1968 n. 482). What is fundamental to its implementation is that it has in-built and explicit loopholes. The first is a so-called "slippage" mechanism by which, in the absence of disabled people in certain of the above categories registered at the UPLMO, companies can take on other categories of disabled people in their place. The employment minister's statistics for 1983 detailing those disabled people actually employed, by category of disability, reveal an insidious (un)popularity poll of the seven categories of disabled people and the percentage of that category allocated employment, with 97 percent of "war invalids" allocated employment as compared to less than 40 percent of "civilian invalids" being called to work. The statistics show that for every 16 disabled people called to work only one is a "civilian invalid".

The second legalised loophole is that a company can be partially exonerated from having to employ disabled people as 15 percent of its workforce due to special conditions, which are: the danger of the work, the poisonous nature of substances employed in the work process, the "insalubrious" nature of the work environment, the "irksomeness" and difficulty of the work, the technical nature of the work and/or the degree of trust required, and the traditional and/or major presence of women in the workforce. In addition to these special conditions, each sector of industry (e.g. manufacturing, construction, distribution, agriculture, commerce, transport, security, etc.) has a percentage reduction of between 25 and 60 percent of the employment obligation. Thus, if a manufacturing firm of 100 employees has a 60 percent exemption, this means that the 15 percent quota is applicable only to 40 percent of its workforce (i.e. six people). These exemptions are "bought" at the price of the obligation to employ orphans or widows instead of "real" disabled people. If a company does not employ these orphans or widows in principle their exemption falls. However, while the Ministry of Employment easily grants exemptions, it neither follows up companies' employment records nor rescinds exemptions.

The application of this law, too, reveals further lack of interest on the part of the state and opposition from employers, both private and public. Under the law companies should provide the UPLMO with 6-monthly returns indicating the overall number of employees and their percentage "quota". On the basis of these returns the UPLMO checks the number of places available against its register and sends out the "nullaosta" (which, as noted above, entails an automatic withdrawal of the disability pension) to the appropriate number of registered disabled people. However, no attempt is made, either on the part of the UPLMO or by the employer, to match the person to the job. The UPLMO official does not know the company, the sector, the disabled person or her/his needs. The company at best does not care and at worst is positively hostile when faced with this "obligation", and most often the disabled individual who presents her/himself at work finds situations such as: that the company offers her/him a financial incentive ("oblation") to give up the post; that the company puts her/him in a difficult work situation such that s/he is discouraged (or encouraged to give up); that the company after an initial trial period sacks her/him; or, perhaps most insidious of all, that the company applies to the Regional Administrative Tribunal (TAR) for a ruling to avoid taking on the allocated disabled person. This TAR in effect decides betweeen the company and the individual on the basis of damage suffered: by weighing up the damage to the company of having to employ a disabled person and to the individual of not having work. This recourse to the TAR is not only a blow to the individual but also a financial penalty in that, if the disabled person has a disability determined as more than two-thirds, the monthly invalidity pension is suspended from the time that the TAR accepts the company's application. This process of recourse, investigation, claim and counter-claim can last for up to 2 years. In 1985 the TAR for Lombardy received 707 such recourses.

The explanation for such a highly antagonistic and conflictual relationship has its root in the necessary (for capital) division and sub-division of labour: the constitutional right to work is tempered by the economic and political reality of unemployment – at present 11.5 percent of the active population. This, combined with an unwieldy bureaucracy of laws, circulars and forms, together with a healthy and historic suspicion of state interference, aggravates the able/disabled divisions between people.

The circulars

It is clear that this law does not promote the right to work of disabled people, and various governmental circulars since, operating in response to economic interests, have clearly reflected the handicapping nature of political and legal institutions. The circulars of the Ministry of Employment (which take their name from the respective Ministers of Employment) particularly hit people who are both physically disabled and have learning difficulties, who, it is claimed by employers, do not come within the scope of this law (1968 n. 482), despite the fact that Article 5 defines as a "civilian invalid" "anyone who suffers from physical impairment". Clearly, a physically disabled person's mental impairment is considered reason enough to exclude her/him from the job market; and, indeed, successive ministerial circulars have clarified the application of the law and worsened conditions for people with learning difficulties, thus:

1 Circular Scotti 1979 n. 85 introduced the "called nomination" by which a company could exercise an option to choose a person with learning difficulties (or not).
2 Circular Foschi 1980 n. 101, contrary to the Scotti circular, asked the UPLMO to give an extensive report and interpretation on the application of the law as regards the obligatory employment of disabled people on the basis of a unified concept of both physical and mental disability, which would be in line with the Constitution and which would end the unjustified discrimination then noted.
3 Circular De Michelis 1985 n. 109, contrary to the Foschi circular, directed the UPLMO not to process the nominations of disabled people with

mental impairment and only to send those already registered to companies who expressly ask to employ them.

The politicians

A move was made (twice) by the last Craxi government [1983–1987] to abolish the "slippage" mechanism in that, given a less than full complement of disabled people in any one of the seven categories, companies would not be obliged to make up the numbers from another category. A whole year of debate was necessary before this amendment was dropped.

Not only was the government negative as regards this history of the obligatory allocation of work to the disabled, but it also positively obstructed any attempts to reform the law. This political and parliamentary obstructionism was so marked that the Christian Democrat Senator Bombardieri, who had been given the task by the Senate Commission on Employment of putting together an agreed text on the reform of this law, when faced with a package of spoiling amendments from his colleague the Minister of Employment, said that the government's behaviour was in danger of politically embarrassing the government itself. With the notable exception of Democrazia Proletaria (Proletarian Democracy) (DP), which supports and collaborates with the work of the League, politicians' thinking on this issue reached new depths when a Bill (entitled "The exclusion from the obligation of employment of invalids for non profit-making organisations, no. 3321/4.12.1985") was introduced and supported right across the political spectrum. This was particularly designed to include (and therefore exclude from this obligation) political parties and trade unions. Fortunately, due to massive protests and political opposition from the "base group" organisations and from those who had been involved in drafting the reform Bill (shelved with the fall of the government in May 1987), this exclusion Bill was set aside, although how permanently remains to be seen. While the other major political parties such as DC, the Italian Communist Party (PCI) and PSI have their respective social security offices/commissions and therefore tend to refer to them on what are seen as social welfare matters, Proletarian Democracy refers directly to the League.

The politics of work

In Italy the right to work is seen as fundamental, indeed, as noted, it is enshrined in the first Article of the Constitution: "Italy is a democratic Republic, founded on work". The fact too, that Italy has a system of proportional representation, which, despite its faults, produces a wider parliamentary political spectrum than, say, in Britain, together with the fact that the vote, following the still recent memory of the fascist regime, is seen not only as a right but as a duty, gives a certain parliametary and legislative orientation to social and political work and movements. That, in Italy, voting is viewed as a civic duty is evidenced by the fact that the lowest electoral turn-out in the ten post-war national elections was 88.7 percent (in June 1987). Reference to consitutional rights can be a weapon, in the same way that legislation can be used as a means to achieve an end – in this case an equality of citizenship – rather than an end in itself. The League has played a central and co-ordinating role in setting up a national assembly of organisations of disabled people to draft and present a reform law on the "obligatory calling" to work of disabled people, thus aiming to put into practice this fundamental right.

This equality of citizenship is particularly important for disabled women. It has been estimated that women comprise only 35 percent of the active population. Many women work in the shadow economy as, for example, informal and low-paid domestic labourers. Disabled women are, therefore, doubly discriminated against, and often denied a reproductive role as well as a productive one. The League's demands then, while clearly reformist in a society whose distribution system is based on work (rather than need), nevertheless aim to bring those sectors of the population traditionally marginalised from work, by disability and gender, into economic activity and recognition. The policies of the right to work is less convincing when applied to elderly disabled people (in Britain, at least a significant proportion of disabled people). In Italy the annual fiscal crisis of the state insurance scheme, which is unable to meet the financial needs and pensions of an ageing population, has led to recent moves to raise the retirement age from 55/60 (woman and men, respectively) to 60/65 and beyond.

The present arrangement whereby some state employees can retire after 20 years' service (sometimes at the age of 45) is also being reviewed. Thus, the concept of a voluntary retirement age and income policy, and, for the League's argument, linked to the right to work, appears less likely or central. However, the principle of the right to work and the consequent rights to decent wages and related pensions still brings elderly disabled people into the market, and the politics of the right to work and "retirement".

The attack on disabled people: marginalised from the market

It is, the League argues, precisely because work is seen as a fundamental right that, when a sector of the population is denied it, the double handicap of being disabled (impaired) and excluded from society at all levels (handicapped) becomes even clearer. In recent years the number of disabled people in work in Italy has fallen by 40,000 – over 10 percent. This is exacerbated by the increasing use of the policy of reducing jobs by paying workers a kind of temporary severance pay ("cassa integrazione guadagni"), which often becomes permanent and which hits disabled people to a greater extent (rather like the "oblation").

The difficulty of the process of registration for work under law 1968 n. 482, combined with the fact that this process in Milan, for instance, takes up to 2 years and in other parts of the country even longer, plus the fact that once you are registered at the UPLMO you are one of 369,268 disabled people registered and waiting for work (July 1986 figures), discourages many people from registering at all. In this society disabled people are denied work and consequently denied access to the market – the labour market and the market of exchange, of selling and buying – and therefore become dependent on assistance. This has detrimental effects economically, in being dependent on the state, the family, etc.; socially, in not being seen as a full citizen, or worse, being regarded as a burden; and politically, in being denied the possibility of full participation. In fact, from an economic point of view, there is an obvious advantage to the state in having another economically productive worker rather than another unproductive welfare client.

The work of the League

The fightback: "the right job for the right person"

For these reasons the League prioritises the politics of the right to work of the handicapped, and, indeed, "Il posto giusto per la persona giusta" is one of the League's main slogans. Work is the key to economic independence, social mobility, and political participation. Work is not only a right, but should be seen as a positive experience both for the disabled person her/himself and her/his colleagues. Furthermore, disabled people have a positive contribution to make to the struggle for better work conditions, considering that the bad state of the work environment is used as an excuse for not employing a disabled person. The League therefore works closely with the trade unions in highlighting these issues, which constitute an attack on all workers.

Trade unions in Italy are organised principally along traditional lines of political loyalty (and then sectorally) thus: La Camera Generale Italiana del Lavoro (CGIL) (Central Italian Chamber of Work), which is predominantly aligned to the PCI/PSI; La Confederazione Italiana Sindacali dei Lavoratori (CISL) (the Italian Confederation of Workers' Trades Unions), which was very oriented towards DC, although it has in recent years been more open to other elements of the political spectrum and, consequently, to more internal debate; and l'Unione Italiana dei Lavoratori (UIL) (the Italian Union of Workers), which is aligned to the PSI; in addition to which are the non-aligned Left autonomous groupings.

On barriers

The second major aspect of the League's work concerns the abolition of architectural barriers, both in terms of raising public consciousness on the issue and in making specific practical proposals. These barriers are not a problem for or of only one section of the population, that is, disabled people; rather they related to a general need to make the environment functional for all. It was this issue that led to what was perhaps the League's most publicised action when it took to court the Milan Transport Board (ATM), which runs the Milan Underground system, after the ATM had issued a circular which explicitly banned the use of wheelchairs from the Underground. This decision was contrary to a Presidential Decree (DPR) 1978 n. 384, which had outlined the general principles and technical details for implementing law 1971 n. 118, designed to help overcome architectural barriers. Referring to this DPR, the League applied for an overruling of the ATM circular, which it obtained within a month, thus claiming a significant victory.

In both of these major aspects of its work – on law 1968 n. 482 and on architectural barriers – the League works with various professionals: social workers, doctors, architects, academics, as well as other bodies, groups and organisations, such as Medicina Democratica (Medical Democracy), a group and a magazine of radical health workers (see Medicina Democratica, 1985). The League has organised demonstrations, lobbies, seminars and conferences at local, regional and national levels; it has formed a joint trade unions/disability associations co-ordination, and the National Assembly for the Reform of Law 1968 n. 482; and it has actively challenged institutions from local authorities, to the state railways and regional governments.

On theory

The League follows the WHO's distinctions between: invalidity as a functional limitation of an individual caused by physical, mental or sensory impairment; disability as the restriction or lack of capabilities (due to impairment) to undertake tasks which an able-bodied person can; and handicap, which is used to describe the loss or limitation of the opportunity to participate fully in society due to social, cultural, economic and environmental barriers.

Disabled Peoples' International (DPI) distinguishes between disability as a functional limitation located within the individual, and handicap as the loss or limitation of opportunities effected by society. The adoption of this distinction came through theoretical debate developed in Britain by UPIAS and taken through the British Council of Organisations of Disabled People to DPI where it is enshrined in DPI's constitution (see Union of Physically Impaired Against Segregation and The Disability Alliance, 1976; Union of Physically Impaired Against Segregation, 1981).

The League understands oppression as the expression of power in relationships between a society which handicaps and disabled people who are handicapped, either by omission (architectural barriers) or commission (segregated institutions). This power is expressed both impersonally through economic, political and social structures, and personally through oppressive interpersonal relations. This oppression derives from society's need to control its workforce – whether productive, reproductive or non-productive. As we have discussed, one way in which this control is mediated is through the welfare state. Although the precise development of the Italian welfare state is the subject of some debate (Ferrera, 1980; Ascoli, 1984), its function is much the same as that of other countries: a medically based management of illness and disability in which doctors, other medical workers and tribunals make decisions and judgements about levels of disability, claims for benefits, aids and equipment, and about where and how disabled people live and work.

The League's political position and programme then is extremely clear: to promote through activity the complete social integration of handicapped people and to expose all forms and aspects of marginalisation. Its focus on legislative and parliamentary processes is tactical: the League insists on equal rights of disabled people before the law and Constitution and in doing so exposes the limitations of those institutions. The contradictions of a "liberal" state promoting the constitutional right to work and full employment while managing an economy, boasted to be one of the most stable in the world having passed Britain in what was referred to as "il sorpasso", based on unemployment are thus made clear. The League does not allow the parliamentary road to distract from its perceived role as a mass organisation organising at local, regional and national levels.

These politics inform and are informed by a strong theoretical current, which underlies the League's practice of insisting on making the links between all marginalised sections of the population (and with professionals). As capitalist societies develop their economic structures become less concentrated on traditional industrial forces and less focused on the worker only as the central force of manufacturing production. At the same time there has been an expansion of the tertiary (or service) sector, which leads, ironically, to those people in the service "industries" "depending" for their work on society's marginalised "problem" groups. The increase in numbers of what has been called "the new poor" means, paradoxically, that marginalised people themselves become a resource. This resource is, however, only a resource for capitalism as these marginalised groups are further divided and remain the object of state and private (or subcontracted) intervention. If it were possible to overcome isolation, individualism and sectoralism, this resource would be a potential force, a source of practical and further theoretical strength: practical in the sense of practical connections between groups, for instance, between disabled people and pensioners campaigning against architectural barriers; theoretical in the sense that the new (and ever-increasing) marginalised people (also referred to as secondarily handicapped in not being disabled but handicapped by society) could influence the analysis of the experience or subjectivity of disabled people – which, in turn, would lead to a more complete understanding of disability and handicap.

On "technicians"

The League works closely with professionals and "experts" (literal translation: "technicians") and indeed they are welcome and eligible to join the local groups and to participate in the work of the League at all levels as equal and full voting members. This position has been the subject of some debate within the League and, on a wider international level, within the DPI. The League argues that its aims include the full autonomy and self-determination of disabled people and only people who subscribe to this aim, able-bodied or not, are eligible to join the League. In any case there is, for all potential members, an associate period during which both the associate and the League will clarify positions, principles, politics and programme. The League's position on this derives largely from the fact that historically many workers or "technicians" have been crucially involved in "social" struggle: it was, for instance, principally workers in the psychiatric field who were prominent in the movement for reform of law no. 180/1978, which closed psychiatric hospitals. In Italy there is a level of radical organisation, not only in terms of traditional trade unionism, but which is also concerned with the content of work. This tendency was represented in Britain in the 1970s in the Fightback organisations – Health Fightback, Education Fightback and so on – whose slogans "Defend our services, services worth defending" made explicit three ideas of defending services under attack; the common, public ownership of those services; and the idea that it is crucial for workers and consumers to debate the nature and content of such services.

In Italy these politics and alliances have a longer and stronger tradition. This is not to say that all professionals work in the interests of disabled people and, indeed, the League is the first to criticise the power and patronising attitudes of some professionals. These antagonistic social relations are based on the antagonistic economic relations between the "normally adapted" and disabled people. In order to confront this antagonism the League argues for complete integration of disabled people and does not propose a kind of positive discrimination, for example, in terms of how it organises. The League collaborates with those professionals, trade unionists, administrators, etc. who respond to the League's aims to pre-figure non-antagonistic economic relations (of a future society organised more equitably). These "technicians" have worked closely with the League in all aspects of its work on the obligatory allocation to work and on the abolition of architectual barriers.

On international work

The League had, until recently, only informal contacts with disabled people in other countries. Over the past 2 years the League has made contact with DPI both at a European level and with its headquarters in Sweden. This in turn has led to contacts in Britain, with the European Economic Community, and an invitation to a conference in Czechoslovakia. This is an important and exciting development as Italian organisations have to date not been very involved in international exchanges. Such international contact is not only a forum for developing theoretical perspectives and exchanging practical knowledge, but is also an opportunity to challenge the English-speaking hegemony. The fact that some international conferences still do not employ simultaneous translation is a treble insensitivity, given the position of disabled people in relation to educational opportunity, and given the position of non-English speaking disabled people in relation to educational opportunity, in addition to which international perspectives will thus inevitably have an Anglo-Saxon/American and, with reference to DPI, a Scandinavian bias.

DPI is an international organisation of national disability organisations which represent their country's organisations of disabled people. At every level these organisations are controlled by disabled people. Historically, DPI was founded as an alternative to Rehabilitation International (RI), which is controlled by professionals acting for, or on behalf of, disabled people. DPI is therefore different in kind from RI and many of its members are understandably and rightly suspicious of professionals and "technicians", for it is they who often patronise and oppress disabled people.

The League is also an organisation which is in practice controlled by disabled people, but one which insists on maintaining a dialogue with professionals. This theory and practice is something which a group which visited Cuba found when disabled Cubans talked about non-antagonistic relations with doctors, rehabilitation workers, state workers, etc. (Hunt, Leaman, Tudor, & White, 1988). Italy and Cuba are obviously theoretically and practically, economically and socially, as well as geographically, miles apart. This analysis and practice, however, appears significantly different from that experience of handicapped people in other western capitalist countries, at least at a European level. However, the League is determined to take its perspectives forward and, I would suggest, it has both a lot to offer and a lot to gain from full participation in international settings, particularly within DPI.

On organisation

The League is a national association, legally recognised as such, with a written statute, consisting of 14 "base groups" all over Italy – in (from north to south) Trento, in the region of Trentino: Brescia, Milan and Pavia in Lombardy; Turin in Piedmont; Genoa in Liguria; Florence and Arezzo in Tuscany; Fermo in Marche; Rome in Lazio; Caserta and Naples in Campania; Melfi in Basilicata; and Catania in Sicily, although its main activities are concentrated in the north and centre of Italy. The group in Genoa produce independently from the League an occasional magazine *Gli Altri* (The Others – for all society's marginalised people), which nevertheless is available for publishing the League's material, information, news, etc. The League's national office is in Milan – at Via Morigi 8, 20123 Milano, Tel: +39 (02) 869 3973 – and consists of two rooms in a ground-floor flat in an occupied listed building in an old part of central Milan. It is open 5 days a week. The League consists of: a general meeting, which meets at least once a year and which decides policy; an elected executive secretariat/council of between 5 and 9 members, balanced so as to be geographically representative, which meets at least once every 3 months and which carries out the League's policy; an elected national secretary, at present Gloria Stea Carboni, who works from the national office and who represents the League on a day to day basis; and an auditing committee. At present the League has a seconded full-time worker, a seconded part-time worker and 2 part-time volunteers, although it is the national secretary who in effect does most of the League's daily work – and there's a lot of it!

Membership is open to base groups, associations and individuals. Each base group pays a subscription fee towards the running costs of the League. The national secretary is unpaid and the League's only sources of external funds are donations and money from seminars, conferences, etc. Other money, for example for attending international conferences, has to be raised.

The League aims to be an organisation which addresses and promotes its political programme through confrontation with the state and institutions; and, in relation to its campaign against architectural barriers, through initiatives which confront authorities both in order to implement existing legislation and in order to obtain the passing of specific new enabling legislation. The League also carries out research and collects and distributes information; collaborates with "technicians"; has a social service and advocacy role both on behalf of individuals and at a campaigning level as a part of which it acts as "active" secretary to the National Assembly for the Reform of Law 1968 n. 482, and promotes social and cultural activities. Through its organisation and against sectoral or corporative interests, the League seeks to represent the interests of all disabled people in Italy, through its local groups, regionally, nationally and, lately, internationally.

The League nourishes rich theoretical debate, which has recently included a re-analysis of its priorities. The priority of the right to work and the reform of law 1968 n. 482 is seen as having a dual purpose of putting forward the centrality of work for disabled people, as well as putting disabled people and the League on the political map. This has already changed the attitude of politicians, legislators and employers. On the other hand, disabled people have only been partially accommodated: in Rome, for instance, by the building of 40,000 housing units for the homeless and handicapped in a run-down area on the outskirts with no service facilities; in Naples by the manufacture of "handicapped homes", that is, units specifically designed but for only one kind of disability; and again in Naples, by giving money (under certain conditions) to individual disabled people for taxis as a response to campaigns for accessible public transport.

Albeit that the climate of assistentialism in the 1960s changed to one of "rights" in the 1970s, now – so the argument within the League goes – we need to ensure that these rights – of access to education, work, housing, the environment, etc. – are rights to complete integration and not technical segregation. In order to continue the League's historical development from the prioritisation of work as a principal role people play and as a claim to full citizenship, through the culture of "rights", to its present politics and culture of equal opportunity, it is now considered necessary to put forward more "cultural proposals", that is the drawing out and together of the wider social aspects of the League's political proposals such that "technicians" will not design, fund, build or organise handicapping ghettos. The consequent link with other social political movements has not yet been made to any great extent: initiatives are isolated and sporadic and this, according to the League, is partly due to the corporate nature of the old associations. It is only the League which is placing its politics in the wider context.

Conclusion

It is said that Italy has one of the best written constitutions in the world as well as some of the best welfare legislation in recent years. While this may be true – and it certainly is true in relation to the integration of disabled children in schools and psychiatric patients in the community – it is also said in Italy "Fatta la legge, trovato l'inganno" ("Once you make a law, you find an illusion"). The application of most social welfare legislation leaves much to be desired, and there is a lot wrong with the lack of political will, bureaucratic obstruction, and the static nature of the helping professions at all levels. Added to which there is remarkable regional rivalry (amounting at times to serious internal racism); economic differentiation; political "partocracy", i.e. government and "interests" lying with the strength and influence of the party; and social conservatism.

Italy is a beautiful and frustrating country: where a constitution and laws full of "rights" are rarely realised; where cars are parked and people gather anarchically on pavements, making an already inaccessible environment even more difficult to negotiate; where people stare intently, but not unkindly, and are more than prepared to lend a hand if asked and have a chat; where able-bodied, "normodotato" machismo helps and hassles disabled women; where fashion and the body beautiful weigh heavily on those not considered beautiful, and yet where disabled people can shout with pride: "Siam belli, siam brutti; lavoro per tutt" ("We're beautiful, we're ugly; work for all"). Yet in this Mediterranean and political climate, the struggles and movements of workers and the unemployed working class have, from the 1840s on, a history perhaps richer and more imaginative, radical and productive than in any other European country. I am thinking here of the resistance to the various imperial powers who ruled Italy in the nineteenth century; the workers' occupation of the factories in the 1910s and 1920s; and the resistance under fascism; to the more recent struggles of the 1960s and 1970s, which are described analytically and graphically in *Red Bologna* (Jaggi, 1977) and *Working Class Autonomy and the Crisis* (Red Notes and Conference of Socialist Economists, 1979).

In this country – Britain – in which there is no anti-discrimination legislation as regards disability and where the employment quota system is tokenistic, we could do worse than look to Italy and the struggles there, and, within the movement of disabled people, the leadership of the League in confronting the state both in terms of legislative proposals and extra-parliamentary activity. In the Italian context it is no accident that an organisation such as the League has emerged at the forefront of the struggle of disabled people handicapped by society and with its politics of integration: at work, with the access to economic independence and integration this brings; through accessibility, in breaking down architectural barriers; and in the way it organises, by breaking down antagonistic barriers between people divided by society.

PART II

THE 1990s

Employment, other work, professional qualifications, accreditations/registration and memberships, academic qualifications, recognitions, and award

Ongoing	Self-employed counsellor, and, 1987–1994 psychotherapist in training
1990	Management Centre, King's College, University of London, senior research fellow
1990–1992	London Borough of Hillingdon Social Services, development and training officer (mental health), a job share with Christine (Louise) Embleton
1991–1996	Management Centre, King's College, University of London, honorary research fellow
1992	Moves to Sheffield
From 1992	Self-employed supervisor, researcher, trainer and consultant
1992	Marries Christine (Louise) Embleton
1993	Saul (son) is born
	Temenos is established
1993–1999	Accredited counsellor (British Association for Counselling)
1993–2010	Temenos, Sheffield, co-director
	British Association for the Person-Centred Approach, member
	Association of Therapeutic Communities, member
1994	Diploma in Psychotherapy (Metanoia Institute), London
From 1994	Certified transactional analyst (European Association of Transactional Analysis [EATA])Registered transactional analysis psychotherapist (United Kingdom Council for Psychotherapy [UKCP])
1996	MSc in psychotherapy (with distinction) Metanoia Institute/ Middlesex University, London
	Mental Health Promotion: Paradigms and Practice (Tudor, 1996b) wins The Bruce Burns Annual Mental Health Promotion Award, The Bruce Burns Trust, Solihull, UK

1996–1999	Registered independent counsellor (United Kingdom Register of Counsellors)
1996–2000	Sheffield Women's Counselling and Therapy Service, associate therapist
1997–2004	Provisional teaching and supervising transactional analyst (EATA)
From 1999	Liverpool John Moores University, honorary research fellow
1999–2008	Registered group psychotherapist and facilitator (UKCP), and Association of Humanistic Psychology Practitioners, full member

CHAPTER 4

COMMUNITY CARE AND MENTAL HEALTH (1990)

Retrospective introduction

In some ways the articles reproduced in this and the previous chapter may be considered a pair: both are concerned with social policy, and were published in *Critical Social Policy*; both draw on Italian experiences; and both demonstrate a certain and developing characteristic detail in my analysis, in these cases, of different social legislation and policy. There are also differences between them: the first (Chapter 3) focuses more on the situation in Italy and is more of a case study; the article reproduced in this chapter is more concerned with the situation in the UK (at that time), and refers to the Italian experience of mental health reform as a way of contrasting models and philosophies of community care. In this respect I think it demonstrates a development in my thinking (which is more integrative) and writing (which is more integrated): I particularly like the point I made, albeit briefly, about policy (in this case, community care) as pathology. This chapter also introduces and references a specific analysis and methodology which, subsequently, has had a profound influence on my thinking and work (see Chapter 7 and Tudor, 1992, 1996c, 2010e).

When I returned from Italy in 1987, I had taken up a job as a psychiatric social worker, based in Hammersmith Hospital, west London; I also began my training in psychotherapy at the Metanoia Institute in Ealing, also in west London. As part of my interest in mental illness, and the practice and politics of psychiatry, I had read about radical psychiatry (Radical Therapist Collective, 1971; Steiner *et al.*, 1975; Roy & Steiner, 1988) and "the Italian experience" of psychiatric reform. In 1989, I returned to Italy to spend some time in Trieste where Franco Basaglia had implemented the significant reforms that he had originally instigated in Gorizia, and which symbolised the praxis of the reform of the Italian psychiatric system (Basaglia, 1968, 1981). I stayed in the old psychiatric hospital as that was where they hosted professional visitors! Whilst visiting, I met people in the community mental health centres; and was given access to publications and papers (which I could read as then my Italian was reasonably fluent). I began writing the article in Italy during my visit, and completed it back in Britain (1989–1990). I have a similar critique to that of the previous article (Chapter 3) in that it is a little too long and (now) a little dated. My critique of the medical model, sadly, has not dated.

Part of my work as a hospital social worker involved liaising with colleagues and projects in the community – and, indeed, breaking down the artificial community/hospital divide. One of the closest projects to me, both geographically and politically, was the White City Mental Health Project, which had been founded by Sue Holland, an inspiring therapist and political activist who I had previously met some 5 years earlier when I was a youth counsellor (see Chapter 2). I got to know Sue, her colleagues, and their work well; I worked with some of the women's male partners; between us we kept some people out of psychiatric hospital; and I learnt a lot, for which I am still most grateful. Sue introduced me to paradigm analysis, based on the work of Kuhn (1962/1996) and its development by Burrell and Morgan (1979) (see Holland, 1979, 1985, 1988a, 1990), to which I refer only briefly in this article.

In 1990 I was working part-time as a development and training officer (mental health) in Hillingdon Social Services Department, and part-time as an honorary research fellow in the Management Centre at King's College, University of London, where I was supervised by Ray Holland (Sue's husband), who had also developed Burrell and Morgan's work (see Holland, 1987, 1990a, 1990b). This research led, after some time, to the publication of my first book, *Mental Health Promotion: Paradigms and Practice* (Tudor, 1996b; see also Chapter 7), and, eventually, to my doctorate (see Chapter 10). As people who were each and both very influential in my intellectual development, I dedicate this chapter to Sue and Ray Holland with great respect and affection.

The [British] government [1987–1990] has, not uncommonly, managed to upset almost everyone across the political spectrum by first trying to railroad the implementation of proposals contained in its White Papers Working for Patients and Caring for People and more recently, by postponing major parts of their implementation until April 1993. For an explanation and understanding of this "Ready, steady – stop" approach (Downey, 1990) we need to refer briefly to the political and financial context of these policies.

The political and financial context of community care

In 1986 the Audit Commission (1986) reported critically on local government and health authorities and the "role confusion" between these two agencies in the provision of community care. The government's response was to ask Sir Roy Griffiths, then managing director of Sainsburys, "to review the way in which public funds are used to support community care policy and to advise ... on the options for action that would improve the use of these funds as a contribution to more effective community care" (Griffiths, 1988: iii). Trevillian (1988/1989) suggested that Griffiths was able to build on essentially Thatcherite notions of community outlined in the Barclay Report (Barclay, 1982). One of the "keystones" of the Griffiths Report was a reorientation of the role of social services to ensure that individual needs are identified, "care packages" drawn up, "care managers" assigned, and co-ordinated services:

> provided within the appropriate budgets by the public or private sector according to where they can be provided most economically and efficiently. The onus in all cases should be on the social services authorities to show that the private sector is being fully stimulated and encouraged and that competitive tenders or other means of testing the market, are being taken.
>
> (Griffiths, 1988: vii)

One reading and reaction to Griffiths was that, in its recommendation (1.5.1) on the transfer of resources from central to local government, it was somehow challenging government attacks on the power of local authorities. That this is a superficial reading of Griffiths, we can see both from Griffiths itself and in the government's subsequent White Papers: central government's notions of community and community care belie an essentially fiscal policy of monetary control of local authorities and the regulation of the community.

As far as "services for people with mental illness" are concerned, in Caring for People the government sets out three key initiatives. The first, "Continuing Health Care", is concerned about collaborative arrangements between health authorities and social services on a patient's discharge plans. This extends the principle and practice of co-operation between district health authorities, local social services authorities and relevant voluntary agencies to provide after-care services for patients detained under certain sections of the Mental Health Act 1983 ("the Act") outlined in Section 117 of the Act. The second, "Capital for Building New Facilities", is about selling off existing health authority assets in order to provide capital for new projects. Interestingly this notion of asset stripping has already backfired in some areas due to the slump in the property market affected in turn by the [same] government's high interest rates. Thus, in some instances, regional health authorities (RHAs) have committed themselves to spending on new facilities on the basis that they will generate a certain income from land and hospital sales. The depreciation in property prices has already jeopardised some of these projected new facilities. The third, "Provision of Social Care" proposes a "specific grant" to social services authorities and that this grant is payable through RHAs "on the basis of plans for the development of social care agreed between social services authorities and the matching district health authorities" (Department of Health, 1989: 57). This goes some way to answering the Royal College of Psychiatrists' criticisms of Griffiths (under the guise of care and concern for the funding and organisational difficulties in social services):

> the mentally ill of all ages require a great deal of continued input from the psychiatric services whether at home or in some sort of sheltered accommodation. The Health Service contains by far the largest fund of expertise in the assessment and care of the mentally ill and an evaluation of services. In our view, Social Services Departments are not the appropriate organisations to provide or to bear the responsibility of developing community care for the mentally ill. This responsibility must be invested mandatorily in the Health Authorities.
> (Royal College of Psychiatrists' Council, 1988: 386–387)

The predominance of the medical model in this statement and in the recommendations of the Royal College, which [aim to] reduce the role of social workers to assistants, is clear. As Nocon (1990) pointed out, the White Paper arrangement whereby health authorities hold the purse-strings

> may allow health authorities to determine priorities in social care for people with mental health problems. It would thus undermine the ability of local authorities to plan services in an area in which they have both experience and expertise.
> (p. 27)

Noonan also made the more general point that:

> future national policy is to be based on planning agreements rather than joint plans ... in the field of joint planning, it will mean a focus on the purchase of cost-effective (i.e., cheap) services. Pragmatism and opportunism will dominate

> the field while the ideals of strategic planning are relegated to the historical backwaters of the supposedly misguided 60s.
>
> (p. 27)

Currently such joint planning is taking the form of, at best, long drawn out and bureaucratic joint meetings between local authorities and health authorities in which the onus is on the local authority to design care "packages" which the health authority will approve in order to release the specific grant; and, at worst, political and administrative in-fighting with health authorities refusing to release the specific grant and, in some instances, threatening to "take over" or "buy out" local authorities' social services' mental health services.

Caring for People, the fiscal policy on which it is based and the consequent regulation of the community is based on "managerialism and the denial of inequality" (Trevillian, 1988/1989: 67). Women are expected to be the "care(rs) in the community". Four out of every five of an estimated 5.5 million people caring for elderly or disabled relatives at home are women (Finch, 1986). At the same time women are more likely to be admitted to a psychiatric hospital and admission rates rise steadily for women aged between 35 and 44 (Department of Health and Social Security, 1986). Women are also twice as likely as men to be diagnosed as suffering from "clinical depression" (Department of Health and Social Security, 1986) and between two and three times more likely to be prescribed minor tranquillisers. More research in recent years has highlighted the inequalities of the "treatment" of black people within the psychiatric system. Serious questions have been raised about the use of Section 136 of the Mental Health Act 1983 by the police to detain predominantly young Afro-Caribbean men (Rogers & Faulkner, 1987). A number of black people have died "in care" (Tudor, 1989). There are disproportionate numbers of black people within the psychiatric population (Francis, David, Johnson & Sashidharan, 1989); one piece of research found that Afro-Caribbeans were ten times more likely to be given a psychological diagnosis as white people (Harrison, Owens, Holton, Neilson, & Boot, 1988). There is widespread psychiatric misdiagnosis of black people (Gabriel, 1987; Fernando, 1988; Harrison *et al.*, 1988). Black people receive on average larger doses of medication than white people and, crucially for our current concern about community care, have less access to alternative treatment (Littlewood & Cross, 1980; Littlewood & Lipsedge, 1982).

The government has been concerned about the escalating costs of care provision in the community, e.g. social security costs of income support claims towards accommodation and care costs in private care and nursing homes. In the field of private residential care for the elderly and disabled people costs increased from £10 million to £878 million over the 10 years to 1988 (Viney, 1990). With an increase in the proportion of elderly people in the population these costs are predicted to rise further. Under the White Paper proposals the government will transfer the present social security payments to local authorities through the revenue support grant. Such grants will be cash limited (and they are unlikely to exceed the current social security payments), thereby transferring the responsibility to local authorities to limit care according to finance, rather than providing care according to needs. Specifically, local authorities will become responsible for the shortfall (known, incorrectly, as the "care element") between the housing benefit and income support a resident receives and the rent they must pay. This additional cost to local authorities will inevitably be reflected by the placement of fewer people in residential accommodation – thus "care in the community"! Trevillian (1988/

1989) predicted "rigorous means testing" by local authorities in order to eke out government grants: Viney (1990) illustrated the financial penalties which will operate throughout government finance and housing benefit regulations; and Harris (1990) argued angrily that such proposed funding arrangments will make community care "little short of impossible":

> All of this is made worse by the Government's rejection of a central plank of Sir Roy Griffiths' proposals – that the money for community care should be clearly identified and ring-fenced. The money for community care will therefore be lost in the general pool of local authority grants.
>
> (p. 8)

There is nothing like the prospect of a general election to concentrate any government's attention on the effects of its more unpopular policies and such a prospect has recently brought into focus the political and financial background to the issue of "community care" more clearly and explicitly than this government has admitted before. When challenged in the House of Commons, the then Deputy Prime Minister Sir Geoffrey Howe said that the implementation date and the pace of the reforms "must depend on the scale of the resources available" (quoted by Travis & Brindle, 1990: 2). This postponement is in order to stem the rise in next year's poll tax bills.

> It would cost £830 million to introduce the programme next April. Some £370 million would be transferred from the social security budget to local authorities, but an extra £460 million would be needed from the Treasury. Postponement could save nearly £15 a head on poll tax bills.
>
> (ibid.: 2)

The community care policies contained in the NHS and Community Care Bill will now be phased in over a 3-year period beginning on 1 April 1991, although four specific mental health initiatives will nevertheless proceed from this date.

Two more years

The new timetable can be viewed in three phases. Phase one (from April 1991) includes the introduction of a specific centrally funded mental health revenue grant (of £21 million for 3 years) "for a planned improvement in the quality of provision" (Department of Health, 1990); the introduction of a specific training grant for training social services staff; and the continuing development work (already started) on planning arrangements; assessment and case management procedures, purchases and related budgetary and information systems, all of which is to be implemented within existing resources. In phase two (April 1991–March 1992) local authorities are to publish their first care plans (on 1 April 1992): to continue phase one development work; and to "top up" the government's care grant with £9 million. Sayce (1990) has pointed out that, in comparison with the £2 billion spent by the National Health Service (NHS) on mental health, "the specific grant itself is powerless to correct this major imbalance between hospital treatment and social, community-based services" (p. 5). From April 1993 onwards (phase three) resources are to be transferred whereby local authorities take on full responsibility for funding care services.

Cervi (1990) has summarised the shock-waves which the government's delay of the community care reforms have caused – with confusion, disappointment and anger from virtually all sectors of care, levels of management and shade of political opinion – the continuing ripples of which continue to be reported in the professional journals and magazines.

The "Italian experience" – 20 years after

Heginbotham (1990) suggested that the NHS and Community Care Bill is "pre-eminently a piece of strategic law rather than one of detailed provision" (p. 25). This is in marked contrast to Italian Law 1978 no. 180 ("Law 180"), which was a piece of enabling legislation which precisely *enabled* health and social service authorities politically, strategically and financially to develop community mental health care facilities and support networks. It is worth looking briefly at the provisions of Law 180 as they reflect the philosophy of de-institutionalisation and community care of the original reformers and it provides a useful yardstick against which to measure the Mental Health Act 1983 (England and Wales) and the current "community care" legislation.

Law 1978 n. 180 (the "Basaglia Act")

Three important principles underlie Law 180.

The first is that the Law, whose Article is entitled "Voluntary and compulsory health treatment", is concerned not with definitions or classifications of disease but with the forms of and reasons for treatment.

Second, Law 1978 n. 180 emphasises patients' rights, already guaranteed under Italy's written constitution (Articles 13 and 32), but specifically as regards personal freedom and the right to treatment (Law 1978 n. 180, Art. 1). In the context of compulsory health treatment for *general* illness (confirmed by Law 1978 n. 833 on the organisation of health and social services, Articles 33 and 34), Law 180 clarified the conditions under which compulsory treatment could be applied to those with a "mental illness" and that this is the only category to which compulsory treatment is applicable (Law 1978 n. 180, Art. 2.1). The emphasis on treatment gives rise here to an important distinction: that between compulsory *treatment* in Italy and compulsory *hospitalisation* in England and Wales – Mental Health Act 1983, Sections (§s) 2.(2)(a) and 3.(2)(a). In Italy the moral and legal emphasis is on treatment in the community, under the auspices of the local Community Mental Health Centre (CSM).

The third important principle of Law 180 was its shift in emphasis from the behaviour of the "mad" person to the importance of the provision of appropriate services. The previous 1904 law had legalised compulsory admission to the asylum of a person due to her/his dangerousness as certified by a doctor or legal ordinance. Law 180 dropped this notion of social dangerousness.

The reactions to Law 180 were many and varied. One, as Dell'Acqua, Mezzina and Cogliati (1986) pointed out, was a certain polarisation:

> It seems to us that in Italy such application [of the law] has given attention exclusively and in an absolutely *ambiguous* and perverse way, on the one hand to the guarantee of personal freedom (non-intervention) and, at the other extreme, to compulsory treatment.
>
> (p. 5; my emphasis)

This led, on the one hand to a scarce realisation of integrated, local resources, and, "at the other extreme", to a proliferation of "diagnosis and cure" emergency services (SPDC) within general hospitals. Crepet and De Plato (1983) suggested that: "These two negative aspects of the reform – compulsory treatment and psychiatric service in the general hospital were intended by this law to constitute the exceptional and short-term instruments. Instead, they have become almost the norm" (p. 127). However, between the passing of Law 1978 n. 180 and 1986 there were in Trieste only 31 orders for compulsory treatment – an average of under four per year – of which 70 per cent were managed directly by the local CSM and 30 per cent were admitted to the Trieste SPDC (quoted in Dell'Acqua & Mezzina, n.d.).

It is not the purpose of this article to review the literature on the Italian reform movement and current services – I have done this elsewhere (see Tudor, 1988) – suffice it to comment that much of the literature available in English is written from the authors' implicit "positions" on psychiatry, mental health and the process of institutional and individual change, and therefore their pre-theorised and prejudiced views on the theory and practice of the reform. "Conclusions" are presented thus: "It doesn't work because it doesn't work throughout Italy" (Jones & Poletti, 1984), although at least they declared their scepticism before they "cut a path through Italy (ibid.: 10) declining to visit Trieste "where the movement has been well-documented and has clearly had some success" (ibid.: 10). Other "conclusions" vary from "It doesn't work because it's too radical" (Papeschi, 1985; Jones & Poletti, 1985) to "It doesn't work because it's not radical enough" (Banton, Clifford, Frosh, Lousada, & Rosenthal, 1985). A second shortcoming in the literature in English on "the Italian experience" is a number of serious misconceptions about the background to and history of the reform, e.g. that Law 180 came before or indeed initiated the reform movement (Heginbotham, 1984; Becker, 1985; Davies, 1990, among others) – which it did not. Benigni, Ciappi, Germano and Martini (1980), Onnis and Lo Rosso (1980), and Piro and Oddati (1983) have been more useful and accurate commentators on various aspects of the reform, while Maranesi and Piazza (1986) provided the first statistical survey since the passing of Law 180 of the effects of the reform and the (then) current state of psychiatric services and mental health resources.

Law 180 also explicitly marked the process of de-institutionalisation and the establishment of the community-based services, a process which had begun 10 years earlier with Franco Basaglia's experiments in de-institutionalisation in Gorizia, a town in the north-east of Italy on the Yugoslavian border. On de-institutionalisation Law 180 states that: no new patients were to be admitted to state psychiatric hospitals (Articles 2.2 and 8.5); the consultant psychiatrist of a psychiatric hospital had to justify the need for continued in-patient treatment of existing patients (Article 8.2), and continued treatment was subject to the procedures described above (Article 3.5); only existing patients could be re-admitted to hospital and that only on a voluntary basis and only until December 1980 (Article 8.5); there was to be no building of new psychiatric hospitals, no use of existing ones as specialised departments or units of general hospitals (Article 7.6); and "compulsory special centres", i.e. psychiatric beds, were to be provided in general hospitals – at the rate of not more than 15 per admission/catchment area "with the purpose of guaranteeing the continuity of the health service for the protection of mental health" (Article 6.4). Importantly, the law also addressed resource provision and stated: that community-based facilities and centres were to be set up for a prescribed geographical area (Articles 6 and 7); that the administrative functions of the mental health services were transferred to the national health services, organised regionally; and that all facilities were to be staffed by existing health care personnel (Articles 7.8–11). Later that year (1978) the Italian health and social services were administratively, financially and organisationally amalgamated.

The legal prescriptions for the transfer of administration, finance and personnel had enabling and far-reaching consequences, for instance in the easy transfer of money from medication budgets to community resource budgets, and the transfer of nursing staff from the institution to the community. Indeed, it is the nursing staff that form the backbone of the staffing resource in the CSMs, fulfilling a function somewhere between that of a community psychiatric nurse and social worker in Britain.

The 1983 Mental Health Act [England and Wales] may have emphasised patients' rights and a philosophy of the least restrictive alternative, but its Italian predecessor was a far more radical and practical piece of legislation.

From "freedom" to services

In reviewing "la politica" (which translates both as policy and as politics) of the Italian reform I concentrate on its development in Trieste for similar reasons Jones and Poletti (1984) gave for avoiding it: precisely because in Trieste the reform movement is well documented, it is successful, *and*, importantly, it was in Trieste that the dialectic between de-institutionalisation and de-hospitalisation was first realised. It is thus a pertinent example for our current consideration. Others have documented aspects of the reform elsewhere in Italy: Ramon (1983) in a Tuscan town; Becker (1985) in Piedmont and Mosher; and Mosher & Burti (1989) in Genoa, Arezzo and Verona.

Giovanna Gallio (1983) described three historical phases of de-institutionalisation of the psychiatric hospital in Trieste.

The first phase of de-institutionalisation, 1971–1974, was characterised by the slogan "Freedom is therapeutic", one which still adorns the walls of ex-psychiatric hospital wards. This period is one of intense activity: the recruitment of new workers and volunteers; the division of the hospital into five teams, each of which corresponded to an area (zone) of the Province of Trieste – population: 280,000 in an area which encompasses some of the countryside immediately surrounding the city.

In the hospital patients were assigned to wards according to the area they came from and no longer on the basis of their diagnosis or behaviour. These teams also corresponded with zones in Trieste in which they were to establish mental health services and centres. All shock therapies were abolished and over a 2-year period all means of restraint – isolation rooms and restrain beds – were dropped. Work therapy was abolished; patients set up a work co-operative, which contracted to do the hospital cleaning at competitive rates. In addition to mixed wards, small groups of patients were formed and, using accommodation within the hospital, the first family-homes were established. Such schemes were the first attempt at encouraging a more autonomous life for patients, and pre-figured the later group-homes and flats in the community. Wards were opened and daily patients/staff/workers meetings were organised.

Although, in this phase, the work and reform was centred on the hospital, the movement was strongly from the hospital into the community with the re-establishment of daily contact with patients' families, outings and, where possible, re-integration at home and in the workplace. The city, too, had contact with the hospital through festivals, concerts and other cultural initiatives. This was a period of effervescence, of anti-psychiatry, of "everything is possible". Perhaps the most famous and public metaphor in this period was Marco the Horse, built inside the psychiatric hospital in Trieste and then paraded, like its Greek/Trojan counterpart, around the streets of the city, symbolising the theoretical view of Franco Basaglia (1981) that illness was located (and hidden) in the external world:

> the conflicts which had previously been regarded as internal to the patient, or at least to the asylum, are thrown back on the wider society from whence they came – for the illness is seen essentially as a distorted representation of specific contradictions of the subject in his social relations.
>
> (p. 190)

As more people, including other professionals, became drawn to this practice, so the need to organise the emerging movement became more pressing. In 1974 Psichiatria Democratica (PD) was founded. This movement became a reference point for political parties, trade unions and activists. Its initial aims are worth noting:

> to fight against any form of segregation and institutional repression, in favour of improving on the present legislation concerning mental diseases; to fight against noxiousness in factories and in the district; to fight against selection and isolation as practices by educational and assistance authorities; to fight for the democratic co-operation of social assistance services, no longer mystified by the corporative, speculative, and bureaucratic logic typical of the current health system; and the need to establish in practice a new work method in the field of health, which will give priority to prevention, in co-operation with worker organsiations.
>
> (Minguzzi, 1974, quoted by Crepet and De Plato, 1983: 123)

PD contains diverse views; in the early years there were those who favoured an autonomous, anti-institutional approach, and those who believed in the need for an alliance with the institutions and parties of the Left. It was the latter grouping that sought legislative acknowledgement in order to promote the practices of alternative psychiatry.

The years 1975–1978, from the opening of the first mental health centre to the passing of Law 180/1978, were characterised by the establishment of an emergency welfare network. It was during this phase, on 24 January 1977, that the project of closing the psychiatric hospital was announced. As the CSM established themselves in their local areas, as the welfare network was extended, and as more alternatives to asylum were developed, so more patients left the hospital; thus the slogan of this second phase became "From defense to the contract" – the contracting of civil rights and resources. Towards the end of this phase the institutional crisis of identity and purpose (and not only for the institution, but also for the staff) reached its height: caught between an institution that did not exist and an organisation not yet recognised or legitimised. This crisis was epitomised when, in 1978, in the face of a cooling of political and administrative support and the bureaucratic blocking of the establishment of services and especially a lack of house provisions, the seaman's hostel in Trieste was occupied by supporters of the reform, an occupation which was forcibly ended by police.

The crisis of the psychiatric institution cannot be viewed outside the context of Italian politics at the time. In the 1970s there was a mass movement to the Left, which in its parliamentary expression gave the Italian Communist Party (PCI) a majority and a governmental role for the first time since the [Second World] War, in the famous "Historic Compromise" with the Christian Democrats (DC). It has been particularly since this period that the question of constitutional and institutional reform, what is referred to as the "crisis of the institutions", has been on the parliamentary political agenda – with little or no resolution. At this time "anti-institutional experience became an organic part of the actual change process" (Crepet & De Plato, 1983: 122).

Through a moving description of one woman's psychiatric history over 13 years Gaglio and Sarli (1977) synthesised the political analysis and practice of the early CSM in Trieste. The key elements of the early years in Trieste are summarised: the social construction of "Anita's" "madness" in her unhappiness and conflict with the traditional female role; self-criticism of the psychiatrists' hesitancy to confront this contradiction; and an analysis of the wider social forces which impinged on her life, e.g. her husband's demand for her to be cured and returned to him "better, like other times". There is a startling honesty about the effects Anita and her developing autonomy had on the inter-disciplinary team, with reference to an extra-marital relationship she had – "the paradox of the crisis" – during her contact with the CSM. The conclusion is equally quintessential: a rejection of psychiatric and medical norms in favour of an analysis of political, social, cultural and psychological contradictions in a class-divided society:

> What seems relevant to us is that now, and different from the past, Anita has been offered the opportunity to recognise and face the mechanisms which have impoverished and destroyed her; all this, without necessarily continuing to lose either in herself or in others in the closed circles which up to now she has known.
>
> (Gaglio & Sarli, 1977: 74)

The third phase of de-institutionalisation, from the passing of Law 180 on 13 May 1978 to the present has been marked by the widening and consolidation of a network of services and organisation as an alternative to the asylum which, in Trieste, was officially closed in 1980.

Praxis

The importance and significance of these phases was that de-institutionalisation *preceded* the process of de-hospitalisation and that there was a developmental relationship between these two processes.

> The humanization of asylum life was not seen as an end in itself, but only as a first step: the ultimate goal was the abolition of the asylum itself. Thus the project was not seeking simply to make the asylum "work better", but to lay the groundwork for its total destruction.
>
> (Basaglia, 1981: 184)

In this Basaglia rejected the essentially reformist approach of the therapeutic community movement propounded by Maxwell Jones, with whom he had worked in Britain. While the therapeutic community broke down an unconscious complicity between the professional medical staff and "the sick" the institutional barrier remained and, Basaglia maintained, was made more elastic by the fact that the patients/residents appeared to play a more active role. Basaglia developed his politics of abolition as he viewed the central contradiction of psychiatry as a social institution as being that between treatment/cure and custody/control. He saw a dialectical relationship between his two conclusions – of abolition of the institution and re-integration into the community of the individual – and, although in practice this was a gradual process, Basaglia's theory and language was at times as violent as the institution he wanted to destroy. On this relationship, he is reported to have said at a dinner for professionals and politicians held soon after his arrival in Trieste that "with the very presence of 'mad' people on the streets of Trieste, my aim is to put the psychiatric institutions themselves into crisis".

That this process – from de-institutionalisation to de-hospitalisation – was not a hierarchical or bureaucratic one is important to note:

> Administration and regulation at Trieste always followed real changes, and the closure of the hospital was not a bureaucratic operation but the collective effort of patients, psychiatrists, nurses, and the public, all of whom worked together in a project of emancipation and the social reproduction of those with little or low contractual powers. It is in this that the difference lies between the de-institutionalisation of Reaganomics and the practice and projects of de-institutionalisation which reaches out to liberate resources, power, subjectivity and autonomy.
>
> (Del Giudice, Evaristo, & Reali, n.d.: 9)

Policy as pathology

This project of abolishing the institution of psychiatry and the psychiatric hospitals as we know them is some way from the Royal College of Psychiatrists' formulation of community care.

The practical point of asylum is to remove "mad" people from their community. One theoretical implication is that "madness" too is "removed" from the community: in other words, when "madness" is excluded we do not have to think about, feel or act in relation to our own distress. Banton *et al.* (1985) made the point that "distress, however, is not a private matter at all, but is generated in and through the social domain" (p. 188). The policy of community care, of placing people back in the community (and not always their own), without de-institutionalisation, with addressing notions of "madness", "mental illness" and mental health, is simply an inversion of the exclusion or sanctioning of "the insane". As such, inversion disrupts, and can indeed provoke (often adverse) reaction from the community. As such, and as a policy of community care, it can be seen as pathological: as an example of distorted thinking, disturbed perception, and irresponsible and unpredictable behaviour – all symptoms of schizophrenic psychoses according to the World Health Organization's (1978) International Classification of Diseases (version 9). Such policy inversion, however, does not challenge notions of mental illness and health, rather it perpetuates them. Thus, community care as proposed in Britain becomes an extension of the psychiatric hospital – as the quote from the Royal College of Psychiatrists' Council (1988) (p. 45 above) virtually acknowledged.

Community mental health

Community mental health is an ambiguous phrase, particularly so as the context in which it is used is often one of illness and disease and a medical/psychiatric model of emotional and mental distress. The hospitalisation of the community is already in progress and exists in the form of the many so-called community health centres (CMHCs), which are largely funded and managed by health authorities with the co-ordinator/manager role often taken by the psychiatrist or psychologist. Sue Holland (1988a) suggested that "the CMHC forms the stepping stone onto which psychiatry has made its territorial move out of the hospital and into the community" (p. 127). Smith (1984), in an original article from the States developing "a geography of mental health", presented a number of alternative conceptual models of community and their implications for CMHC services; and Sayce (1989) reviewed the rhetoric and reality of CMHCs in Britain.

Here CMHCs are too often imposed on communities with little or no consultation or sensitivity, and propagate a medical model of mental ill-health and disease. In one case I know of the launch of a local CMHC that was sponsored by a drug company. When this was questioned the psychiatrist involved remained (or chose to remain) blissfully ignorant of the implication or "message" to the community, professionals and potential users that such sponsorship conveyed. Despite the fact that psychiatry

> has had to adopt the language of social causal models such as "psycho-social transitions" or "life events" ... none of the issues concerning the effects on mental health of the environment, work, housing, poverty, racism, sexism, ageism [are] considered to be appropriate subjects for preventive action.
>
> (Holland, 1988a: 127)

Indeed, many psychiatrists do not appear to accept that preventative action works or even exists as a scientific truth; at least one consultant I know of has blocked financing of research into mental health prevention and promotion because of concern that he will lose psychiatric hospital beds, budgets and therefore power. Equally, when CMHC services are withdrawn from the community, environmental and social factors are ignored. Smith (1984), in a survey and analysis of service provision, noted the differential effect on women and Hispanic men of the closure, or "recentralisation", of CMHC services:

> although longer distances, need to cross major routes, and unfamiliar public transport were relevant to this, they appeared less important than crossing of community boundaries, loss of cultural supports through the move, uncertainty of travelling in unknown areas, and identification of the new service with another community and racial group.
>
> (p. 141)

Sayce (1989) suggested that "the promotion of positive examples of community provision ... was a key part of the rationale for setting up a study of community mental health centres" (p. 160). However, the conflict, as Sayce suggested, between treatment and social reform is a false dichotomy. The conflict is rather between, on the one hand, a medical/psychiatric model and view of mental illness and health, theories of society, community, individuals and change; and, on the other hand, many other "models" of illness, health, society, etc., or, more accurately, paradigms or sets of different theories and practices.

Paradigm and strategy

From Burrell and Morgan's (1979) paradigm analysis, Ray Holland (1987, 1990b) has developed a "paradigm map", which identifies different approaches to theories of society – from social regulation to radical change – and theories of knowledge – from objective to subjective – on two axes. The resulting grid provides four quadrants: functionalist, interpretive, radical humanist and radical structuralist. In this analysis the traditional medical/psychiatric model with its emphasis on identification of scientifically "objective" symptoms and of individual "patients" would fall within the functionalist quadrant of the paradigm. The implication of this paradigm is that there are at least three other quadrants, each representing sets of theories with which we can understand "mental illness". There is an increasing use and application of this paradigm map to describe and locate both theory and practice in social work theory (Whittington & Holland, 1981), health education theory (Caplan, 1986), health education teaching (Holland, 1987, 1990b), and theories of knowledge (Holland, 1990a). Also, Sue Holland (1979, 1985, 1990) has described her work on a multi-racial housing estate in west London "using psychodynamic counselling as a tool for action, rather than as an end in itself" (p. 256) and, importantly and developmentally, suggests a movement around the paradigm map from individual and individualising "symptom" to collective social action. Her work in the well-established White City Mental Health Project offers a critical example of the promotion of mental health in the context of social action precisely because it has helped to move depressed women from being passive recipients (functionalism); through an understanding of their personal pain (interpretive); through desire, i.e. a desire for personal change (radical humanism); through to collective action (radical structuralism), and the establishment of an independent sister organisation, Women's Action on Mental Health, a title, concept and organisation within which the women who run it promote vigorously. Their history and this movement represents the way ahead for community mental health work, thinking and reflection: a movement, as it were, from psyche to society. Elsewhere (Tudor, 1990a) I have been developing this paradigm map to identify and describe different approaches to community mental health promotion (see Figure 4.1).

Such thinking, reflection and action is not just desirable, it is necessary if we are to avoid the worst excesses of the medicalisation and hospitalisation of the community. Unless hospitals and the people involved in and with them – psychiatrists, managers, "patients", families, social services and the voluntary/independent sector – critically challenge the ideology of current psychiatric and social work practices, "community care" will inevitably mean that in addition to the asylum (usually outside our communities) we will only further the hospitalisation of the community.

As a theoretical and practical strategy we can use the paradigm map in this task: first, by analysing, as I have done, the origins of the "community care" initiatives and the location of the psychiatric response – within a functionalist paradigm, which is concerned with social regulation and "objective" (scientific) reality. Second, we can offer a critique of such "objectivity" and social regulation from a number of perspectives. From a radical structuralist perspective I have referred to inequalities within the psychiatric system; from a radical humanist perspective I have

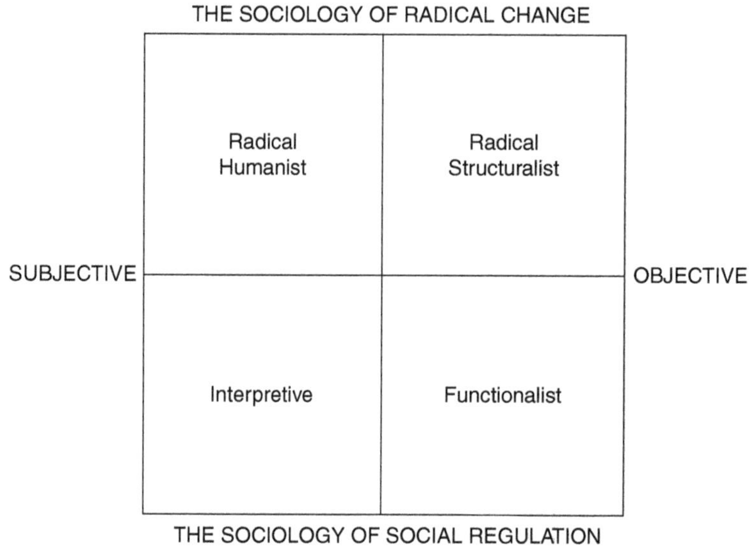

Figure 4.1 Four paradigms for the analysis of social theory (Burrell & Morgan, 1979: 22)

commented on people's subjective experience of change, for instance, with reference to "the Italian experience"; from an interpretive perspective I have questioned the meaning of certain policies and actions. Third, we urgently need to develop more critical practice in mental health from perspectives other than a functionalist one. Fourth, following Sue Holland (1988, 1990), we can develop a theoretical and practical movement around the paradigm map from functionalist/symptom (fiscal policy, "community care", the institution of psychiatry, etc.); through interpretive/meaning (e.g. psychotherapy, some CMCH work); through radical humanist/desire (e.g. anti-psychiatry as a theoretical perspective, and on a practical level the user/advocacy movement); to radical structuralist/action (Basaglia, "the Italian experience", de-institutionalisation). This analysis and movement can (and should) involve everyone concerned with mental health, the community and the closure of psychiatric hospitals, in every forum: committee and policy meetings, local authority/health services, joint planning meetings, staff groups, ward rounds/case conferences, community forum and other local meetings, etc.

Conclusion

In reviewing what has come to be known as "the Italian experience" with reference to recent policy and political developments here in Britain in respect (or disrespect) of mental health I have suggested that the current "care in the community" initiatives are fatally and theoretically flawed, and as such have a particular discriminatory effect on women and provision for black people. I have argued, from the "Italian experience", that in order for "the community" to develop awareness of and responses to mental illness and mental health we first need to challenge and change the theoretical foundations and practices of the asylum, and to bring the community into those challenges and debates directly. A rare example of this in embryonic practice is reported in Doyle (1989) – an adult education course as a part of which the public spent structured time on wards in a local psychiatric hospital. Only then can we move people out of the asylum into their communities which will be ready to receive them rather than reject them. I have drawn on Burrell and Morgan's (1979) sociological paradigm and mapped out a theoretical field as well as a strategy for practical intervention in policy and practice.

De-hospitalisation without de-institutionalisation will change nothing. Those of us in the field, managers and policy makers – across disciplines and authorities – must make use of the time before April 1993 to look critically, radically and structurally at current notions and assumptions of community care. Without this time of reflection and action, community care, as the editor of the magazine of the same name suggested, will be "a policy set to advance from anarchy to chaos without the redeeming interregnum of rational thought" (Philpot, 1990: 13). Such chaos will entail large numbers of distressed and disturbed adults leaving institutions which have been homes for them, some for many years, badly prepared and ill-equipped, on both social and psychological levels, to live in the community – a community neither prepared nor adequately resourced to receive them. As far as the "elderly mentally ill/infirm" (often referred to as EMI) are concerned, local authority bureaucrats try to design schemes that will attract the so-called "dowry money" released by health authorities for EMI patients to be cared for in the community, in reality another institution or "home". The scandal of private nursing homes, set up by (ex) health authority or social services employees with inside information on patients and the collusion of psychiatrists and management is only just emerging.

In parts of Italy where the process of reform was blocked or only partially put into practice, such people are referred to as "gli abbandonati", literally, the abandoned ones. Here in Britain if we do not engage in the urgent theoretical and practical task I have suggested, the consequences will be the abandonment to objective, regulatory models of disease and mental illness of individuals and of notions of positive mental health care in the community.

CHAPTER 5

ALIENATION AND PSYCHOTHERAPY (1997)

Retrospective introduction

This chapter reproduces an article originally published in *Changes*, an international journal of psychology and psychotherapy that was founded in 1983 and ran until 2001 when it was renamed more explicitly as *The Journal of Critical Psychology, Counselling and Psychotherapy*, with which I have been associated since its inception as a member of its editorial board.

By the time of writing this article, I had been influenced by Marxism for some 20 years, i.e. since 1976 when I had been radicalised by my experience as a temporary probation officer, a radicalisation that was informed and developed by my social work training (1977–1979). When, in the mid 1980s, I was considering a full training in psychotherapy, as a political activist I was concerned to train in an approach and in an institute that accounted for the social/political world. I had read some of the literature on radical psychiatry; and been inspired by Sue Fish whom I'd met when living in a collective house, to the adults in which she acted as a group therapist. Amongst other things, Sue was a trained transactional analyst, and a co-founder of the Metanoia Institute in west London. I began my training there in 1987 and passed my international qualifying examination as a certified transactional analyst in 1994. Although my training was by no means radical, I continued to search out and learn from radical practice (see introduction to Chapter 4) and to study the literature on radical therapy, especially in the humanistic tradition.

In 1990 I had been asked to teach on a person-centred training course at Metanoia, an invitation that marked the beginning of a long association with and commitment to the person-centred approach and with Mike Worrall, with whom I wrote a book advancing the theory of person-centred therapy (Tudor & Worrall, 2006). An important aspect of the book was that we framed psychopathology as alienation, about which I was particularly passionate. In this article I developed that work in a way that made more explicit reference to the Marxist concept and analysis of alienation and to class-conscious therapeutic practice. This was important as within the critical tradition in psychology and psychotherapy, there was – and still is – comparatively little that addresses class. My own critique of the article was that this aspect of the piece is still underdeveloped. However, as part of a recent process of going through old files in the context of writing this book, I came across the original, extended version of the article, which included a whole section on class and consciousness as a background to class-conscious practice. I have, therefore, taken this opportunity to reunite the two parts of the original whole. In the original (long version of the) article, I acknowledged and thanked my comrade and friend, Ben Lowe, for his contribution to the first part of the article.

The chapter includes a reference to John Major, British Prime Minister 1990–1997, who, on taking office in 1990, had said that he wanted "to see us build a country that is at ease with itself", which he defined as being a country "that is confident ... able and willing to build a better quality of life for all its citizens" (quoted in Butler & Butler, 2010: 296). He had said this (in a speech made on 24 November 1990) in the context of standing for election to the leadership of the British Conservative Party and his declared ambition to make changes which would make Britain "a genuinely classless society". The title of the original article was a direct reference to Major's phrase, whilst the article itself addresses the naïvity of his perspective.

Re-reading the original article, three aspects strike me, each of which prefigure concerns that I have subsequently developed. The first is the theme of polarities, in this case ease and dis-ease, a subject I subsequently explored in a keynote speech (Tudor, 2007c), and in my doctorate (Tudor, 2010e; see also Chapter 10). The second is the issue of the state registration of psychotherapists, which as I put it in the article, I viewed as an "unnecessarily professionalised and bureaucratic superstructure", a subject about which I have taken a strong stance for some 20 years (see Tudor, 1999c; 2011e, 2013b; Smith & Tudor, 2015; and Chapter 11). The third is the question of our alienation from the Earth, which, whilst I acknowledge in the article, I did not develop, 'though to which I have subsequently returned (see Tudor, 2013c; Clare & Tudor, 2016a, 2016b).

Class, consciousness, and psychotherapy

There is a fundamental fault running through most attempts to deal with the interplay between Marxism and psychoanalysis and other psychotherapeutic theories (Marcuse, 1968; Mitchell, 1975) and, alternatively, in using Marxism as a tool in developing theories relevant to psychotherapy (e.g. Reich, 1934/1972b). The fault lies in the acceptance of the Marxist tenet that class consciousness is a given and that it is a central element in an inevitable transition from capitalism to socialism. To break from this fault provides a route to a new, living Marxism for the next [i.e. this] century, one which takes account of the economic, the political, *and* the psychological.

Following an introductory summary of the psychological relationship between individual and society, class and class consciousness are defined and analysed. The connections between consciousness and the unconscious are explored with specific reference to the family. Two key concepts in Marxist method, historical materialism and dialectic method, are briefly reviewed and applied to the field of psychotherapy. In the second part of this chapter, a Marxist understanding of alienation frames discussions of class-conscious psychotherapeutic practice.

Individual and society

Traditional psychology and psychological theories have isolated the individual, refusing to see her/him as a social entity or in a social context. In his work exploring the Marxist theory of personality, Brown (1979) pointed out "the false divorce between the personal and the political ... [and the consequence of] not developing an analysis of the individual, a science of biography" (p. 6). Marxist and other radical structuralist accounts of society rightly criticise traditional theories of psychology and development for their individual, individualising and pathological perspectives. Equally, materialist accounts – and some of the radical organisations which draw on such accounts – need to be subjected to the same rigorous analysis with regard to their lack of insight into individual psychology. It is perhaps significant that Reich, who visualised himself as a Marxist psycho-analyst, was rejected by both communist and psycho-analytic organisations.

From these mutually critical starting points, Leonard (1984) suggested that "two alternative ways forward are presented" (p. 39). One is to attempt to transform psychological theory, and, specifically, psychoanalysis, from a materialist standpoint. This way is represented by the work of Reich (1933/1972a), Marcuse (1968, 1969), and Mitchell (1975). This project is, however, subject to Jacoby's (1977) criticism that "a harmonious synthesis of Marxism and psychoanalysis presupposes that society is without the antagonisms that are its essence" (p. 73). The other way forward, according to Leonard, is "beginning to build, on the basis of the principal concepts of historical materialism, an entirely new psychology of the individual" (p. 39). This possibility is reflected in the work of Sève (1975, 1978), Brown (1979), Roy and Steiner (1988), and this present work.

Class and class consciousness

In Marxist theory, classes only exist as a social relation, i.e. when there is more than one class in society. Classes are by their nature antagonistic and, through their mutual hostility, create a dynamic which plays a fundamental role in historical change. Classes depend on the division of all labour – master and slave, feudal lord and serf, capitalist class and working class – divisions defined by the predominant method by which goods are produced, thus, craft and agricultmal labour under feudalism, industry under capitalism.

Marxist notions of class can be conceptualised in three ways: an essentialist view; those based on class analysis; and those on an historical/political analysis.

Marx's essentialist view is a subjective one: a class only exists when it is conscious of itself and its role in changing society (Marx & Engels, 1846/1964), a view which implies an "essence" or essential understanding and consciousness of class. This notion is predicated upon the view that the working class has a historical role to overthrow capitalism and assumes that it has an intuitive understanding of that role. Occasionally, workers develop a consciousness of their own strength, whether as a craft union, a more general union, a racial or religious force, or even a defender of a gender position. However, history is short on examples of when a whole working class in any one country has risen up and acted as though it had any sense that it was in the position to take power with an alternative vision of society.

Marx's class analysis of three classes in capitalist society, i.e. wage labourers, capitalists, and landowners (Marx, 1894/1962), remained incomplete. Contrary to Marxist thinking, the working class shows no sign of ever becoming a majority of the population under capitalism and actually represents a relatively small and shrinking fraction across the global capitalist world. Moreover, far from being supposedly concentrated in ever larger factories, as Marx expected, the working class is, in fact, becoming ever more dissipated as smaller and globally sub-divided units. In Britain, most tellingly, those who have sought to uphold working class solidarity, such as miners' leaders, have been among the most accurate prophets of the demise of the working class as we knew it; our children will barely be aware that coal mines, once the major employer of working class people in Britain, any longer exist.

Marx's third view of class focuses on the working class and its historial/political role in changing society. Marx developed a rather schematic, but convenient, stagist view of history, whereby one class structure gave way to another as (predominantly European) history evolved. Thus, there was slavery under the Romans, later feudalism, and then capitalism. Whilst it is accepted that social classes have an important role in the dynamics of a society and that the collapse of a ruling class can help explain change to a new system, it is impossible to accept that an oppressed class will ever take power from its oppressor when there is no historical evidence of this having occurred in human history. In Ancient Rome the slaves did not take power and their "historic role" was to disappear as a class; as for the feudal serfs, they, like their lords, have gradually devolved into the new capitalist classes during the transition through the centuries from feudalism to capitalism.

A fourth Marxist notion of class is a psychological one. Marx was quite specific that an individual's personality (i.e. character structure) was influenced, first and foremost, by her/his class position: "we do not mean to be understood ... that, for example, the rentier, the capitalist, etc. cease to be persons; but their personality is conditioned and determined by quite definite class relationships". (Marx & Engels, 1846/1964, p. 76). The clear implication for psychotherapists is that an understanding of every individual's personality is dependent on an analysis and understanding of their class position and relationships.

"The concept of class consciousness occupies a central place in the socialist movement and its politics ... becoming class conscious [is] the most urgent precondition of the revolutionary overthrow of the present social system". (Reich, 1934/1972b, p. 284). The fact that the working class has never acted in accordance with its supposed historic role, or been "class conscious" in the strict Marxist sense, has preoccupied much Marxist writing of relevance to psychotherapy. The Marxist concepts of fetishism and alienation are seen as the most useful tools in understanding this, and in developing a Marxist theory of personality (see Brown, 1979), and are ones which I develop in this present work.

Class consciousness tends to imply a subconscious collective perception of one's class, whether in its historic role of acting as the main agency of social change to a new economic system, particularly in the context of a pivotal histolic moment (e.g. the bourgeoisie in 1789, during the French revolution), or as the self-appointed representative of the interests of the whole of society after the creation of a new economic system. This collective perception is generally advanced through actual processes such as shared economic conditions, cultural or local affinity, etc. There is a strong sense, too, in which it is a role driven by deeper historic forces which impact upon the subconscious (and unconscious) of members of a given class at a given moment.

Consciousness and the unconscious

For Foreman (1977), who attempted to synthesise Marxism, feminism and psychoanalysis, the concept of fetishism in Marx offers the potential for a theory of the unconscious. She viewed the weakness of Marxism as lying in its failure to develop a theory of the unconscious, and to incorporate this into a strategy for political action. Thus, in Marxism, ideology tends to be seen as a set of wrong ideas (e.g. false consciousness), whereas a Freudian-influenced psychotherapy relates ideology, at least in part to lived experience (e.g. the family). Foreman (1977) argued that fetishism or (she preferred) reification (because things are given the attributes of human relations) "structurally excludes a level of reality from thought" (p. 108). The implication of this is that we only have access to a *subconscious* perception of reality through some form of analysis of our *unconscious.*

Reich was probably the first psychoanalyst to connect class consciousness with its impact on individuals' psychological or character structure and to outline the different tasks of sociology, economics and psychology:

> every social organisation produces those character structures which it needs to exist ... hence, natural scientific psychology and characterology have a clearly defined task: they have to put their finger on the ways and mechanisms by means of which man's social entity is transformed into psychic structure and, thereby, into ideology.
>
> (Reich, 1933/1972a: xxii–xxiii)

The principal vehicle by which the individual's class-derived character structure is transmitted through the generations is "the family", which itself is unique, at least in its present form, to the capitalist system. In recent decades Marxist feminists in particular have sought to understand the specific role and importance of this social entity as both a capitalist and a psychological phenomenon. Following Reich's tasks, I briefly consider the social entity of the family, and the ideology of the family, and how the former is transformed into the latter.

The social entity of the family

Foreman (1977) argued that the nuclear family is a specifically capitalist phenomenon which serves particular functions for this socio-economic system (the reproduction of labour, ideological conformity, etc.) while, crucially, imposing an ideological construct on the role of women in society. Barrett (1980) showed that the capitalist nuclear family was developed by middle class, or "bourgeois" households during the era of mercantile (trade-based) capitalism which pre-dated the industrial revolution of the late eighteenth century. As the bourgeoisie gained ascendancy in the wake of the industrial revolution, it used its power over the media and government to advance its family model as the norm. With the bourgeois ascendency assured, alienation gradually becomes a factor in child development with, typically, the "dehumanised", mind-damaged father absent and the oppressed mother unable either to offer the nurturing role she had in earlier societies or to meet the model of the committed maternal role to which the ideal typical middle class family aspires.

Another dimension to alienation developed by feminists argues that the woman working in the home as mother and housewife is alienated from her husband and from the outside world (Mitchell, 1975; Foreman, 1977). The strength of much of this writing is to seek to integrate a theory of patriarchy with the Marxist analysis of capitalism and Freudian psychoanalysis. Thus, the division of labour which lies at the root of alienation within capitalism is traced back, with reference to the work of Engels (1884/1972) to the sexual division of labour, which division, of course, predates class society.

The ideology of the family

Barrett (1980) viewed the development of the nuclear family more as "a struggle between the familial ideology of the emergent bourgeoisie and the practices of other classes, than in terms of a strictly necessary logic of capitalism" (p. 202). Further, she questioned whether the nuclear family, in its ideal capitalist form, has ever operated for the great majority of the working class, given that divorce, women in paid work and single parent families are becoming more the norm rather than the exception. However, Barrett did view the family-household model, the nuclear family, as being essentially a capitalist phenomenon and considered that this is the point at which Freud and Marx merge:

> it is not necessary to accept the entire corpus of psychoanalytic theory to argue that gender identity and the definition of masculinity and femininity that pervades our culture are pre-eminently constructed within the ideology of the family. Furthermore, it is here more than anywhere else that we see most clearly an ideological process by which supposedly "natural" relations between parents and children, men and women, are struggled for. "The family" provides the nexus for the various themes – romantic love; feminine nurturance, maternalism, self-sacrifice; masculine protection and family support – that characterise our conception of gender and sexuality. It is, however, an ideological nexus rather than any concrete family system which is involved here and there are many connections between these processes within and outside the locus of the family home.
>
> (ibid.: 205)

This extraordinary passage stands in stark contrast to the writings of many other authors considered here precisely because it contains both a bringing together of Freud and Marx and a proper use of Marx's dialectical method. The crucial, if simple, phrase "struggled for" instantly separates Barrett from so many Marxist feminists in refusing to accept any "reality" and putting the emphasis on a process of *becoming*, brought about by the collision of conflicting and interacting forces.

Trauma, formation and transformation

This struggle also provides an integration between the three elements of Reich's task (as above) as the physical or emotional abuse or trauma (*formation*) presented to psychotherapists, is often the practical and often painful result of collision or conflict (*ideology*) within the family (*social entity*). The family is not just an ideological construct but a lived experience for people, one which, as Barrett makes clear, cannot be wholly separated from social and biological pressures and an internal (family system and individual) psychological dynamic.

Different psychological theories have their own, different notions about how precisely transformations (or deformations) – from family as social entity to family as ideology – are characterised and enacted. Traditional (Freudian) psychodynamic theories locate such formation as being consolidated within the superego. Jungian analytic psychology views family and collective cultural formations as something from which the mature individual needs to individuate. Reichian and neo-Reichian therapy describes how deformations become structured in the "character" of the body. Various forms of family therapy have developed sophisticated methods of intervention which confront "sick roles" within dysfunctional families and which support healthy family structures. Each of the various schools within the humanistic/existential "third force" of psychology also has its own perspective: the person-centred approach, for example, views such formations as external conditions of worth mediated and/or reinforced by the family, whilst transactional analysis analyses family formations in terms of individual, family, inter-generational and cultural scripting. All these represent some different concepts, in different languages, to describe unconscious and subconscious phenomena.

Marxist method

Marx introduced two important methods in scientific enquiry: historical materialism and dialectical method.

Historical materialism is an approach to history which studies social life and "social problems" in relation to the ways in which people produce their means of subsistence. It also explains the cause and nature of social change:

> at a certain stage of their development, the material productive forces of society come into conflict with the existing relations of production. ... From forms of development of the productive forces these relations turn into their fetters. There begins an era of social revolution.
>
> (Marx 1858/1971: 21)

Thus the motor of social change is the conflictual – and dialectical – relationship between the forces and relations of production.

Marxism, however, is not simply a science of history; it is a method which constantly analyses society's structure-in-process as it develops through the production and reproduction of material life:

> Dialectics makes it possible to think of a materialist process since it aims at the simultaneous recognition of "things" as both objects and processes. In other words, dialectics aims at ... grasping things immediately in their full relation to other things, and finally grasping the unity and disunity of both.
>
> (Coward & Ellis, 1977: 84)

The dialectic in Marx's method is about interconnections and dynamics, not about understanding what is, but what is becoming. It is about everything bearing a relation to something else and being directly or indirectly affected by that relation. It is about material developments acting as the fundamental but not the sole dynamic, nor one unaffected by other dynamics, such as the effect of ideology, or an ideological construct like the family. It is, above all, about understanding the human world as one, in all its complexity, and about making sense of how that world has evolved and is continuing to evolve. For psychotherapy, it provides a material-historical context for the very family/household which is seen as acting as the principal determining element in a child's psychological development, and a schema whereby the family and its members can impact upon the wider world beyond them.

Marcuse (1968) gave a more Freudian slant to Marxist method in attacking what he called the Freudian "revisionists", through which he was particularly concerned to spell out the difference between "understanding relationships", on the one hand, and developing a dialectical analysis on the other. In doing so he acknowledged the superficial truth that man appears as an individual who integrates a diversity of inherited and acquired qualities into a total personality with the result that the personality develops in relating itself to the world. However, he insisted that:

> this personality is pre-formed down to the deepest instinctual strncture, and this preformation, the work of accumulated civilisation, means that the diversities and the autonomy of individual growth are *secondary* phenomena. How much reality there is behind individuality depends on the scope, form and effectiveness of the repressive controls prevalent at a given stage of civilisation.
> (Marcuse, 1968: 175)

Whether or not one agrees with Marcuse's particular perspective (on the preformed nature of the personality), his method – of detennining the relation between primary underlying dynamics and their relation to secondary phenomena – epitomises dialectical analysis.

Being at dis-ease with ourselves

The central thesis of a Marxist approach to the individual is that of alienation: the notion that as individuals within a conflictual society which operates and maintains oppressive power relations by class, race, culture, gender, ability and so on, we are alienated from nature, from ourselves and others. For Marx, alienation is the conceptualisation of four basic but closely related social relations within capitalism: man's [sic] relation to his product; man's relation to his productive capacity; man's relation to other people; and man's relation to his species.

Whilst: "genuine disalienation is ... impossible without a total restructuring of socio-economic realities" (Bulhan, 1980: 260), the rest of this paper considers disalienation in terms of psychological realities. This is not an "either or" argument or one about prioritising the intra-psychic world; it is, in the Marxist tradition, one which proposes a dialectical method and dialogue between socio-economic realities and their impact on our psychological experiences and realities, and is the thesis, for instance, of radical psychiatry (Roy & Steiner, 1988). [Here] each concept of alienation is summarised and discussed in relation to psychotherapeutic practice.

Man's relation to his product

Before capitalism, products were generally produced for direct sale by the producer. Under capitalism, the worker has no direct connection with the product's sale, nor with the product. Work is no longer the satisfaction of a need, nor voluntary, but is something coerced by one's class position. As such, it leads to denial of self and of one's basic nature or "species-being" – which is, by implication, a pre-historical, almost mythical, "pure", unalienated, and free-spirited being.

This analysis is based on work and employment: "the first historical act is ... the production of the means to satisfy these needs, the production of material life itself" (Marx & Engels, 1846/1964: 165). The primary way in which "man" is alienated derives from the need to work. The more specialised the division of labour, the more alienated the work and the worker (Marcuse, 1969). In addition, as economies have changed so have patterns of employment; permanent unemployment has resulted in a permanent and alienated underclass, particularly amongst black youth. The gendered nature and division of labour, e.g. the reproduction of labour through the family, has challenged the concept of the "product"; and the white heat and exponential growth of new technology also challenges man's relation to the "product". Of course, psychotherapy, like many other social and welfare services, is itself a product and the psychotherapist also has a relation to this product. As with any other work, the setting, organisation and social relations of psychotherapy are also subject to critical class analysis. A current issue for such analysis is that of the organisation and [state] registration of psychotherapists, about which there is a debate between those for registration, represented by those within the United Kingdom Council for Psychotherapy (and the British Association for Counselling [BAC]) and those against (e.g. Mowbray, 1995). These positions represent, respectively, Rousseauian and Hobbesian views of society (Tudor, 1997c). A Marxist view of registration would be in favour of psychotherapy being accountable and, at the same time, critical of unnecessarily professionalised and bureaucratic superstructure on/in what should ideally be a public service industry.

The implications of this analysis for class-conscious psychotherapy include the psychotherapist's awareness of the client's economic position, of their "product", and their relation to these – as well as their own relation to each of these and to those of their client's. In an international survey on political material brought into the clinical setting (Samuels, 1993), "economic issues" (e.g. distribution of wealth, poverty, inflation) was the second most frequent specific political theme (after gender issues for women) discussed by clients in psychotherapy. It is important that psychotherapists do not pathologise such material(ist) concerns.

Man's relation to his productive capacity

> The fact that labour is *external* to the worker, i.e., does not belong to his essential being [means] that he therefore does not confirm himself in his work, but denies himself, feels miserable and not happy, does not develop free mental and physical energy, but mortifies his flesh and ruins his mind.
>
> (Marx, 1932/1975a: 326)

Although most references in this article cite Marx's early writings, he retained these concepts through his life to his last notebooks (see Carver, 1975). In *Capital*, and based largely on empirical evidence, Marx (1894/1962) referred in detail to the way in which work causes stunted size, bent backs, gnarled fingers, damaged lungs, etc. He also made general comments about the worker's mind, referring to delusions, decaying will-power, wide-ranging ignorance and mental inflexibility as evidence of alienated labour.

By placing material development at the root of their understanding of history, (in direct contrast to the dominant perspective current in the early nineteenth century), both Marx and the German philosopher Ludwig Feuerbach (1804–1872) paved the way for a new way of thinking about history and for understanding the development of the human being and her/his psyche [Feuerbach, 1841/1854]. Marx's understanding of human development in the context of man's productive capacity and her/his relationship to objects, together with his placing of "capitalist man" in a specific socio-historical context, is an important insight that has influenced much of the most important historical, economic and psychological work this century.

One of the first examples of what we might identify as class-conscious therapeutic initiatives was Reich's sexual hygiene clinics for workers and employees, six of which were opened in the early 1930s in Germany. Boadella (1985) presented some of the areas in which Reich faced problems: the interruption of pregnancy – contrary to conservative medical opinion of the time, Reich argued for a woman's right to choose in the matter of abortion; contraception – Reich promoted giving advice about contraception to young people; sex-affirmative education – Reich advocated counselling that focused on the quality of adolescent love-life. In establishing the sexual hygiene clinics for workers and employees, Reich and others were making political statements about the people they worked with, the subject/s on which they concentrated, and the way in which they worked.

In terms of psychotherapeutic practice, Perls, Hefferline, and Goodman (1951/1973; the latter, an anarchist) discussed alienation in psychological terms (in the context of the malfunctioning process of projection):

> Alienated from his own impluses, yet unable to obliterate the feelings and acts to which they give rise, man makes "things" out of his own behavior. Since he then does not experience it as himself-in-action, he can disclaim responsibility for it, try to forget it or hide it, or project it and suffer it as coming from the outside.
>
> (p. 259)

Thus gestalt experiments which invite clients "to own" their impulses and behaviours, to experience themselves as themselves-in-action in the social world are practical psychotherapeutic forms of disalientation.

In an attempt to help focus on the social as well as the psychological, Banton *et al.* (1985) proposed a "subjectification" of people's experience: "through some forms of therapy people can be brought to experience themselves as 'subject' … both … to the unconscious and to the forces of the social world" (p. 153). Radical psychiatry is a form of therapy founded on the belief that "personal and political change are interconnected: personal 'growth' cannot occur without changes that transcend the individual, and social change is a drama of real people, actors in an historical play which is written by those who perform" (Roy, 1988: 3). Radical psychiatry develops the concept of alienation, which is defined as "*the result of oppression about which the oppressed has been mystified or deceived*" (Steiner, 1971c: 5, original emphasis) and expressed as "Alienation = Oppression + Mystification + Isolation" (Roy, 1988). This formula and its antithesis "Liberation (or Power in the World …) = Awareness + Contact + Action" (Roy, 1988) have both been developed from the praxis of radical theory and practice: the concept of internalised oppression is used to counter mystification, awareness is developed through psychotherapy, contact is encouraged through groupwork which also helps overcome isolation, and people are supported in taking action in their lives and in the world, which is an expression of their productive capacity.

Man's relation to other people

> If the product of labour does not belong to the worker and, if it confronts him as an alien power, this is only possible because it belongs to *a man other than the worker* … If therefore he regards the product of his labour, his objectified labour, as an alien, hostile, and powerful object which is independent of him,

> then his relationship to that object is such that another man – alien, hostile, powerful and independent of him – is its master … Every self-estrangement of man from himself and nature is manifested in the relationship he sets up between other men and himself and nature.
>
> (Marx, 1932/1975a: 330–331)

Man and woman, women and men, are thus alienated from their bosses because they are alienated from their product. It is no less the case that relations *between* workers are also alienated relations because the very position of a worker is unnatural, forced and alienated. Indeed, all relations between people in capitalist society are alienated: i.e. fraught with hostility, false perceptions and sublimated personas. The concept of alienated relations, whilst helping to understand the worker's position in capitalist society, at the same time points to a dynamic working against a class alliance between workers. These contradictions are represented in the case of trades unions (TUs). The historical need for and role of TUs arose in response to structural conflict and exploitation; they have been and continue to be crucial not only in defending workers' rights but also in advancing positive contributions to industrial relations. They are thus important at an organisational level. Beyond this, in modelling collective and co-operative organisation and action, they are, at best and at a psychological level, a method and a means of disalienation. The fact that many active trades unionists experience alienation from their own union hierarchies is a reflection of the lack of Marxist analysis and understanding amongst the leadership of TUs and is an argument for the restructuring of traditional forms of socialist organisation (Howell, 1981). This aspect of alienation contributes to a materialist/psychological understanding of the relative timidity of workers in relation to their employers and the lack of ultimate solidarity between workers. One working class psychotherapy client, a committed and active trades unionist, spent most of her initial time in psychotherapy expressing her anger about her boss, on behalf of her TU comrades and against "the system" in general. The psychotherapist (who had herself previously been a shop steward) acknowledged her client's anger and the genuine causes of it *and at the same time* helped her to acknowledge how her anger alienated her from others, her self-estrangement, and how both affected her relationships both at work and in the rest of her life.

Later Marxists (for example, Lukács, 1971) have developed the conundrum of alienated relations between people into a theory of false consciousness, deriving from what Marx called the "fetishism of commodities". This signifies the reification of products under capitalism, so that they take on a life and character and value of their own, independently of the people who produced them. Thus we do not think of the worker who put value into a car through her/his labour; we think of the car's value as defined by market competition. We subconsciously deny or distort the role that fellow workers have played in bringing products to the market, and in giving them value, and we allow this to undermine solidarity between working people. Further, and most importantly, we see money as the creator of wealth, rather than as the outcome of our own wealth-creation. Money thus becomes the ultimate fetish, rather than the mark of exchange value. The exchange value of money for psychotherapy is an ill-considered and under-researched matter in psychotherapy training and practice. It is a commonplace argument that it is important that clients pay for, and therefore (literally) value their therapy, an argument which is also used to justify the payment for missed sessions in private practice. The high rates of attendance for public sector psychotherapy belies this argument. Significantly, the BAC's *Code of Ethics and Practice for Counsellors* (British

Association for Counselling, 1992) stated that "the communication of terms and any negotiations of these should be concluded *before* the client incurs any financial liability" (B.2.2.11; author's emphasis). This places a clear requirement on counsellors to offer free initial consultations and, by implication, not to charge for those subsequent sessions in which the terms and conditions of counselling are discussed. Class-conscious psychotherapists will be aware of the financial context of their clients and of psychotherapy; those working in private practice need to develop conscious and creative approaches to exchange which may involve accepting barter arrangements or offering psychotherapy through local economic trading schemes (see Tudor, 1998).

Man's relation to his species

"Estranged labour not only (1) estranges nature from man and (2) estranges man from himself, from his own active function, from his vital activity; because of this it also estranges man from his *species*" (Marx, 1932/1975a: 328). For Marx, alienation of man from his product and from his productive capacity also dehumanises him such that "his inorganic body, nature, is taken from him" (p. 329). This may be overstated for effect but is not as arcane a point as at first appears. Freud's "reality principle" also describes a denial of self and of nature in the world of work, although Freud does not attribute this denial solely to capitalism, viewing it instead as running through human history (Freud, 1911/1984).

Psychotherapy's responses to this alienation have been various. Although psychology has often studied and pathologised people as individuals, from the time of Wundt, the nineteenth century philosopher, physiologist and founding father of experimental psychology, there has also been a strong collective and social psychology which has influenced various psychotherapeutic traditions. Freud's work on civilisation (Freud, 1930/1961), Jung's notion of the collective unconscious and Reich's classic text on the *Mass Psychology of Fascism* (Reich, 1933/1970) are all early examples of the application of psychoanalytic thinking to the problems of the social world.

Perhaps the earliest of these was the psychodrama, and later sociodrama, of Moreno (1946/1964), which subsequently inspired the *Theatre of the Oppressed* (Boal, 1979). Schutzman (1994) reported a further development of this tradition in a workshop which helped "to identify and embody oppressive territory rather than the more dichotomous oppressors and oppressed, and, in so doing, provided us with a map for dealing with our non-prescriptive, unchosen social positions within that oppressive territory" (pp. 144–145). Such theatre and experimentation provides a collective tool both for exploring "behavioural options *at the moment of discrimination*" (p. 145), and for political organising. Within the psychodynamic tradition, a number of radical practitioners have been involved in establishing projects which have (or had) an integrated strategy of intervention which is both political and therapeutic. The work of the Battersea Action and Counselling Centre (Holland & Hoggett, 1977), the White City Mental Health Project and its sister organisation Women's Action on Mental Health (Holland, 1979, 1985, 1990), Nafsiyat (Kareem, 1992), and Shanti (Mills & Topolski, 1996) all help people move psychologically from individual psychotherapeutic space to one of collective identity and action. Radical therapists and psychiatrists have also worked with patients in groups in the residential setting of the therapeutic community (see Edleson, 1970). In an attempt to synthesise Marx and Reich, Collingwood (1991), a counsellor and a revolutionary socialist, develops a four-dimensional model of individual and social change which echoes a Marxist theory of alienation: the foundational, the relational, the representational and the fusional. Within the humanistic/existential tradition the radical psychiatry of early transactional analysts (as discussed above) is the most explicit example of a class-conscious psychotherapy, whilst the influence of Rogers on education (Rogers, 1969, 1983) and on power (Rogers, 1978) is widespread. The four-fold dimensions of human existence of existential therapy – the physical (*umwelt*), the social (*mitwelt*), the psychological (*eigenwelt*) and the spiritual (*ueberwelt*) (see van Deurzen-Smith, 1996) are also useful in considering alienation from our species and species-being.

Conclusion

From this analysis, it follows that four conceptualisations of disalienation – or five, if we accept Roy's (1988) further conceptualisation of man's alienated social relations with the Earth – are useful in promoting a class-conscious psychotherapy. Psychotherapy and psychotherapists also need to develop an anti-oppressive stance whether through the pedagogy of the oppressed (Freire, 1972), the theatre of the oppressed (Boal, 1979), or a psychotherapy of the oppressed in which psychotherapy is viewed as "a form of psychopolitical enlightenment" (Holland, 1992: 143). Fromm (1971) suggested that "the destruction of illusions and the analysis of consciousness ... are the conditions for social change" (p. 76). The destruction of illusions and the analysis of consciousness (and false consciousness) might equally be considered as a condition for psychotherapeutic change. Following our Marxist schema, and no doubt disillusioning John Major, being truly "at ease with oneself" is being connected to oneself, to one's product and productive capacities, to others, and to the world. It is also having a consciousness of and identity with our class. Laing (1967) wrote in terms of the inevitability of alienation: "we are born into a world where alienation awaits us" (p. 16). Shenker (1986) viewed alienation as "a condition wherein a person is unable to maintain a sense of identity" (p. 20) and that identity means that the individual: operates a coherent system, has meaning in terms of themselves and their environment, is stable, feels "at home" in the world, and is a discrete entity in the world. Shweder (1990) defined and discussed cultural psychology, arguing that we are – and need to be – culturally intentional beings, i.e. conscious of our own culture. In this tradition Singh and Tudor (1997) have explored the culturally intentional conditions of therapy, including class as a variable of culture. Equally, we are – and need to be – intentional beings in class terms. Through disalienation, the destruction of illusions, the analysis of consciousness and anti-oppressive practice comes the achievement of a political – and psychological – communism, that is:

> The positive supersession of private property as human self-estrangement, and hence the true appropriation of the human essence through and for man; it is the complete restoration of man to himself as a social, i.e., human, being ... it is the genuine resolution of the conflict between man and nature, and between man and man, the true resolution of the conflict between existence and being, between objectification and self-affirmation, between freedom and necessity, between individual and species.
>
> (Marx, 1932/1975a: 348)

CHAPTER 6

THE PERSONAL IS POLITICAL – AND THE POLITICAL IS PERSONAL (1997)

Retrospective introduction

This chapter reproduces an article that was originally published in *Person-Centred Practice*, the journal of the British Association for the Person-Centred Approach (BACPA), of which I was a member for a number of years (1993–2010). The journal, which ran from 1993 to 2004, was edited by Tony Merry, who, sadly, died in 2004. Tony, with whom I had written a *Dictionary of Person-Centred Psychology* (Tudor & Merry, 2002), had invited me to edit a special issue of the journal, to which I responded by offering one on the theme of "The Person-Centred Approach and the Political Sphere". Three other members of the BAPCA responded: Anne Kearney, herself the author of a book on *Counselling, Class and Politics* (Kearney, 1996), wrote an article on class and politics in relation to the training of counsellors (Kearney, 1997); Rose Cameron offered a re-reading of Rogers in the context of (then) current criticisms and, in doing so, reclaimed the political relevance of key concepts of the person-centred approach (Cameron, 1997); and, drawing on the work of Fujio Tomoda, who translated much of Rogers' work into Japanese, Judy Moore discussed the concepts of "reality" and "the self" from a cultural perspective (Moore, 1997). Tony was pleased with the issue and obviously liked the article as he later reproduced it in a collection of articles from the journal (Merry, 2000). Tony was a big man, both physically and psychologically, and, although, I didn't know him for very long, I enjoyed and appreciated the contact we had, especially over the dictionary, as well as a number of long and lively discussions with him, usually over some pints of real ale! To him I dedicate this chapter with profound appreciation for his contribution to the person-centred approach, and love.

My own contribution in this piece was to develop a person-centred analysis of the political sphere. I was – and am – aware that, historically, social and cultural commentators have drawn more on psychoanalysis than other forms of psychology, and I was keen to apply person-centred concepts to the social/political world. Thus, I used first, person-centred personality theory (Rogers, 1951) to consider aspects of the 1997 British general election; second, the person-centred theory of human development (Rogers, 1959) to look at the then recent referenda on devolved powers to a Scottish parliament and a Welsh assembly; and third, Rogers' theory of the (six) necessary and sufficient conditions of therapy and personality change to reflect on the responses to the death of Diana, Princess of Wales. Drawing on Totton's (2000) four categories of what he has referred to as the "interplay" between psychotherapy and politics, i.e. psychotherapy *in* politics, psychotherapy *of* politics, politics *of* psychotherapy, and politics *in* psychotherapy, the article offered a person-centred psychotherapy or understanding *of* politics, an example of what Totton defined as "a range of attempts to *understand* and to *evaluate* political life through the application of psychotherapeutic concepts". (p. 6). The title echoes the feminist slogan of the 1970s, and, thereby, acknowledges the influence of feminism on my thinking about personal politics, and politics in general.

As for the article itself, I still like it, 'though in some ways, given the specificity of the examples, it is arguably the most dated of this selection. My comments regarding Tony Blair should not be taken as any support for him or his policies (see also Chapter 8); indeed I remember waking up on 2 May 1997 feeling somewhat out of kilter or synch with a number of my friends in not being at all excited about the incoming "new Labour" government. As this book was going to press shortly after the 2016 Brexit vote, I find my comments about devolution somewhat poignant as I suspect that there will be more conversation about, and a need for greater analysis of, the psychopolitical forces for separation, dissolution, and devolution, as well as for union, association, and federation. While, again, I was working to a specific word-length and was – and still am – quite pleased with how I was developing the necessary editorial muscle to do this, I would now probably look to expanding the examples to give greater detail. In this sense, I think the article is more indicative than comprehensive. Although I was on to something with my reference to two directions of movement, i.e. the politicisation of the personal and the personalisation of the political, with the benefit of Totton's taxonomy, now I would look to use this to develop a more thorough analysis of the interplay between person-centred psychology and the political sphere. Re-reading the article, I was also interested to see the reference to Rogers' 1973 paper, one to which I returned a couple of years ago in writing an article in which I reviewed and renewed his "new challenge" (Tudor, 2013a; see also Chapter 11). In terms of editing, I have reversed two paragraphs (on p. 000), and introduced some sub-headings.

A person-centred approach to the political sphere

This article describes the meeting of two spheres: the therapeutic sphere with its focus on healing the psyche, i.e. the internal, intra-psychic world, and the political sphere of the external, social, civic world. In describing this encounter between the psyche and the social, the article develops two directions of movement: the politicisation of the personal and the personalising of the political. This provides a frame for discussions developing a person-centred approach (PCA) to understanding the relation between these two often separated spheres and, particularly, to understanding the impact of local, national and international events.

The personal is political

This early feminist slogan summarised one of the concerns of the women's liberation movement to highlight issues which had previously been seen as personal and private. Relationships between women and men, sexuality, abuse, childcare, housework, etc. became the subject of public debate. Later, other movements put issues of race, culture, sexuality and disability on the agenda – issues which now affect personal beliefs, attitudes, feelings and behaviour as well as public policies and popular culture. Here the *focus* of enquiry is on the *personal* whilst the *direction* of concern and debate is towards the *political*, for instance by subjecting particular (hitherto) "personal" conflicts, say between a heterosexual couple, to a political analysis using concepts such as those of patriarchy and class relations. Generally, this has an effect of widening our understanding from the particular to the general: in the above example, to understand a personal conflict as an example of distorted gender relations.

This sphere includes the politics *of* psychology and of therapy. This is based on a belief that therapy as an activity is *itself* political: as a social phenomenon it is inevitably political. For those who believe and claim that therapy is – and should – not be "political", a few comments on the history and organisation of therapy may place this in context. Historically, psychoanalysis became seen as a branch of science within medicine and psychiatry. One implication of this is that psychoanalysis in particular and psychotherapy in general has developed an (unhealthy) obsession in psycho*pathology* – the origins of the *illness* of the psyche – rather than an equal concern with what might be referred to as psycho*sanology* – or the *health* of the psyche (see Tudor, 1997b). Another implication of this incorporation into the medical/psychiatric establishment was the search for respectability and acceptability in the way in which psychotherapy was/is organised and psychotherapists were/are trained. The struggle against the hegemony of the medical model, of fixed ideas about human nature and change, and of closed, self-generating training institutes (institutions) forms a crucial, if largely ignored, part of our collective psychohistory.

The person-centred tradition has made a particular contribution to the politics of therapy, founded on a politics of the person. In a challenging address to the American Psychological Association (APA), Rogers asked if they (we) dared to develop a *human* science, to be whole people, to be designers rather than repairers – in all spheres of life – and to do away with professionalism: "as soon as we set up criteria for certification … the first and greatest effect is to freeze the profession in a past image. This is an *inevitable* result" (Rogers, 1973b/1990a: 364). In his ideas about education Rogers (1983) challenges traditional theories of "top-down" education and training. Rogers' regret at his involvement in establishing a board of examiners within the APA is paralleled by Thorne's (1995) more recent concerns about the vicious circle of accountability and the lack of soul in, effectively, the developing closed shop of the British Association for Counselling individual counsellor accreditation. Kearney (1996) offered a critique of counselling based on considerations of (the absence of) class and politics and, in this issue, extends this to the training of counsellors (Kearney, 1997). Rogers applied his ideas to the field of personal politics in his book *Carl Rogers on Personal Power* (Rogers, 1978), subtitled *Inner Strength and its Revolutionary Impact*, in which he discussed the organismic tendency towards fulfilment as a constructive basis of human motivation and for "a harmonious politics of interpersonal relationships" (p. 243) in relation to the helping professions, the family, partnership, education, administration, oppression and intercultural tension. Recent work on and in large groups is an example of the therapeutic application of the PCA in developing a person-centred politics of community and the social world (see Caspary, 1991; Lago, 1994; Wood, 2008).

Others too have challenged the received theories and practices of the various traditions and schools of psychotherapy ever since Freud first coined the term a hundred years ago. For example, in the early days, those on the radical Left such as Reich and Adler attempted to account for social as well as psychological realities. More recently, the establishment in 1995 of the organisation Psychotherapists and Counsellors for Social Responsibility (PCSR) and its journal *Transformations* is a sign that a significant number of therapists are interested in the social sphere. Two recent books have also contributed to political understanding of the personal sphere: Mowbray (1995) puts the case against psychotherapy registration and House and Totton (1997) argue for pluralism and autonomy in the *activity* (as distinct from the profession) of psychotherapy and counselling.

The political is personal

Here the *focus* of enquiry is on the *political* sphere whilst the *direction* of understanding is towards the *personal* and therapeutic, for instance the impact of politics and the political world on "personal" life. This is the therapy of politics: the healing power of the political (the way civic society is organised, particular policies, etc.) as well as its potential for denying personal experience and distorting the way we understand ourselves. Traditionally, some political systems have impacted more than others on people's personal lives. Generally, socialist governments influenced by Marxist analysis have tended to emphasise the social by favouring planned economies and societies and developing certain social policies, which legislate in the personal sphere such as fertility, abortion, childcare and parental responsibilities. Generally, conservative governments tend to emphasise the individual – epitomised by Margaret Thatcher's famous comment that "there is no such thing as society" (Keay, 1987) – thus promoting the philosophy of the free market, both economically and socially, often leaving themselves open to accusations of a lack of caring about issues such as poverty, homelessness, mental illness and distress. In such societies, the emphasis is, respectively, on the community and the individual.

From the early days of psychoanalysis, therapists have been concerned with and have used their analytic insights to understand the wider social/political sphere. Freud published his book *Civilisation and Its Discontents* in 1930; at the same time Reich was applying his theories on human character structure to analysing *The Mass Psychology of Fascism* (Reich 1933/1970) and Jung (1936/1959) was writing about the unconscious connections between peoples across cultures and time. In the 1960s a number of humanistic psychiatrists and therapists were actively involved in political movements and struggles, viewing this *in itself* as radical therapeutic practice. More recently, in its organisation of topic groups, PCSR clearly views therapy as concerned with the politics *of* … disability, ecology, economics, gender, race and culture, sexual diversity, etc.

The person-centred tradition has made its own contribution to this direction of enquiry, particularly through Rogers' development of the notion of personal rather than institutional power and his emphasis on the emerging person rather than organisations or political parties as the spearhead of "the quiet revolution". His work with groups in conflict and in what he referred to as some of the world's "hottest" areas of tension (Northern Ireland, Central America and South Africa) reflects the development and practical application of the PCA to the political sphere.

> Politically, then, if we are in search of a trustworthy base to operate from, our major aim would be to discover and possibly increase the number of individuals who are coming closer to being whole persons – who are moving toward a knowledge of, and harmony with, their innermost experience, and who sense, with an equal lack of defensiveness, all the data from the persons and objects in the external environment.
>
> (Rogers, 1978: 250–251)

This elaborates Aristotle's dictum that "man [sic] is by nature a political animal": our organismic tendency and the basis of human motivation is towards actualising ourselves *and others*. Here, Rogers is also elaborating the need for harmony both with our inner (intra psychic) *and* our external (extra psychic) worlds. Yet, despite Rogers' own work and other notable examples, and despite the depth of its theoretical understanding of the person and her/his environment, the PCA has not developed a widespread understanding (even analysis) of the external environment/world outside therapy and its impact on people – a gap in application which this article seeks to redress.

Developing a person-centred analysis of the political sphere

Historically, psychoanalysts using psychoanalytic and psychodynamic concepts have been at the forefront of developing analysis of society and social events – most popular psychological commentators and columnists, too, are more or less explicitly influenced by psychoanalysis. Although the person-centred approach has necessary and sufficient concepts with which to understand events in the social sphere as well as their impact on people's lives and internal worlds, it has not been as developed or applied to the political world. To illustrate this I discuss briefly three recent events in the British political sphere in terms of the PCA: the general election (in terms of person-centred personality theory); the recent referenda on devolved powers to a Scottish parliament and a Welsh assembly (in relation to human development); and the death of Diana, Princess of Wales (with reference to Rogers' six conditions).

The British general election May 1997

Many will view the British general election in May 1997, rather than the founding of the Social Democratic Party 16 years earlier, as breaking the mould (in both senses [of the word]!) of British politics. Rather than focusing on the nature of the electoral system, the votes cast, particular political personalities, etc., here I am more concerned to understand what the result represents. In all elections, when it is apparent which party has won, an interesting transition takes place: in this case the political and partial (Labour) Party becomes the government; the leader of the opposition becomes prime minister. The government led by the prime minister becomes the government of *all* the people, even those who did not vote for them and, indeed, those who did not vote at all. The defeated party bows to the will of the people – generally with the grace not to tell us that we made a mistake. In May this transition took on a different (political) hue. ... In Blair's subsequent statements about the third or middle way of politics, in the government's proposals for constitutional reform as well as reform of the voting system, and in its invitation to the Liberal Democrats to sit on a cabinet committee on such reforms: the government appears to be espousing "one nation" consensus politics. This may be understood in terms of Rogers' (1951) personality theory in which the total personality comprises two overlapping circles which, in a state of psychological tension, represent experience and self-structure (see Figure 6.1).

Experience, "the immediate [phenomenological] field of sensory and visceral experience" (Rogers, 1951: 525), suggests that there are situations, issues and problems in the social world and responses and solutions to these phenomena. The concept of self-structure, "the configuration of concepts which has been defined as the

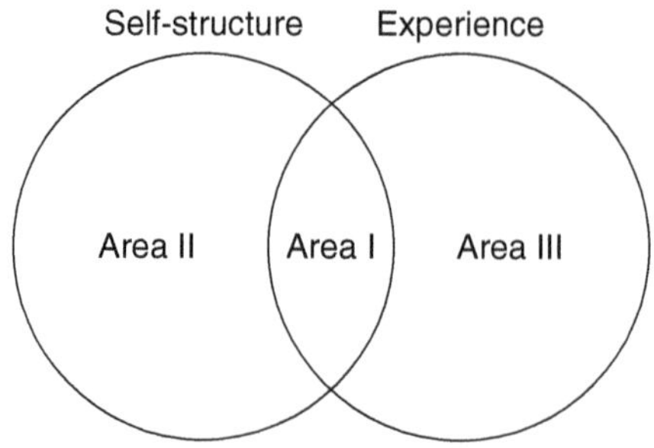

Figure 6.1 The total personality (Rogers, 1951)

structure of the self [which] includes the patterned perceptions of the individual's characteristics and relationships" (ibid.: 525) may be applied to an organisational structure such as that of a political party. Person-centred personality theory may thus be applied to the personality of the body politic.

Area II. Social and other experiences are distorted and values are perceived as experience. Most politicians claim that they have the truth, that all their policies are right, that all the other parties' policies are wrong – and that the public perceives this to be the case and supports them (if only we knew all the facts). Thus most political issues – the economy, tax and spending policies, education, health, etc. – become polarised *and distorted* as for/against, us/them and good/bad.

Area III. Experiences are denied to awareness because they are inconsistent with the self (organisational) structure. Some within and outside the Labour Party criticised Tony Blair for consulting Margaret Thatcher about his first "Heads of States" conference. In effect, they denied her experience as it is inconsistent with their criticism of her – and inconsistent with much of their organisational structure and culture which has, over the years, been defined by their opposition to her. (One of the problems of the British Labour Party has been that, over the last 18 years, its identity has been defined only by opposition.)

Area I. The concept of self (i.e. organisation) and organisation-in-relationship is congruent with our experience. No one and certainly no one political party has the monopoly on the truth. Thus the British government is open to political partnership; the Liberal Democrats state that they will provide a "constructive opposition", supporting the government on policies on which they agree and maintaining their opposition to policies on which they disagree. Thus, in political life, experience becomes congruent with the structure (organisation) of politics – and vice versa. One example of this is the way the business of the House of Commons is organised and conducted. Recent changes (to prime minister's question time and the reorganisation of committee meetings and times) are designed to reflect life in the twentieth – and twenty-first – centuries, thereby making this political life more accessible to those with families (rather than maintaining a structure which reflects the needs of eighteenth century landed gentry).

Such analysis also has its application in therapy. One client who generally viewed her life as a battle between two oppositional aspects of herself talked about being surprised at her own excitement at the result of the election. As she discussed this in therapy, she talked about the new government as representing a new politics of consensus (area I) rather than the old politics of adversarial positions and polarities. Subsequently she drew on this as a potent metaphor for the resolution of her personal conflicts.

The referenda on devolution September 1997

The recent referenda on devolving powers to a Scottish parliament and a Welsh assembly, which resulted in "yes" votes (overwhelming in Scotland and more muted in Wales) is an example of people voting for more devolved local powers and responsibilities. This may be viewed in terms of individual – and, more generally, national – self-development and differentiation as well as devolution. For Rogers (1951), the self is "the awareness of being, of functioning" (p. 498) and is synonymous with self-awareness and self-experience. Widening this to a "we" self-concept (Nobles, 1973), a sense of family, collective, tribal and even national identity in an awareness of and desire to be and to function as "we" is understandable. Developmentally, the self is a differentiated portion of the perceptual field (Rogers, 1951, 1959). Again, on a wider level, this provides an understanding of increasing moves on the part of identified and identifiable parts to differentiate from larger wholes, particularly when those "wholes" are countries, nations, "blocs" or geographical areas, which have been united by conquest (as in the case of Wales by England) or artificially amalgamated by historical expedient or treaty (as in the case of Scotland and England – and, for that matter, six counties of the island of Ireland). From our understanding of development and differentiation, it is perhaps not surprising that, at the same time as the European Community is expanding and certain powers are being centralised, many peoples throughout Europe are expressing their desire for the powers and responsibilities of government to be experienced and expressed more directly and personally.

The death of Diana, Princess of Wales, August 1997

The death of Diana, Princess of Wales – and, perhaps more significantly, the impact of her death – appears to have taken the public, including republicans and commentators, by surprise. As with the other examples, whatever one's own opinions and partiality, Diana's impact on people may be understood, appropriately enough, in person-centred terms. As an integrative model, Rogers' (1957/1990b) six conditions of interpersonal relationships is especially well suited to application to relationships in the wider social/political sphere. Diana clearly made *psychological contact* with people she met – and, arguably, with people she did not meet: "probably it is sufficient if each makes some 'subceived' difference in the experiential field of the other" (p. 221). This perhaps accounts for the number of people who were surprised at the strength of their reaction to her death. In her work with the homeless, those with AIDS and leprosy, and with victims of landmines – "the constituency of the rejected" as Diana's brother Earl Spencer put it in his funeral address – she had an acute sense of *the vulnerability of others*. In this sense, and especially in recent years, she appeared *congruent*: often communicating her awareness of self and others on a range of personal and social/political issues. She showed compassion and love (*unconditional positive regard*) towards the people she met through her charitable work, despite perhaps not having the same regard for herself – in his address her brother commented that her desire to do good for others had the effect of releasing her from "deep feelings of unworthiness". Significantly, the reading at her funeral service, 1 Corinthians 13, ends with the famous phrase about faith, hope and charity – which translates as love. Similarly, Diana appears to have expressed her *empathic understanding* for many people's experience, again perhaps borne out of her own vulnerability and difficulties. Finally, people she met said that they had felt her regard and empathy and many thousands, even millions, of others report having felt touched by (having *received*) her love and understanding. Diana's impact may thus be viewed as having fulfilled the necessary and sufficient conditions by which interpersonal relationships are enhanced – even at a distance.

Conclusion

These are but three topical examples of how the PCA may be used and developed as a framework for understanding the wider world and its impact on our personal worlds. Rogers' basis for harmony between innermost experience and the external environment requires us to be at ease with, and in, both the personal and political spheres and the movement between the two: to develop our congruence with ourselves as individuals-in-political-context. In his ground-breaking work covering issues such as masculinity, nationalism and political material in the clinical setting, Samuels (1993), drawing on analytic (Jungian) psychology, successfully moves in both directions at the same time. This article is a contribution to developing a *person-centred approach* to understanding the political nature of the personal and, particularly, the personal nature of the political.

PART III

THE 2000s

Employment, other work, professional qualifications, accreditations/registration and memberships, academic qualifications, and recognitions

Ongoing	self-employed counsellor, psychotherapist, supervisor, researcher, trainer, and consultant
	United Kingdom Council for Psychotherapy (UKCP), registered psychotherapist
	European Association of Transactional Analysis (EATA), certified transactional analyst
	Temenos, co-director, 2004–2009 director of education and training, and director, postgraduate diploma/MSc in person-centred psychotherapy and counselling, and 2004–2010 staff member
	Institute for Transactional Analysis, UK, clinical member, from 2004 training member
	EATA, clinical member, from 2004 teaching member
	International Association for Transactional Analysis, clinical/regular/CTA member, from 2004 teaching member
Ongoing–2002	Liverpool John Moores University, honorary research fellow
Ongoing–2004	EATA, provisional teaching and supervising transactional analyst
Ongoing–2008	Association of Humanistic Psychology Practitioners, full member
	UKCP, registered group psychotherapist and facilitator
Ongoing–2010	British Association for the Person-Centred Approach, member
	Association of Therapeutic Communities, member
2000	Esther (daughter) arrives
2000–2006	Sheffield Natural Health Centre, proprietor, 2005–2006 centre manager
2002–2004	Metanoia Institute, London, course tutor, MSc in transactional analysis psychotherapy

2004–2011	EATA, teaching and supervising transactional analyst
July 2009	Emigrates to Aotearoa New Zealand
From 2009	Auckland University of Technology, (2009–2010) senior lecturer, (2009–2014) programme leader, (from September 2009) certified postgraduate supervisor
	Ngā Ao e Rua, member

CHAPTER 7

MENTAL HEALTH PROMOTION (2004)

Retrospective introduction

In 1990 I obtained a senior fellowship at King's College, London to research the subject of community mental health promotion. This position had been established by the good offices of Russell Caplan of the Health Education Authority (HEA), and Ray Holland, a senior lecturer in the Management Centre at King's College. The fellowship was part-time for a year, which I undertook alongside my work as a psychiatric social worker, thereby working with and in both mental health (well-being) and mental illness (psychiatry). At the end of the year I produced a report which, after some consideration and time, was rejected by the HEA. After some more time and with the help of Ray and Russell, the HEA released the copyright of the report; I undertook further research in my own time, and made it into a book which was published by Routledge in 1996.

The book, the first on the subject, was well reviewed and well received. It won that year's Bruce Burns Annual Mental Health Promotion Award. Bhugra (1998) summarised it as "a thought provoking, well written book in an area which needs novel ideas and the application of these ideas in relation to social policy and community mental health organisation" (p. 249); and Thomlison (1999) described it as "an impressive book from many perspectives ... From a scholarly perspective, the book presents a coherent critique and integrative view of empirical and theoretical literature in mental health promotion". (p. 478). The holistic, multifaceted view of health outlined in the book was cited by the About NHS Evidence website, hosted by the National Institute for Health and Clinical Excellence (2009). The conceptualisations set out in the book had a direct impact on the development of a national strategy in Aotearoa New Zealand, called *Building on Strengths* (Ministry of Health | Manatu Hauora, 2002), an influence which was acknowledged by Briggs (2001). The book has been cited in two publications on mental health and its promotion produced by the World Health Organization (Herrman, Saxena, & Moodie, 2005; Friedli, 2009). The book has led to various invitations for me to speak at a number of international conferences, and to act as a consultant to two governments: Health Canada/Santé Canada in both Ottawa and Toronto; and the Scottish Government in Edinburgh, specifically regarding its National Programme for Improving Mental Health and Wellbeing (see www.wellscotland.info/mental-health/national-programme.html). In 1999, in recognition of my work in this field, I was made an honorary lecturer in the School of Health at Liverpool John Moores University. My development of the two continua concept (Minister of National

Health & Welfare, 1988) has been influential in supporting the rationale for the development of mental health indicators for adults in Scotland (see Parkinson, 2007). Writing about the influence of my work and that of Keyes (2007) on the Scottish Government's National Programme, Smith-Merry (2008) commented that: "The work of both Tudor and Keyes brings with it a policy strategy for health promotion" (p. 7), and that:

> This approach underpins all of the policy aims envisaged for the next stage of the National Programme. Through the introduction of this new language the Scottish Government aims to address the criticisms of both the 2004 and 2006–7 reviews that there was not a clear and well-understood definition of what constitutes positive mental health.
>
> (p. 7)

The following year (2009) I was asked to comment on the mental emotional, physical and social wellbeing aspects of the Curriculum for Excellence being developed by Learning and Teaching Scotland. I have had a specific influence on the development of mental health promotion/improvement in Grampian:

1. In 1998 I developed contacts with both universities in Aberdeen and in 1999 wrote two distance learning papers on mental health for the Faculty of Nursing, Midwifery and Community Studies, University of Aberdeen (Tudor, 1999b, 1999d).
2. For some 5 years, between 2000 and 2004, I had a contract with Health Promotions, Aberdeen to deliver training courses for a variety of public sector workers on the subject of mental health and its promotion, in the course of which I trained and influenced nearly 500 people. One of the people who commissioned these courses, now a development officer for mental health and emotional wellbeing at Learning and Teaching Scotland, recalled participants' responses to the training (S. Leslie, personal [e-mail] communication, 3 February, 2009): "The evaluations were all very positive with staff finding the training very helpful in terms of aiding their understanding of mental health and implications for themselves as well as their work with children and young people".
3. In 2005 I was involved in drafting Grampian's regional policy on mental health improvement (Tudor & Begbie, 2005).

Elsewhere in the UK, others have used the book as the basis of training on mental health and its promotion; as Thomlison (1999) acknowledged: "The book serves as an impressive reference for those teaching in the field of mental health" (p. 478).

In 2003 Ian Norman and Iain Ryrie approached me to contribute a chapter to their extensive textbook on mental health nursing, an invitation I was delighted to accept as it provided me an opportunity both to update and condense my ideas into one chapter. The chapter framed mental health in the context of a number of problematic assumptions in contemporary debates about health, and then presented theories and models for understanding health and psychological health, and mental health in terms of concepts, paradigms, elements, and empirical research. As my work and this chapter distinguished mental health from mental illness, I critiqued two (then) contemporary and influential social policy documents which conflated the two: The *National Service Framework for Mental Health* (Department of Health, 1999a) and *Making It Happen* (Department of Health, 2001).

With regard to the original chapter, in the section on "Mental health and mental illness" (pp. 98–101 below), I have included some material from my PhD (Tudor, 2010b) (marked in square brackets [...]), which adds to the conceptual and philosophical argument about the advantages of the two continua model; I have also deleted a short section which was written for the particular context of the book (and which I thought was the weakest section of the original piece): two edits that address my own critique of the original publication. In the chapter I refer to the then current, fourth edition of the American Psychiatric Association's (2000) *Diagnostic and Statistical Manual of Mental Disorders* (*DSM-IV*). Although I was – and am – critical of this taxonomy of and approach to mental disorders and, more broadly, mental illness, I did appreciate its multiaxial system of and perspective on diagnosis and, thus, have not updated this in terms of *DSM-5* (which has dropped the multiaxial system of diagnosis). During the production of the original book, when I saw that the chapter was due to appear somewhere towards the end of the book, I wrote to Ian Norman to ask him and his co-editor to consider placing the chapter earlier in the book, to make and reinforce the point that positive mental health was not so much an application of "mental health" (generally taken as meaning illness), but, rather, a positive approach to the whole field. To their credit – and my appreciation – they accepted the argument and placed this chapter as Chapter 2 in the book. In my original acknowledgements, I thanked Fiona Begbie (Scotland), Natacha Joubert (Canada), Elizabeth Morris (UK) and John Raeburn (New Zealand) for their support and their comments on earlier drafts of the chapter.

Introduction

> "Health is more difficult to deal with than illness".
> (D. W. Winnicott)

It is a commonplace that "health", both as a word and as a concept, is often used to stand for "illness". Nowhere is this more true – and detrimental – than in the field of "mental health". The ubiquitous term "people with mental health problems" disguises the actual referent, that is: people diagnosed with a mental illness or personality disorder (or both). Leaving aside the deconstruction of "mental illness", such definitions by substitution do no favours either for those with a diagnosed mental illness or for those defining and promoting positive mental health. Despite the fact that the distinction between mental health and mental illness – and understanding of that distinction – has been around for, arguably, over 100 years (since the early days of the international mental hygiene movement), policy makers, politicians and practitioners almost wilfully continue to conflate and confuse the two terms. The latest example of this is contained in and indeed represented by the *National Service Framework for Mental Health* (Department of Health, 1999a) and *Making It Happen* (Department of Health, 2001) which, whilst talking the walk (referring to the promotion of mental health in its aim), certainly does not walk the talk as, within four sentences, it refers to assessing performance of its aim with reference to the National *Psychiatric* Morbidity Survey!

Taking Winnicott's statement as a challenge to "deal with" health, the first part of this chapter concentrates on health in its own right, certainly as more than the absence of disease and in a number of ways beyond the medical model. Following this, in the second part of the chapter, the focus shifts to understandings of *mental* health, including a discussion of the relationship between mental health and mental illness and the efficacy of promoting the mental health of the mentally ill. In conclusion mental health promotion theory, policy and practice is summarised and the role of mental health consultation is discussed. Mental *health* is viewed as the concern of all, not some and, therefore, as much the business of mental health nursing as any other discipline or profession. Moreover, just as *mental* health is viewed as criterial to health (an argument referred to in the second part of this chapter), so an understanding of mental health is central to nursing – and, in this, the role of the mental health nurse as consultant, advocate and facilitator is critical.

Health

There are a number of problematic assumptions in contemporary debates about health and health care. Doyal and Pennell (1979), writing about medicine and health, identified three such assumptions:

1 That the determinants of health and illness are predominantly biological.
2 That medicine is assumed to be a science.
3 The belief that scientific medicine "provides the only viable means for mediating between people and disease" (p. 12) (– and, for that matter, health).

In addition, I see two further assumptions which underlie – and undermine – discussions about health and mental health (as distinct from illness):

4 The dualistic split between mind and body.
5 The defining of health in terms of illness.

Despite at least 20 years of critical thinking and practice in health care, these assumptions are alive and kicking and influencing public "health" policy such as *Our Healthier Nation* (Department of Health, 1999b) and the *National Service Framework for Mental Health* (Department of Health, 1999a). In the first part of this chapter, responses to these five assumptions frame an exploration of *health* beyond illness. (A response to a sixth assumption – that government, in this case the British government, its advisors and advisory bodies have the monopoly on the ideology or economics of health – is held over to the second part of the chapter on mental health.)

Health as beyond the biological

The assumption that the determinants of health (and illness) are predominantly biological implies that patterns of health, the prevalence of health (health status), as well as patterns of disease (morbidity) and mortality, all have little to do with the social and economic environment in which they occur. Moreover, solutions to "health" problems are seen as lying exclusively within the domain of modern medicine. Over 25 years ago, the Lalonde Report, (the report in which the term "health promotion" first appeared) (Lalonde, 1975), offered a new perspective on health, arguing that causes of death and disease could be attributed to inadequacies in health care provision and environmental pollution as well as to lifestyle, behavioural and bio-physical characteristics. Following this, a World Health Assembly (meeting in Alma Ata in 1977) incorporated into its declaration a commitment to "community participation" and, following the Ottawa Charter (World Health

Organization, 1986), which amongst other things, defined health promotion, two further international conferences emphasised the need for "healthy public policy" (in Adelaide 1988) and on "supportive environments" (in Sandsvall 1991). Shifting the emphasis from biological determinism to social/environmental factors does not simply shift the blame from the individual to society; rather it acknowledges the impact of social determinants such as poverty and exclusion and helps focus the hearts and minds of health workers and policy makers on the bigger picture. It also acknowledges that health is for all and concerns all (not only medical practitioners). In his research on *Population Mental Health in Canada*, Stephens (1998) identified the determinants of mental health (qua *health*) as: demographic characteristics (age, household type, etc.), social conditions, social status (income, activity, education) and working conditions, as well as personal health practices and physical health. This perspective is particularly pertinent in the field of positive mental health as people who promote it are open to the accusation that it is at best irrelevant and at worst self-indulgent in the light of such big issues as poverty, unemployment, homelessness and other forms of social exclusion. However, it is precisely these "big issues" that have such a deleterious impact on our mental health (and as well as mental illness). Recent policy developments in Britain such as the identification of action zones (on health, education and unemployment) and the new deal for communities are creating common ground for health and social care agencies to work together to bring about regeneration and to tackle social exclusion. Whilst the primary focus of these developments is on reducing incidence of mental illness and social exclusion, some initiatives have combined promoting positive mental health (e.g. self-esteem and community capacity) by addressing the social determinants of mental ill health (see McCulloch, 1999). Postmodernist perspectives on health also contribute to the deconstruction of biology and the biological as well as to the co-construction of health and illness (see Fox, 1999).

Medicine as more than science

Following on from this first assumption is a second that assumes medicine as a science:

> the way medicine is presented, and society's acceptance of its claim to authority and resources, rests to a considerable extent on its definition of itself as a natural science ... and medical progress is said to be based on the use of "scientific method" which supposedly ensures certain and objective knowledge.
>
> (Doyal & Pennell, 1979: 12)

Nowhere is this more true than in psychiatry which has often been viewed as medicine's poor relation (or Cinderella). In response, psychiatry has sought respectability in "science" – from phrenology to diagnostic manuals of mental disorder. Whilst medical diagnosis has its uses, not the least in providing the relief of a certain kind of knowledge of "what's wrong", it is also highly problematic; as Steiner (1971c) put it: "*Alienation is the essence of all psychiatric conditions* .... Everything diagnosed psychiatrically, unless *clearly* organic in origin, is a form of alienation" (p. 5; original emphasis). Moreover "objective" medical diagnosis is not the only form of knowledge relevant to a person's illness; what someone knows about themselves and their illness *subjectively* is, arguably, equally if not more relevant to diagnosis, treatment, cure and care. In her seminal work on "fundamental patterns of knowing" in nursing Carper (1978) described empirical knowledge as: "knowledge that is systematically organized into general laws and theories for the purpose of describing, explaining and predicting phenomena of special concern to the discipline of nursing" (p. 14) – and went on to observe that: "one is almost led to believe that the only valid and reliable knowledge is that which is empirical, factual, objectively descriptive and generalizable" (p. 16). Carper suggested that, in addition to *empirical knowing* there are three further patterns or ways of knowing, relevant to the nursing task and role – *aesthetics*, *personal knowing* and *ethical knowing* – which both challenge and ameliorate the dominance of empirical knowledge in medicine and nursing. Although Carper described these patterns of knowing as distinct but interrelated, Johns (1995) argued that, in practice, the aesthetic way of knowing is core, as it is within this way of knowing that reflection on the other ways of knowing takes place. In this sense aesthetics may be understood as "meta" knowledge, with reflection as a meta-skill. Table 7.1 outlines Carper's ways of knowing and applies them both to mental illness and to mental health.

Beyond scientific medicine

The third assumption identified by Doyal and Pennell (1979) is the belief that scientific medicine mediates between people and disease, and either that it is the only viable means, or that it is necessarily the best; medicine is seen as good and that the only problem is that there is not enough to go around. Indeed, arguments about resources form the basis of most current political discussion on health care – and, as Doyal and Pennell (1979) point out succinctly: "this assumption, is, of course, dependent on a broader conception of the nature of capitalism – specifically on a belief in its capacity to solve social problems through economic growth" (p. 13). One of the consequences of this assumption is that the patient (who is expected to wait patiently) is seen as the passive victim of her/his illness, disorder or disease, while the doctor – and, traditionally, to a lesser extent the nurse – are seen as the experts. In the field of mental illness, historically it was far from certain that medicine (scientific or otherwise), would be the principal mediator of madness. Indeed, in Britain, until the nineteenth century, "madness" was mediated:

1 through the expression of feudal paternalism, by means of trusteeships decided by *the judiciary*;
2 in criminal trials through the defence by an *advocate*;
3 through the domain of *public order legislation* (see Porter, 1990).

None of this involved medicine or doctors; indeed, according to Porter (1990), "mad doctoring" only came of age (on 5 December 1788) when a specialist "mad doctor", Francis Willis, was called to attend to George III.

In the two centuries since Dr Willis was called to cure the delirium of George III, we have more understanding of madness and the mind, science and medicine, and of the nature of knowledge and theory, authority and expertise. In a present era in which there has been an exponential growth in medical technology that in many ways mediates the relationship with our own bodies, their limitations, breakdown and even failure, there has been a parallel growth of scepticism (even cynicism)

Table 7.1 Ways of knowing, mental illness and mental health (developed from Carper, 1978)

Ways of knowing (Carper, 1978)	*Definition*	*Application to mental illness*	*Application to mental health*
Empirical knowing	Knowledge that is systematically organised into general laws and theories for the purpose of describing, explaining and predicting phenomena.	Most research in psychiatry and the organisation of research in, for example, the *Diagnostic and Statistical Manual of Mental Disorders* (4th revised edition) (*DSMIV-TR*) (American Psychiatric Association, 1994).	Research such as Stephens (1998) which defined positive mental health status and considers the determinants of mental health.
Personal knowing	"Concerned with the knowing, encountering, and actualizing of the concrete, individual self" (Carper, 1978: 18).	Found in accounts of users and survivors of the psychiatric and "mental health" system; also the (rarer) reflections by professionals on their own response to and relationship with madness.	Reflection on any practitioner's own mental health in terms of, say, coping, stress, self-concept, etc.
Ethical knowing	Involves a process of deliberation and reflection, informed by ethical principles mediated by the practitioner's own values and by "situational ethics".	...with reference to legislation (i.e. mental health acts), codes and policy as well as relevant professional codes of ethics, practice and conduct (doctors, nurses, social workers, etc.).	...with reference to legislation and professional codes relevant to the particular practice under consideration.
Aesthetics	The practitioner's response to a particular situation; it involves a *process* of perceiving, interpreting, envisioning and generating possibilities, responding and reflecting.	E.g. in a "mental health assessment" (under the Mental Health Act 1983), in which the parties to the assessment, at best, perceive, interpret, envision and generate possibilities (based on the principle of the least restrictive alternative), respond and reflect in dialogue with each other.	Reflective – or reflexive – practice as regards any mental health consultation (see Tudor, 1996b).

with regard to "scientific medicine" and the doctor as expert. There are a number of factors that support this scepticism or critique:

- The resistance and more recent rise in popularity of medicine and health care complementary to the allopathic medical model.
- The development of public health psychology, community health psychology and critical health psychology.
- The growth and expression of civil rights, as reflected in the consumer movement and, for example, in "patients' charters". The term "expert patients" has even appeared as part of the "Healthy Citizens Programme" promoted by *Our Healthier Nation* (Department of Health, 1999b).
- The increasing interest (both in the broader philosophical sphere as well as in health psychology and care) in constructivist, narrative and postmodernist critiques of theory and practice, e.g. viewing illness as metaphor (see Fox, 1999).

Sacks (1991, 1995) has documented the refusal of medical and medicalising definitions of health and illness amongst his patients; and Fox (1999), in his postmodernist critique of health and illness, has questioned "cures" which cut across people's subjectivity, with no acknowledgement of our right to "otherness".

Holistic health

The roots of the English word for health, in Old English and Old High German, link it to wholeness and healing: "etymologically speaking ... to be healthy is to be whole or holy, which clearly embraces both spiritual and physical features rather than merely the latter" (Graham, 1992: 53). The grammar of health, then, is one that implies a holistic or integrative structure to our health and to our understanding of health. Thus, health may be taken as referring to mind (including thoughts, beliefs and feelings), body (including behaviour) and spirit. This common sense wisdom has prevailed for most of human history; Marks (2002) argued that it can be traced to the earliest period of history around 10,000 BCE. It is only the comparatively recent Cartesian dualism of the seventeenth century that had the effect (if not the intention) to conceptualise a split between the mind and the body, a split which ultimately gave rise and succour to the practice of referring to whole, if ill, people as "the appendix in bed four". It is a short step from bed four to the back ward and to being referred to – and, perhaps more perniciously, referring to oneself – as "*the* schizophrenic", as if that is all one is. This reductionism of person to symptom and/or behaviour is not only limited and limiting, it is inaccurate and, ultimately, anti-human.

A holistic approach to the person, which "embraces and affirms complexity, inclusion and diversity and resists reductionism" (Clarkson, 1989: 8), also locates the person/organism within their environment. Half a century ago, Lewin (1952) argued that it was impossible to view a person except in the context of their environment or "environmental field" (hence field theory) – and, of course, the viewer/researcher/doctor/nurse/etc. is also a part of this interactional field: "only the interplay of organism and environment ... constitutes the psychological situation, not the organism and environment taken separately" (Perls *et al.*, 1951/1973: 19). In relation to mental health promotion this view is reflected in the notion of mental health as requiring both "individual resiliance" and "supportive environments" (Joubert & Raeburn, 1998), a notion which proposes a necessary balance in focus between individual and environment, and which offers a challenge to promote the mental health both of individuals (at intrapsychic and interpersonal levels) and of environments (workplace, organisation, institution, culture), often through hearts and minds as well as policies and procedures. This interactional view focuses our attention on the health (or otherwise) not only of the subject or figure but also of the other figures in the field and of the environment itself. Thus the health of the doctor and nurse and whether the general practice or hospital is a healthy environment, or similarly the health of the child and the school, become as much the subject for concern and critical enquiry as the health and illness of the patient. Lest holism leads us to some spurious unity, the Zen Buddhist Master, Shunryu Suzuki (1999) in the spirit of "no dualism" offered a reminder of the complexity – and simplicity – of the relationship between mind and body:

> our body and mind are not two, and not one. If you think your body and mind are two, that is wrong; if you think they are one, that is also wrong. Our body and mind are both two *and* one.
>
> (p. 25)

In this sense holistic expansions of the mind/body duality (as above) are but stepping stones to a postmodernist commentary (meta-analysis or meta-text) on health and context, biology and culture (see Fox, 1999).

Health beyond the absence of illness

The often quoted WHO (1948) definition of health as "not merely the absence of disease and infirmity" also defines health, somewhat ambitiously, as "a state of complete physical, mental and social well-being" (p. 3). There are three implications of this:

1. Health is seen as *a state*, perhaps even a steady state to be achieved, rather than a *process* to be lived and thus something which fluctuates over time – and that illness is to be eschewed.
2. The ambition of *complete* health perpetuates a grandiose and perfectionist view of the human condition, one which is implied and exacerbated by the British government's invidious "league table" mentality in health and education and its consequent "naming and shaming" of "failing" institutions. Apart from anything else (such as the psychological reality that no-one makes positive changes in response to being shamed), as complete health and perfect hospitals and schools are impossible, this only serves to set up individuals and institutions to fail – failing, that is, in terms of imposed standards, measures and outcomes and a purely external locus of evaluation and control.
3. The WHO identified "physical, mental and social" as elements or indeed the parameters of health. This not only misses out the spirit (as in mind-body-spirit) or the spiritual, but also does not adequately acknowledge the multifaceted nature of health beyond the absence of illness.

There are a number of models that help in the elaboration of health without necessarily referring to illness. Here, in concluding this first part of the chapter, two models are briefly reviewed and applied to health and its promotion. In a paper on the integration of psychotherapies, Groder (1977) identified, in addition to the affective, behavioural and cognitive dimensions of psychotherapy and human life, the physiological, social systems and the suprapersonal. As a framework this has been found useful, for instance, in designing health education initiatives that, as it were, "touch all bases" or dimensions and which, therefore, are comprehensive and accessible. One sex education programme, working with young Muslim men, had focused on sexual *behaviour* and was foundering: the young men were embarrassed at the presence of plastic models of penises and the workers felt stuck (rather like the unsuccessful attempts to roll on the condoms). A consultant introduced the male workers involved to Groder's framework and discussed the efficacy of discussing values and faith (the *suprapersonal* or *spiritual* dimension) as well as the young men's culture (social systems) before further behavioural interventions. The workers took this back to their work, put the penises away, and later reported lively and useful discussions with the young men about religion, faith, morality, sexuality, culture and racism. (Other specific initiatives that reflect Groder's other dimensions are summarised in Tudor, 1996c.)

Although any such dimensional model is open to addition, it is also open to the criticism (ironically) that it appears somewhat one dimensional and fixed. Another model, based on existential philosophy and psychology, provides a sense of the more dynamic relationship we have with our health and, indeed, our existence:

> the existential approach considers human nature to be open-minded, flexible and capable of an enormous range of experience. The person is in a constant state of becoming ... this impermanence and uncertainty give rise to a deep sense of anxiety (Angst), in response to the realization of one's insignificance, and simultaneous responsibility to have to create something in the place of that emptiness. Everything passes and nothing lasts.
>
> (van Deurzen-Smith, 1996: 169)

Existentialism identifies four basic dimensions to human existence (see Table 7.2) in each and all of which we struggle with the givens of the past and the possibilities for the present and future, and with the meaning of our lives. Table 7.2 applies this conceptual framework to health. Although existential philosophy and psychology do not favour any one dimension, authors and practitioners in the field of health, mental health and its promotion may and do. French and Adams (1986), for instance, asserted that: "the most significant determinant of health is social and economic circumstance" (p. 73), a position which leads them to place a collective action model of health education at the top of their hierarchy of health education models.

In an important study on "emotional labour" in a hospice James (1989) found that: "the social, spiritual, emotional and physical care encompasses elements of care which are usually obscured in medical settings ... and require management and attention in the same way that physical symptoms do" (p. 20).

Mental health

In this part of the chapter some concepts of mental health (*qua health*) are introduced and discussed; then, having differentiated mental health from mental illness, the relationship between the two is explored; finally current social policy concerning mental health promotion is examined – and found wanting. Discussing *mental* health is, at least for this author, strategic: given a holistic appreciation of health,

Table 7.2 Existential dimensions of human existence applied to health

Dimensions of human existence	*Definition*	*Struggles/existential crises*	*Application to health*
Physical (*Umwelt*)	How we relate to our environment and the givens of the natural world, including our body, concrete surroundings, climate and weather, objects and material possessions.	Between the search for dominion and domination over the elements and natural law, and the need to accept the limitations of natural boundaries such as age, ability and fertility.	How we relate to our body, the age, size and shape we are; to what extent we accept who and how we are or rail against this. Health issues include the acceptance of such limitations or the application of medical technology to ameliorate the limitations of, for instance, disability, infertility and old age.
Social (*Mitwelt*)	How we relate to others and interact with the public world, including understandings in terms of class, gender, race, sexuality, etc.	Between acceptance and rejection, belonging and not belonging and isolation, success and failure.	How our health is affected by our status and wealth as well as class, gender, etc. Health issues focus on social health, health status, resources and planning, systems of care, as well as accessibility to services and on health and community (see Money, 1993).
Psychological (*Eigenwelt*)	How we relate to ourselves and our personal (intrapsychic) world: our temperament and personality, our past and possibilities.	Between what are perceived as personal strengths and weaknesses, between a sense of identity and of being substantial and states of disintegration and confusion.	How we relate to and understand our "internal life", our personal development and crises. If not somatised (physical) or acted out (social), health issues are expressed through some form of reflection, e.g. meditation, talking and/or psychotherapy.

(*continued*)

Table 7.2 (*cont.*)

Dimensions of human existence	*Definition*	*Struggles/existential crises*	*Application to health*
Spiritual (*Ueberwelt*)	How we relate to the unknown, and make meaning of it, through ideology, philosophy, religion, etc.	Between purpose and absurdity, hope and despair, being and nothingness.	How/whether we make time for our spiritual health, for instance, through some regular meditative, contemplative or reflective practice. Health issues include how we understand (and make meaning of) some of the struggles and contradictions of our physical, social and psychological existence and worlds.

it would be more accurate and useful if our understanding and discourse included all the elements or parameters discussed earlier (mind, body, spirit, etc.); indeed, in training workshops on this subject I am increasingly using the more generic term "health". Nevertheless, at present, the mental in health needs elaboration and "mental health" needs to be distinguished from mental illness if it is not to be subsumed beneath the conflated term "mental health" or the ubiquitous "mental health problems" – and thereby confused, ignored, misinterpreted and misunderstood. There is also an argument, advanced by Neumann, Schroeder and Voss (1989), that our mind or psyche, as the agent of all health-relevant interactions, is at the centre of all dimensions of mental health and thereby criterial to health. Similarly, in his work on multiple intelligences, Gardner (1993) suggested that the personal intelligences (the *inter*personal and the *intra*personal), which amount to information-processing capacities, and the combination or fusion of which provides a sense of self, are in effect the intelligences with which we reflect on the other intelligences (linguistic, musical, logical-mathematical, spatial, and bodily-kinesthetic).

Mental health – concepts, paradigms, elements, and research

There are no doubt as many definitions of mental health as there are readers of this book. Although some authors offer definitions of mental health, they are inevitably subjective, partial and, at worst, simplistic – *Making It Happen* defines mental health as "thinking, feeling and physical health and well-being" and the relationship between the three described and defined by three double-headed arrows! More useful than any one definition is to consider the elements of mental health common to such definitions – hence the importance of *concepts* of mental health. This approach to the subject was first adopted by Marie Jahoda in 1958 who, in a report to a United States Joint Commission on Mental Illness and Mental Health (readers will note the distinction explicit in its title) identified six major categories of concepts:

- mental health as indicated by the *attitudes of an individual towards themselves*;
- mental health as expressed in the individual's style and degree of *growth, development or self-actualisation*;
- mental health as *integration* of the above (– that is, the individual's ability to integrate developing and different aspects of themselves over time);
- mental health based on the individual's relation to reality in terms of:
    - *autonomy*
    - *perception of reality*
    - *environmental mastery* (Jahoda, 1958).

Whilst these are *categories* of concepts, each one of which represents a literature in itself (which, in the last four decades has obviously expanded with the growth of interest in self-development and popular psychology), nevertheless Jahoda's categories may be adopted by professionals and clients as the basis of a genuine mental *health* assessment. Drawing on an appreciation of the interpersonal field and the significance of the environment or context, mental health may be viewed as relevant at four levels – the personal, the interpersonal, the institutional and the cultural – first identified by Jones (1972) as ones in which racism is expressed; and, in relation to mental health, as with racism, all four levels interact. Applying Jahoda's categories to these levels offers practitioners, workshop participants (and, of course, the reader) a comprehensive and practical frame with which to assess mental health – for themselves, for and with others, and as regards the institution or workplace as well as the broader culture or sub-culture. Table 7.3 lays out this framework with some examples to stimulate the reader to apply their own and to fill in the gaps.

Drawing on the work of Kuhn (1962/1996) and Burrell and Morgan (1979), I followed in this tradition of conceptualising mental health by developing a conceptual framework of mental health through the application of paradigm analysis to the different and differing definitions of mental health and its promotion. Putting together two dimensions as axes – one, concerning assumptions about the nature of science (a subjective–objective dimension), the other concerning assumptions about the nature of society (a regulation–radical change dimension), Burrell and Morgan defined four distinct sociological paradigms (Figure 7.1).

Burrell and Morgan made a number of points about the nature and use of paradigm analysis:

1 That although each paradigm contains a variety of viewpoints, there is essential unity within the paradigm, defined by its external boundaries, Thus, the "essential unity" of notions of mental health within the interpretive paradigm is defined by the boundaries of and adherence to subjective knowledge and social regulation. In this paradigm mental health is viewed in interpretive and relational terms (e.g. Neumann *et al.*, 1989) with a focus on the regulation of the individual to conform to a harmonious and integrated sense of self and society.

Table 7.3 Jahoda's concepts of mental health applied to levels of human experience and context

Personal	*Interpersonal*	*Institutional*	*Cultural*
The attitudes of an individual towards themselves, e.g. self-concept, self-esteem	The attitude of individuals towards each other, including communication and social support, both positive – Birtchnell (1993) described mental health as positive relating – and negative, such as bullying and harassment; hence the importance of emotional literacy	The attitude of the institution towards itself, e.g. the "self"-concept of the organisation	The attitude of the culture or sub-culture towards itself and other groups
Personal growth, development and actualisation	Growth, development and actualisation with others, expressed in group and co-operative initiatives	Growth, development and actualisation of the institution/organisation, including initiatives which promote "workplace wellbeing"	Growth, development and actualisation of the culture, perhaps most explicitly expressed in *The Possible Scot* (Stewart, 1998)
Personal integration (of the above), through forms of personal reflection (therapy, non-managerial supervision, etc.), sometimes referred to as coherence and measurable as such (see Antonovsky, 1993)	Interpersonal integration (of the above), through forms of reflection with others, e.g. group therapy, group supervision, "circle time" in school or "check in" times at work	Institutional integration (of the above), through institutional forms of reflection such as reflective and consultative "review days" or "mental health away days"	Cultural integration (of the above), through initiatives involving cultural groupings and, at a national level, policies and even legislation
Personal autonomy	Interpersonal autonomy, although viewed by some as an apparent contradiction, the arena for discussion between two or more people (say, a couple or a family) and concerned with everyone achieving autonomy in the context of relationships	Institutional autonomy, i.e. the extent to which an institution is autonomous – in the context of other institutions, legislations, etc.	Cultural autonomy, often expressed through the struggle for and the achievement of cultural and/or regional or national independence

(*continued*)

Table 7.3 (cont.)

Personal	*Interpersonal*	*Institutional*	*Cultural*
The individual's perception of reality, the nature and extent of an individual's relationship with consensual reality, as well as how they manage their uniqueness and "otherness"	Interpersonal perceptions of reality, the business of much interpersonal communication	Institutional perceptions of reality	Cultural perceptions of reality, the arena of cultural and intercultural studies and intergroup relations (see Tudor, 1999a)
The individual's environmental mastery, the nature and extent of the individual's mastery of their environment	Interpersonal environmental mastery	The environmental mastery of the institution, e.g. the health promoting hospital and the health promoting school (Weare, 1996, 2000)	The environmental mastery of the culture, expressed in initiatives such as the WHO's "Healthy Cities" project (see Kickbush, 1989) and in health and community (Money, 1993)

2 That "all social theorists can be located within the context of these four paradigms according to the meta-theoretical assumptions reflected in their work" (Burrell & Morgan, 1979: 24). Thus, when Preston (1943) wrote about mental health as consisting of "the ability to live ... happily ... productively ... without being a nuisance" (p. 112), he was clearly reflecting a view of society that is concerned with social regulation, and representing a view of mental health which claims a certain certainty and "objectivity" – and thus, in terms of our analysis, is located within the functionalist paradigm. This is confirmed by an appreciation of the wider historical context of the mental hygiene movement that predominantly portrayed a conformist and functional view of health and productivity: "a healthy worker is a productive worker".

3 That, by definition, the four paradigms are mutually exclusive: "a synthesis is not possible" (ibid.: 25). Paradigm analysis thus describes the conceptual and theoretical assumptions underpinning differences which lead to – and are often demonstrated through – differences in practice and action such as that of the consultant psychiatrist who refused to sit on the same conference platform as representatives of the psychiatric user movement.

Paradigm analysis has thus proved useful in understanding and exploring differences in definition, policy and practice. Caplan (1986) applied this analysis to health education theory – and in doing so, offers a paradigmatic way out of the often futile "health promotion *versus* health education" debate: theory and practice in both is based on underlying assumptions which may be analysed and located within the four paradigms. Developing Caplan's ideas, the present author

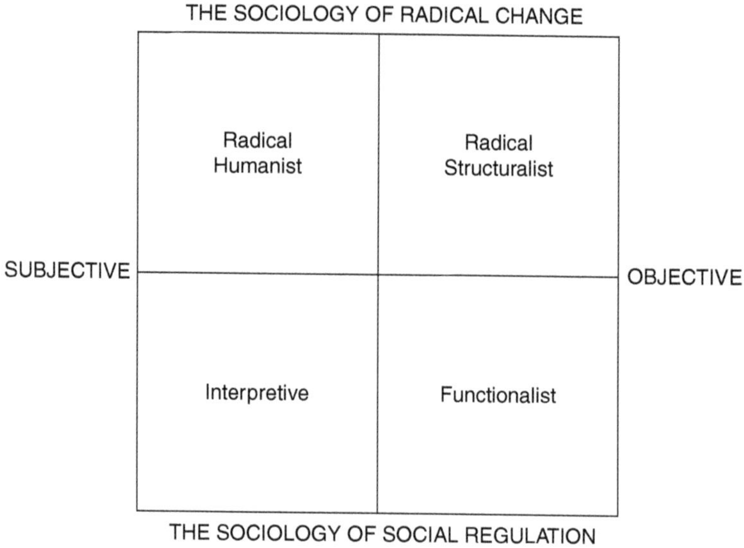

Figure 7.1 Four paradigms for the analysis of social theory (Burrell & Morgan, 1979: 22)

subsequently applied it to the field of mental heath and community mental health promotion (Tudor, 1996b), and in doing so identified mental illness prevention with its focus on identifying vulnerability and causative factors and "targeting" as little to do with mental health promotion.

In elaborating this analysis, as a result of an extensive literature review and in the spirit of Jahoda's work, I identified eight elements (two representing each paradigm: the functionalist, interpretive, radical humanist and radical structuralist, respectively), each of which may be viewed as on a continuum of health – ill-health (Box 7.1).

Box 7.1. Eight elements of mental health promotion (Tudor, 1996b)

Health — Ill-health

Coping
Tension and stress management
Self-concept and identity
Self-esteem
Self-development
Autonomy
Change
Social support

These elements do not stand alone as defining mental health; they are representative of the literature and of the four paradigms. McDonald and O'Hara (1998) also identify elements of mental health, mapping ten, comprising five elements each of mental health promotion and demotion (see Box 7.2).

Box 7.2. Ten elements of mental health promotion and demotion (McDonald & O'Hara, 1998)

Mental health promotion	**Mental health demotion**
Environmental quality	Environmental deprivation
Self-esteem	Emotional abuse
Emotional processing	Emotional negligence
Self-management skills	Stress
Social participation	Social exclusion

McDonald and O'Hara mapped these elements on three levels, a mapping that acknowledges (at least conceptually) the relevance of the individual (micro level), groupings (meso level) and wider, social systems (macro) in terms of taking action on promoting mental health. However, it is not exactly clear in McDonald and O'Hara's model what the relationship between promotion and demotion is. Thus, for instance, emotional abuse is not the opposite of self-esteem or the only element that demotes self-esteem; also, identifying stress as demoting mental health does not account for positive stress (or "eu-stress") (see Seyle, 1956; Antonovsky, 1979, 1987). Finally, the interpersonal aspect of mental health is almost completely missing from this model.

Undoubtedly the most impressive piece of empirical research on mental health is Stephens' (1998) work on population health in Canada. Prepared for the Mental Health Promotion Unit, Health Canada, which, under the directorship of Natacha Joubert, led the field in its advocacy and resourcing of positive mental health promotion, the report is clear in the distinction between mental health and mental illness. From his survey of data and previous research Stephens presented evidence that considered mental health status on the "positive dimension" in terms of happiness, self-esteem, mastery, sense of coherence and work satisfaction, as well as the negative (in relation to depression, distress, child emotional disorders, cognitive problems, hospitalised disorders and suicide). The whole report was set in the context of socio-economic restructuring and health care reform in Canada. Stephens distinguished between *indicators* of mental health status (as above) and its *determinants* (demographic characteristics, social conditions, social status, working conditions, personal health practices and physical health). Whilst the conclusion is that superficially the mental health status of Canadians appears to be reasonably good – three-quarters of the population describe themselves as usually happy and interested in life and 91 percent report some degree of job satisfaction – Stephens (1998) cautioned that:

> comparisons among population groups reveal that both positive and negative mental health are far from evenly distributed in the population: there are sharp differences according to an individual's household type and age, and, to a lesser extent, province of residence and gender.
>
> (p. 40) (see also Stephens, Dulberg, & Joubert, 1999)

From the discussion in this section, a number of points may be made:

1 Particular definitions of mental health are useful, especially for the individual concerned.

2 In order to grasp and indeed develop the field of mental health, it is necessary to think in terms of concepts or even categories of concepts of mental health.
3 All concepts and elements of mental health may – arguably, must – be viewed in *context*. One contextual frame has been presented and applied to concepts of mental health.
4 In order to understand different and differing (competing) definitions of mental health, a meta-theoretical framework is essential with which to analyse the underlying assumptions of particular definitions and their implications for policy and practice. This may, of course, be applied to any and all empirical research in the field of mental health.
5 In terms of forms of knowledge, there are differences between a definition, an element, a concept, a category, research, a model, a theory and a paradigm.

Mental health and mental illness

This chapter has argued for the separation of mental health from mental illness. At present most policy and practice is based on the conflation of the two under the one referent "mental health". In effect this conceptualises the two on one continuum, which I represent as a slide (as that is what people seem to fear) from mental health into mental illness (Figure 7.2).

What this means in practice is that people neither talk about mental health (*qua* health) as they think others are assuming that they are referring to mental illness; nor do they discuss mental illnesses, preferring instead to refer to them with the anodyne phrase "people with mental health problems". Merely substituting the term "mental illness" with this libertarian nomenclature does nothing to challenge the power of the medical/psychiatric model in this field, or to advance a critique of diagnosis, or to change the stigmatising effect of mental illnesses and the general public's attitude to them – exacerbated by the present British Home Secretary, Jack Straw, who consistently conflates "personality disorders" with dangerousness – with serious (and dangerous) consequences for proposed changes to future mental health acts, currently under review (see http://www.doh.gov.uk/mentalhealth/summary.htm and http://www.doh.gov.uk/hspch/visped.htm). Proposing a conceptual separation between the two terms may be represented by *two continua*, first advanced by the Canadian Minister of National Health and Welfare (MNHW) in 1988 (see Figure 7.3).

There are a number of implications – and advantages – to this formulation.

Conceptual

From experience we know that we can be ill and well at the same time such as when we have a cold and feel OK; when we have cancer and are functioning well; indeed, when we are in any way physically or mentally ill and, at the same time, mentally healthy. It is useful, therefore, to have a conceptual apparatus which describes the two phenomena of health and illness, and which supports the distinction between the two, especially given the widespread conflation of the two terms. [The difference between the two concepts is not merely

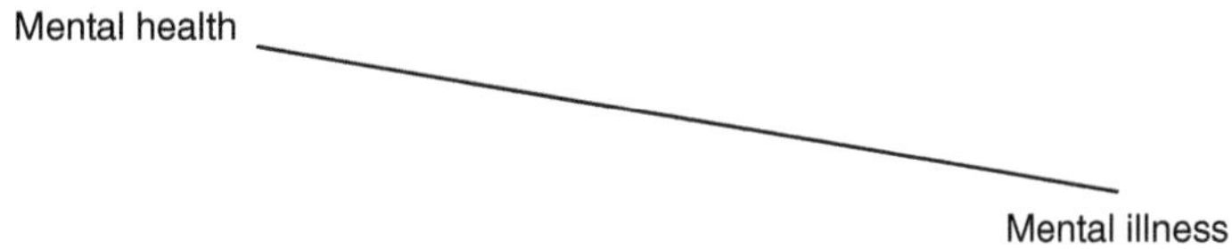

Figure 7.2 The "mental health" continuum

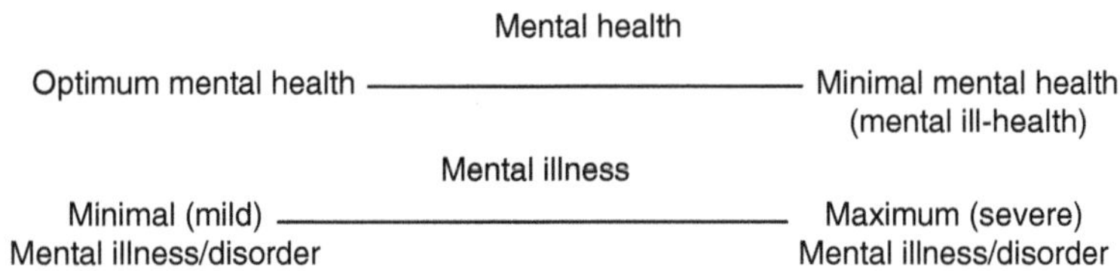

Figure 7.3 The two continua concept (based on the Minister of National Health and Welfare, 1988)

the absence of presence (of illness) – or the presence of absence. As Winnicott (1988: 1) put it:

> the doctor's assumption that health is a relative absence of disease is not good enough. The word health has its own meaning in a positive way, so that the absence of disease is no more than the starting point for healthy life.

Winnicott's work is important in developing a view of health as the continuity of being and, as such, central to human development, growth and maturity – and, indeed, Winnicott was an important figure in developing a psychoanalytic perspective on health, including the importance and contribution of play and creativity (see Winnicott, 1986). Coincidentally, in the same year (1965) in which Winnicott's groundbreaking book on *The Maturational Processes and the Facilitating Environment* was published, another key book on health was published. This book, by Angyal (1965/1973), outlined a holistic theory of *Neurosis and Treatment*. In it, amongst other ideas, Angyal introduced the concept of the ambiguous gestalt, which describes two primary and autonomous organisations within the personality, one characterised as healthy and the other as neurotic, thus: "Health and neurosis are to be thought of as two organized processes, two dynamic Gestalts organizing the same material, so that each item has a position within two different patterns" (pp. 102–103)].

Philosophical

By separating the two fields, the two continua concept opens up the possibility of dialogue between health and illness (which, in its one dimensional approach, the one continuum concept avoids). From this we can then engage in the debates advocated, albeit from their different perspectives, by Fox (1999) and Suzuki (1999). In considering the relationship between the two, Duff (1993) reminded us of the value of illness to health: "illness is to health what dreams are to waking life – the reminder of what is forgotten, the bigger picture working toward resolution". (p. 33). Other examples of the complex interrelationship between illness and health include: [the argument that illness is a part of normal development and health, as Hartmann (1942) put it: "a limited amount of suffering and illness forms an integral part of the scheme of health" (p. 311); the idea of illness as metaphor (Sontag, 1978); the experience of a "healing crisis" familiar to complementary health practitioners (see Fife, 1997); and] the significance of subjectivity and the concept of *arché-health* (Fox, 1999): "the condition of possibility for health and illness" (p. 10).

Practical

It is only possible to promote the mental health of the mentally ill (as *The Health of the Nation* [Department of Health, 1992] first proposed) if we advance the two continua concept, else they are left languishing at the ill end of the one continuum, with no possibility of health. Some forms of occupational therapy, self-development courses, a women's consciousness-raising group, patients' meetings, all within the psychiatric setting, and involving users in their diagnosis and treatment and in the planning of services – are all examples of mental health promotion of the mentally ill and all depend on the view that, whilst having a diagnosed mental illness or disorder, they also have mental health which can be promoted and enhanced. This approach also addresses the critical comment the Standing Nursing and Midwifery Advisory Committee (1999) made in a report on mental health nursing, admitting that "users have no real role in designing and implementing professional education and training" (p. 12).

Clinical

The two continua concept is congruent with the multi-axial diagnostic approach taken by the *Diagnostic and Statistical Manual of Mental Disorders-IV-TR* (American Psychiatric Association, 2000) (an approach adopted in the revision of its third edition in 1987). This multi-axial system proposes five axes or continua which in effect describe a holistic approach to diagnosis (see Table 7.4).

It is a short logical step to propose a sixth axis on mental health and, even more radically, to propose in addition, a dialogic approach to each axis (see Table 7.5).

Indeed this could almost define the role of the mental health nurse in mental illness diagnosis, treatment and care *and* in mental health care and promotion.

Pragmatic

The two continua concept can be (and has been) viewed as pragmatic: it claims mental *health* for all whilst not necessarily challenging the authority or territory of psychiatrists or mental "health" professionals. In this sense the concept may be welcomed by already overworked practitioners in this field with some relief that they do not have to "do" or "take on" mental health promotion; and therefore, that they can welcome the involvement in patient care of workers in health education, health promotion and health improvement.

Political

On the other hand, claiming mental *health* for all may also been viewed as highly political, as the logic of promoting the mental health of the mentally ill may well involve other (non psychiatric/mental "health") professionals and lay people as it were breaking into the asylum. At one point in the "Italian experience" of mental

Table 7.4 The five axes of DSM-IV

Axis I	Mental disorders
Axis II	Development disorders Personality disorders
Axis III	Physical disorders and symptoms
Axis IV	Severity of psychosocial stressors
Axis V	Global assessment of functioning

Table 7.5 The continuum concept applied to multi-axial assessment

Axis I	Mental disorders	______	Mental "order" or integration
Axis II	Development disorders	______	Healthy development
	Personality disorders	______	Personality process (based on a process conception of personality, for instance, Rogers, 1951)
Axis III	Physical disorders and symptoms	______	Physical health
Axis IV	Severity of psychosocial stressors		
Axis V	Global assessment of functioning		
Axis VI	Mental health		

health reform, psychiatric patients and staff in Trieste built a wooden horse (called Marco) which, in the same way that its Ancient Greek counterpart was taken into the city of Troy (only later to reveal its contents), was also paraded around the streets of the city (see Tudor, 1990b; Chapter 4). The approach to mental health promotion advocated in this chapter and other similar work might well be viewed as a subversive "wooden horse": this time putting sanity into the mental hospital and, indeed, seeing sanity in and alongside madness.

"Not making it happen": the failure of mental health policy

A further problematic assumption (in addition to those identified in the first part of the chapter) concerns the monopoly the government and its agents have or claim on health policy. This involves a certain ideology, enacted through legislation and policies such as *The Health of the Nation* (Department of Health, 1992) and *Our Healthier Nation* (Department of Health, 1999b) and backed up with certain economic resources, although not a planned economy of health – or illness.

Elsewhere (Tudor, 1996b) I offered a critique of *The Health of the Nation* and other health policies of the early 1990s insofar as it and they concerned *health* and specifically *mental* health. From the wealth of paper generated by this legislation and related documents (such as the key area handbooks) only two strands emerge which support mental health and its promotion:

1 the aim to improve significantly the health and social functioning of mentally ill people (*The Health of the Nation*); and

2 the development of good practice to improve mental health in the NHS and local authority workplace (*Key Area Handbook on Mental Health*) (Department of Health, 1993).

Despite extensive criticism of this previous health policy, the politicians, civil servants and advisors changed little: *Our Healthier Nation* (*OHN*) suffers from the same confusions and deficiencies as previous policies.

Alongside cancer, coronary heart disease and stroke, "mental health" (predominantly meaning mental illness) is one of four national targets for 2010 identified in *OHN*. From its subsections (modernising mental health services, the NHS plan, the review of the Mental Health Act, etc.) it is clear that "mental health" refers to mental illness. As part of its strategy to modernise mental health services the government has, with the help of an "expert reference group", chaired by a psychiatrist, developed a *National Service Framework for Mental Health* (Department of Health, 1999a). The framework:

- Sets national standards for both health and social care, and establishes performance indicators to measure the progress made by services, ensuring that they meet all basic criteria.
- Addresses the range of mental health service provision, from primary care, where the majority of mental health problems can be managed, through to specialist mental health services.
- Will help to ensure that people with mental health problems receive the service they need, regardless of who they are or where they live (Department of Health, 1999a).

This is clearly about "people with mental health problems" i.e. people with a mental illness. The framework then sets five standards, the first of which covers mental health promotion: "health and social services should: promote mental health for all, working with individuals and communities; combat discrimination against individuals and groups with mental health problems, and promote their social inclusion" (Department of Health, 1999a). In some ways this is positive as the first clause names "mental health for all", although it is still somewhat confusing that the framework uses the same term in the second clause when clearly referring to people with mental illness. More problematic is the separation of the two clauses: it is not clear whether combating discrimination (of the mentally ill) forms part of mental health promotion or whether it is viewed as part of the government's commitment to social inclusion, separate from its understanding of mental health. The subject becomes clearer from the rationale which follows the aim and standard of the *Framework*, which refers to depression (twice), mental disorder (three times) and the ubiquitous "mental health problems" (four times), terms used interchangeably. Moreover, given that this aim was outlined in *The Health of the Nation*, one might be forgiven for questioning why it has taken 7 years for the government to produce a document with the same conflation and confusion of terms.

In order to support local services in a mental health promotion strategy, the Department of Health commissioned the mental health charity Mentality (the mental health interest of the defunct Health Education Authority (HEA) under a new name) to prepare a mental health promotion framework document which was published as *Making It Happen* (Department of Health, 2001). From the perspective advanced in this chapter this is a profoundly disappointing document. Throughout, it confuses mental health and mental illness: the lack of clarity in the

Framework concerning mental health promotion and combating discrimination is echoed throughout *Making It Happen*. Its definition of mental health (referred to on p. 92) is simplistic in the extreme. It refers to only one model of mental health promotion in the now substantial literature on the subject, and invites no critical reflection on the field. It is completely uncritical of the government – on public mental health it simply asserts that "standard one of the National Service Framework presents a significant opportunity for further developing mental health promotion work" (Department of Health, 2001: 16). It is contradictory: at one point it affirms that "reflective practice, the ability and willingness to think critically, is at the core of developing a robust and inclusive evidence base" (p. 93), yet on the next page it summarises the *Framework*'s "grades of evidence" which do not include any reference to reflective, let alone critical practice – and does so without comment or irony! It is also uneven as some of it is about mental *health*; some sections are well researched, e.g. S3.2 on the relationship between physical health and mental health (i.e. illness); and some of the examples of interventions are reflective of mental health promotion. It is nonetheless disappointing. However, given its provenance, this disappointment is not surprising. The HEA had a reputation of marginalising and excluding critical perspectives, and of capitulating to its political paymasters; on one occasion (in)famously, and at great expense, shredding a sex education booklet aimed at young people because Margaret Thatcher did not approve of the language it contained! Mentality appears to have inherited the HEA's conservatism. *Making It Happen* is the latest in a line of lost opportunities in 10 years of public health policy that has failed to develop and advance mental health promotion as a reflective and critical practice, capable of transforming levels of emotional literacy in the population, institutions and in the culture, and of creating a real sense of social inclusion, participation and civic wellbeing. As Campbell (2000) put it in a rare contribution on mental health promotion from the perspective of a "community mental patient": "the current contract available to people with a mental illness diagnosis – both as citizens and service users – appears to be linked to a vision of essentially anti-social contribution and the need for compliance" (p. 96).

For this sense of transformation, we need to look "beyond" the *National Service Framework for Mental Health*, as indeed the subtitle of this book [*A Textbook of Principles and Practice*] suggests we should do.

Promoting mental health

In this third and concluding part, mental health promotion beyond the *National Service Framework for Mental Health* is envisioned.

Beyond the framework

From the review of recent health policy (above), it is clear (at least to this author and practitioner) that in order to promote positive mental health we need to look elsewhere for inspiration in order to advance theory, policy and practice.

Theory

Craib (1987) wrote about "the unavoidability of theory". All action is based on – or may be traced back to – some idea or theory. A simple exercise makes this point (Box 7.3).

Box 7.3. Identifying personal theory

Think about a piece of work you did or an interaction you had with a client about which you were really satisfied, "a job well done" as it were. Write down a simple statement that summarises your feeling about it. Working with someone else, tell them your simple statement. They, in turn, ask you "Why did you do that?" or "What was your thinking about doing what you did?" You answer and they ask you again "What was your thinking about *that*?" and so on until you come to a natural conclusion. This "laddering down" exercise often uncovers the personal theory behind particular actions and interactions.

Theory can be hugely complex (and off-putting) and incredibly simple (and accessible). The personal theory behind the theory advanced in this chapter, as the reader will by now be aware, favours subjectivity over objectivity. This is because I value personal, subjective forms of knowledge, fluidity over fixity and rigidity, multiplicity over singularity, and accessibility and equality – and therefore find, for example, Carper's (1978) patterns of knowing liberating. Beyond a particular theory and application of that theory, paradigm analysis offers a meta-theoretical framework with which to understand differences, based on underlying assumptions.

Policy

It has already been noted that in the field of health promotion from the Ottawa Charter onwards and in the field of policy and research in mental health promotion Canada, and specifically Health Canada, has led the way. New Zealand also has a comparable track record, aided by the work of the psychologist, community development activist and academic John Raeburn (see Raeburn & Rootman, 1998). For thinking about genuinely positive mental health policies in Britain we have to go north of the border to Scotland where, despite the fact that *Our National Health* (National Health Service Scotland, 2001) is as disappointing in relation to mental health as its English and Welsh counterpart, the Scottish Council Foundation (SCF) has published *The Possible Scot* (Stewart, 1998). This document, published by the SCF, which was launched in 1987 with a mission to promote independent thinking in public policy, is, from its inspiring title onwards, innovative in a number of ways. It argues (amongst other matters):

- that *possible Scots* should be involved in decision-making at all levels;
- that reaching one's potential is not the preserve of the affluent but is the birthright of all;
- that health services should not dominate the health policy agenda – and that the health of the Scottish people would be best served by abandoning health policy as a separate entity and embracing "holistic government";
- that the dimensions of health can be measured both subjectively and objectively;
- that if the determinants of health are multiple and interactive, then policy making must be holistic rather than fragmented – holistic government is defined as "incorporating incentives for cross-departmental and cross-tier working and for co-operation with non-governmental actors" (Stewart, 1998: 15).

It is perhaps no accident that *participation* – a central plank of "people-centred health promotion" (Raeburn & Rootman, 1998) – is a feature of *The Possible Scot*, set in the context of the aspiration for a more participative political system since devolution. In the section on life skills for the young, citing Gardner's (1993) theory of multiple intelligences and Goleman's (1996) work on "emotional intelligence", it argues for a shift of focus in education "from content and recall to processes and skills" (p. 25). The SCF has gone on to apply the same principles in a subsequent publication *The Possible Human: America's Approach* (Scottish Council Foundation, 2002). The content, style and tone of both publications are, in contrast to the UK government's policies (as discussed above), exciting, innovative, accessible and inclusive. Policy is also strategic. Elizabeth Morris, principal of the School of Emotional Literacy, has made a similar point in describing the programmes the school promotes: "we have found time and time again that for emotional literacy to have any significant impact on pupils it needs to start at a strategic level ... it has to be written into the policy documents and driven from there" (personal communication, 9 September 2002).

Practice

As mental health promotion is a disputed concept, its practice is not unproblematic. An analysis of three successive annual conferences on mental health promotion revealed that only just over a third (37 percent) of all presentations were directly concerned with mental health – and by no means were all of these concerned with practice (see Tudor, 1996b). Nevertheless, there are examples of good practice in the literature (see Tudor, 1996b; McCulloch & Boxer, 1997; Raeburn & Rootman, 1998; see also www.antidote.org.uk and www.schoolofemotional-literacy.com); some examples in the conference papers from the Annual (now European) Conference on the Promotion of Mental Health (principally collected and edited by Dennis Trent and published by Ashgate, 1992–2000); and some in *Making It Happen* (Department of Health, 2001). More important, however, is the practice generated by the practitioner and the client/s working together. As has been noted, the *Key Area Handbook on Mental Health* (Department of Health, 1993) elaborating *The Health of the Nation* (Department of Health, 1992) advocated the development of good practice to improve mental health in the NHS and local authority workplace. In some ways this may be viewed as a cascade approach to promoting mental health at work: facilitating the mental health of carers in their working environment so that they can go out and facilitate others. Of course, it does not always work like this. The NHS and local authorities are not necessarily the most benevolent or forward-thinking of employers, and carers for their part are notoriously diffident about looking after themselves let alone putting themselves first. One might argue that if, as carers, we cannot look after our own health needs and interests, then who are we to tell others how to do it? The irony of practitioners charged with the task of mental health promotion who are themselves overworked, under-resourced and stressed must not be lost. Elsewhere I have applied a similar analysis to mental health promotion at work (Tudor, 1996a). Undoubtedly the single greatest change will come from the extension of the employers' duty of care under health and safety legislation to include *health* and the promotion of positive workplace health and mental health or wellbeing; and it is possible that European legislation may enable such extensional responsibilities and thinking. In this context it is perhaps not surprising that in recent years there has been increasing interest in the balance between work and the rest of life, sometimes referred to as the work-life balance. There is a National Work-Life Forum (website: www.worklifeforum.com), which, in conjunction with The Industrial Society (now The Work Foundation), produced a *Work-Life Manual* (McCarraher & Daniels, 2000) that encourages innovative work organisation (flexitime, compressed working week, etc.), leave provision, and employee development and support (see also McCarraher & Daniels, 2002).

CHAPTER 8

"TAKE IT"

A sixth driver (2008)

Retrospective introduction

This chapter forms part of a critical reading of transactional analysis from radical psychiatry (see the Radical Therapist Collective, 1971; Steiner *et al.*, 1975; Wyckoff, 1976; and Chapter 9; see also introduction to Chapter 5). The original article was influenced by work I had written with others from within the framework of the person-centred approach to therapy (see Sanders & Tudor, 2001; Tudor & Worrall, 2006), which, like radical psychiatry, is generally sceptical about diagnosis, and specifically as it is conceptualised and practised within the medical/psychiatric model (see Rogers, 1951). For a long time, I have also been sceptical about diagnostic categories and their implicit and even explicit claims to universalism. The article was informed by my own clinical work and, specifically, my reflections on and thinking about the origins of narcissism. These form what is the middle section of the article and this chapter (under the subheading "Take it"). As I was proposing some addition to theory, I then decided that I should argue the case for this and thus wrote the sections on "The Necessity and Sufficiency of Theory" and "Some Implications for Transactional Analysis Theory". At this point I discussed the draft of the article with my colleague and friend Claude Steiner who encouraged me simply to state what I was wanting to say, rather than to include the sections on the nature of theory or relationship of the "Take it" driver to existing theory. In this instance, I did not take his advice, preferring to address what, for me, are important meta-theoretical issues. Given the reactions to the article, however, it would have been interesting to see if a shorter version would have elicited the same amount of heat.

In my original article I specifically thanked Helena Hargaden, especially for the literary references, and Ray Little, Charlotte Sills and Claude Steiner, as well as the anonymous reviewers for their helpful comments on earlier versions of this article and for their engagement with the material.

I have chosen this article not only for the significance of its contribution to theory, but also as it evoked quite a response. In her editorial introducing the issue in which the article was published, Heathcote (2008) wrote that "In his scholarly and politically pertinent article ... Keith Tudor argues convincingly for a sixth driver" (p. 3). Although I don't have the benefit of what you, the reader, think about the article, I thought that I did a reasonable job in terms of a thorough treatment of existing theory, and a reasoned argument about the need for additional theory. Nevertheless, the article provoked particular responses from Taibi

Kahler, the co-author of the original article on drivers (Kahler & Capers, 1974), Steve Karpman, and John Parr, in the form of letters which were published in the *Transactional Analysis Journal* (Kahler, 2008; Karpman, 2008; Parr, 2008) and a personal attack (in some e-mail correspondence) from Steve Karpman who referred to me as a "British carbon-copy PC leftish" (PC presumably referring to being "politically correct") and, along with three other colleagues as "the axis of evil PC-Four" [personal communication, 22 March 2008], and accused me of fasely inventing the driver to justify a rant against America. Their (more considered) objections to the article focused on:

1 my argument that Kahler's theory was – and is – an example of a "self-sealing doctrine" (from Kahler);
2 that "Take it" is not a driver, in that it does not fulfil Kahler's requirements for a driver (Kahler, and Karpman);
3 that I was inaccurate on a number of points (Kahler);
4 that the article was political and not "scientific" (Karpman, and Parr);
5 that the editors should not have published it (Parr).

I was given the opportunity to respond to these criticisms – which I did, also in a letter to the journal (Tudor, 2008c), as did the co-editors of the journal (Cornell, Heathcote, & Heiller, 2008), and, the following year, others who supported both the article's analysis and its publication (Argent, 2009; Cariapa, 2009). Although some of the attacks were personal and hurtful, I was – and still am – more interested in reflecting on the whole picture, i.e. the article, its analysis, the reactions, and the correspondence, as, I think, it demonstrates something about the development of theory and, in some cases, the struggle to develop theory in the context of interests vested in the status quo and, in this case, in marketed brands (see www.kahlercom.com and related websites). Most recently, the article and the responses to it have been the subject of further commentary by Sandle (2015) who has considered – or, more acuurately, imputed – my motivation and the conflict it generated in terms of psychodynamic sexual theory: both Oedipal (an unconscious murderous intent), and repressive (the reactions).

In the previous year in which the original article was published, I had presented at a transactional analysis conference a paper on dogma (Tudor, 2007d) in which I identified a number of ways in which dogma and dogmatism is maintained, i.e. through purity, conformity, priesthood, and certainty. The reactions to this article have only confirmed my thinking about and critique of self-sealing doctrines, closed theory, and kitemarked models, especially given my commitment to free thinking and the freedom to practise. I feel especially strongly about this with regard to encouraging students and trainees to be able to think, practise and associate freely, without the fear of retribution or interpretation.

Abstract

"Take it" is considered as a sixth driver that accounts, both in developmental and social terms, for the introjection by the child of Parental messages to take and own objects in an inappropriate, exploitative, and unsustainable way. As a negative driver message, "Take it" is considered to support the development of narcissism. It also accounts for the integration of messages that encourage the child to impact in a constructive and sustainable way his or her environment. The author reflects on the nature of theory and the impact of a new contribution to existing transactional analysis theory, as well as on a number of theoretical implications of this additional driver. This contribution to the literature is placed in the context of transactional analysis as a social psychology and a radical psychiatry.

Transactional analysis as a social psychology

Transactional analysis is described as a social psychology. This attribution appears, for instance, on the web site of the International Transactional Analysis Association (ITAA) (www.itaa-net.org). Although a number of authors writing within the transactional analysis literature, from Berne (1961/1975a) onward, have interpreted and applied this phrase variously (see Massey, 1996; Price, 1978; Zalcman, 1990), in general terms, "social psychology" refers to the branch of or approach to psychology that concentrates on human behaviour in its relational field and context (i.e. others, groups, institutions, and society as a whole). Given its origins in the analysis of transactions between people, many concepts within transactional analysis support and elaborate a social psychological approach. At the same time, and particularly in its clinical applications (both psychotherapy and counselling), transactional analysis is not immune to the criticism of individualism and narcissism that has been levelled against therapy, notably by Lasch (1979). From a social psychological perspective, then, it is also necessary to subject psychological theory and practice to social, relational analysis. For a number of years, I have been interested in both aspects of social psychology – the application of psychological theory to society and the social analysis of psychological theory – and, specifically, in the interface between politics and therapy (see Embleton Tudor & Tudor, 1994; Tudor, 1997a, 1997d, 1997e; Tudor & Hargaden, 2002).

Radical psychiatry – in many ways the "lost tradition" of transactional analysis – is particularly important and useful in addressing the accusation that therapy promotes individualism and is apolitical. As Steiner (2000) put it:

> Radical psychiatry holds that all functional psychiatric difficulties are forms of alienation resulting from the mystifying oppression of people who are isolated from each other. People's alienation is the result of power abuse and is therefore a political matter. Any person in the practice of psychiatry (soul healing) becomes involved in the personal politics of those he or she attempts to help ... Radical psychiatry is a political theory of psychiatric disturbance and a political practice of soul healing.
>
> (p. 578)

Key concepts underpinning the theory and practice of radical psychiatry include: alienation, oppression, power, mystification, competition, the stroke economy, the Pig Parent, powerless scripts, autonomy, and co-operation. It was through rereading some of the early radical psychiatry literature, against the background of the current war on and in Iraq, that I became aware that the existing identified driver messages do not adequately account for the development of the psychology of competition and oppression in the individual, let alone in and between groups, organisations, and nations, or for the unsustainable greed apparent in so-called "advanced" industrial (i.e. capitalist) societies.

The necessity and sufficiency of theory

I am hesitant to propose additions to theory as, generally, I support the principle of Occam's razor. This refers to ontological economy or parsimony, based on the argument advanced by the fourteenth-century Franciscan philosopher William of Occam that reality exists only in individual things and events. In other words, the simplest explanation that most fully explains the phenomena under consideration is most likely to be useful. An example of this in transactional analysis is Summers and Tudor's (2000) critique of Clarkson's (1990) multiplicity of therapeutic relationships, in which we reduced her five relationships model down to two. Just as "small is beautiful" (Schumacher, 1973/1989), so too is theoretical thrift or parsimony. A theory or model should be both sufficient and necessary to explain a thing or phenomenon – and, as far as Berne was concerned, have a diagram! This perspective informs much of philosophy and mathematics and lies at the heart of Rogers's (1959) famous (and often misrepresented) "conditions" of therapy (i.e. that the therapist is in psychological contact, authentic, accepting and empathic, and that the client is in psychological contact, incongruent, and receiving the therapist's acceptance and empathy). There is also a strong environmental argument for ecological economy. We may take the view that there are too many books and journals – or, at least, bad and unnecessary books and articles – and not enough trees. This places some onus on both author and editor to justify the cost of his or her intellectual footprint. So, here, first, I argue the necessity for an additional driver message.

In response to Gellert's (1975) point that there are more than five drivers, Kahler (1975) argued that "in order to suggest that there are other behaviours that are distinct from these five, a person would first need to be very knowledgeable in terms of identifying each type (driver) as I have labeled it" (pp. 426–427). Kahler's argument is an example of a "self-sealing doctrine" (see Riebel, 1996) and, as such, simply needs to be dismissed as defensive and unscientific. In the course of writing this article, some colleagues suggested that I was taking Kahler's self-sealing doctrine too seriously and questioned whether the whole concept of drivers was worth such "reverent irreverence". I could simply say that the enshrined concept of five drivers is nonsense. Also, from a pragmatic point of view, we can justify any addition to theory simply in terms of experience and observed practice. While I have some sympathy with these perspectives, from a systemic, paradigmatic perspective, the confrontation of old theory and the addition of new theory is a little more complex. As Kuhn (1962/1996) argued, "A new theory, however special its range of application, is seldom or never just an increment to what is already known. Its assimilation requires the reconstruction of prior theory and the re-evaluation of prior fact" (p. 7). Thus, it is important to consider both what in the existing theory is insufficient and why the addition is necessary. In this spirit, I take up the challenge of distinguishing the additional "Take it" driver from the each of the other five identified by Kahler. The addition of a sixth driver has an impact on a number of interrelated theories and models within transactional analysis, in particular, driver messages (Kahler & Capers, 1974) and personality adaptations (Joines & Stewart, 2002; Ware, 1983). In the last section of this article I discuss some of the implications of this addition.

The following sections are introduced by an overview of injunctions, counterinjunctions, and drivers.

Injunctions, counterinjunctions, and drivers

Steiner (1971a) first wrote about injunctions and attributions being the two types of script-implanting transactions between the parent in the child of the parents and the parent in the child of the offspring. He noted that the injunction "is in almost every case nonverbal, [and] not transmitted in explicit words" (p. 58). Steiner originally proposed the term "permission" for the message from the Parent, but Berne adopted the term "counterinjunction" over Steiner's objections (and I agree) that it muddied the waters (C. Steiner, personal communication, 21 April 2007). Berne (1972/1975b) later confirmed this term in *What Do You After You Say Hello?*

In their understanding of psychopathology, Bob and Mary Goulding, founders of the redecision school [tradition] of transactional analysis, emphasised certain pathological messages conveyed from parents to children, which they called "injunctions". Goulding and Goulding (1976) identified a short list of 12:

- Don't Be (exist)
- Don't Be You. Specifically, for the Gouldings, the sex (gender) you are, although I would extend this to include class, race, sexuality, and so on
- Don't Be a Child (e.g. don't have needs)
- Don't Grow. The Gouldings suggested that this injunction includes others, such as don't grow beyond infancy or beyond a certain age, don't be sexual, and don't leave me
- Don't Make It (don't succeed)
- Don't (do anything)
- Don't Be Important
- Don't Be Close (trust or love)
- Don't Belong
- Don't Be Well (or sane)
- Don't Think. That is, don't think about x (a forbidden subject) and don't think what you think (rather, think what I think). The Gouldings also noted that this injunction is similar to Don't Grow
- Don't Feel. Similarly, don't feel x (a particular feeling) and don't feel what you feel (feel what I feel).

Although in their original article Goulding and Goulding (1976) said that this list was approximately the same as one they had devised 10 years earlier, later, in their book on redecision therapy (Goulding & Goulding, 1979), they acknowledged that there are undoubtedly many other injunctions.

Such messages derive from the parents' own unresolved pain and are therefore conceptualised within the Child ego state of the parent/s or carer/s. As Steiner noted in his comments to me, they are often communicated non-verbally and unconsciously and are rarely acknowledged or remembered as such.

The Gouldings went on to define counterinjunctions as "messages from the Parent ego state of parents which are restrictive and, if adhered to, may also prevent growth and flexibility" (Goulding & Goulding, 1979: 38). These were originally referred to as counterinjunctions because Berne believed that they literally countered the injunction in that, for example, someone might save his or her life (Don't Exist) by working hard, even though, in response to the power of the injunction, the person remains depressed. Such messages include the five drivers identified by Kahler and Capers (1974): "Be strong", "Try hard", "Be perfect", "Hurry up", and "Please me". What are generally referred to as drivers refer both to driver messages that were originally external and then and now replayed internally, and driver behaviours that are the external, behavioural manifestations of the internal messages. The reader will note the use of quotation marks with regard to the counterinjunctions but not the injunctions. Although the Gouldings did not explain this, the point of this punctuation is presumably to distinguish the fact that the counterinjunctions or driver messages are often conveyed in actual speech, as in: "Come on, hurry up and put your coat on. I've been waiting and I'm in a hurry". In their work, Goulding and Goulding (1979) acknowledged Mary Goulding's addition of "Be careful" to Kahler and Capers's taxonomy; they viewed this as specifically countering the injunction: Don't. This addition appears to have been lost in the literature as, to my knowledge, neither the Gouldings or anyone else has developed this idea since.

As with a number of debates within transactional analysis, there has been some discussion over the years regarding terminology, definitions, and the meaning of counterinjunctions and drivers and their relationship to script and counterscript:

- Drivers are not-OK counterscript messages (Kahler & Capers, 1974); drivers or driver-related habits can be positive (Hazell, 1989) and represent aspiration (Clarkson, 1992).
- Drivers are like other counterinjunctions (counterscript messages) (Goulding, 1974); drivers are counterscript messages (Kahler, 1974); drivers are not part of the counterscript (Gellert, 1975).
- There are five drivers (Kahler & Capers, 1974); there are more than five drivers (Gellert, 1975; Goulding & Goulding, 1979). In addition to "Be careful", Gellert (1975) considered "Be weak" and "Think" to be other drivers. I acknowledge this in the use of the indefinite article in the title of this article: "*A* Sixth Driver".

In addition, Hazell (1989: 212) substituted "Be right" for "Be perfect" "so that this driver, like the others, will describe a goal that is desirable and possible to achieve, within reason"; and his resolution of the "Please me/Please you" duality was to rename that driver "Be pleasing".

Driver behaviours refer to brief observable behaviours, such as distancing language ("Be strong"), muffled and hesitant tone ("Try hard"), counting points off on fingers ("Be perfect"), agitated and changing posture ("Hurry up"), and exaggerated smiling ("Please me"). Kahler (1974) asserted that such behaviours last no longer than from a split second to between five and seven seconds. For a complete matrix of driver behaviours with regard to words, tones, gestures, postures, and facial expressions, see Kahler (1979), Stewart (1996), and Joines and Stewart (2002). The implicit, psychological driver message is one of conditional OKness: You are only OK if you are strong, trying, perfect, hurried, and/or pleasing. As the word suggests, "driver" carries a sense of drive or motivation. Gellert (1975) thought that there is only one drive, a drive toward self-actualisation (à la Maslow). He argued, therefore, that Kahler had observed and labelled different facets of this one drive. In a similar aspirational vein, Clarkson (1992) pointed out that such a drive or drives can be praiseworthy as well as problematic. She suggested that "being fast, energetic, pleasing, strong, and excellent is not the same as being in driver behaviour. However, these qualities can be mislabeled in such a way as to blunt the distinction between driver behaviour and the autonomous Adult integration of parental values" (p. 18).

Working therapeutically to confront or modify the impact of negative Parental drivers is generally associated more with the redecision and cognitive-behavioural traditions of transactional analysis. These traditional views of drivers, their identification through "detection" and diagnosis, however, do not acknowledge the relational dynamic involved in the behaviours this theory describes. Moreover, other transactional analysis traditions also draw on and develop this piece of transactional analysis theory:

- As has been acknowledged, this present article considers drivers and, specifically, the "Take it" driver from the perspective of viewing transactional analysis as a social psychology and a radical psychiatry.
- From a co-creative transactional analysis perspective, Summers and Tudor (2000) view drivers and their impact as co-created. A message from a father, "Pull yourself together, son", may be matched by his son's response, "Hold me tight (and be there for me always)", a transaction that may represent mutual drives to "Be strong". A mother's encouragement of her daughter to take things from her environment may encourage a sense of right and rights and a certain sense of detachment from a passive environment. This may be echoed by the daughter's request of her mother to "Take me" in a way that co-creates and reinforces the driver message and that renders the daughter a passive subject of "being taken".
- From a psychodynamic perspective, drivers epitomise a drive psychology that, as Pine (1990) put it, "emphasizes the taming, gratification and socialization of drives" (p. 50). In their review of drive psychology in transactional analysis, Sills and Hargaden (2003) suggested that Berne's view of the Parent ego state moved away from a Freudian theory of drive. Yet, as they acknowledge, Berne's (1961/1975a) view of the function of the Parent ego state as energy conserving and anxiety diminishing "by making certain decisions 'automatic' and relatively unshakable" (p. 76) is a double-edged sword. In some ways, working hard may save a person's life; at the same time, it may create other anxieties and pressures that may, in some instances, shorten it. Taking (acquiring) material things may satisfy a need, for instance, for security or self-definition; at the same time, it also stimulates this need and a cycle of demand and supply. The psychodynamic perspective also offers a transferential/countertransferential understanding of drivers and their behaviours. Some people take and disguise their taking, sometimes in a way that others get the blame. The character of Mrs. Coulter in Pullman's (2003–2007) *His Dark Materials Trilogy* is a classic example of this. She is the greediest, most power-hungry character in the trilogy, yet she is accomplished, her behaviour looks good, and she sounds good. In effect, she disguises her "Take it" behaviour perfectly, and it is others who become encumbered with that projection. Often we will pick up and know this driver message intuitively and sometimes in isolation as others may be conned by the projection.

These three perspectives all open up more relational ways of understanding and working with driver messages and behaviours.

"Take it"

My suggestion for the addition of another driver message comes from an interest in identifying the origins of a social psychological process that, in terms of human development and later socialisation, encourages greed, competition, and power seeking (i.e. power "over" people and adversarial transactions). Zuboff and Maxmin (2004) suggested that 50 percent of human intercourse is adversarial and that, in the context of the individual's relationship with organisations, we assume that our experience of consumption will be largely adversarial. I am also interested in the interrelationship between processes that encourage adaptation to a competitive frame of reference and those that support physical and economic domination, from psychological bullying and violence, the policies and politics of international capitalism, and, ultimately, wars that represent such processes and "interests". In this context, the five drivers identified by Kahler and Capers (1974) do not appear to describe adequately a developmental process whereby an infant is encouraged to take from his or her environment inappropriately, whether it be food, a toy, or something from others. In this way, the conditional OKness of "Take it" conveys the message "You're only OK if you take it and make it". It is thus distinguished from "Try hard" because, as Joines and Stewart (2002) observed, "The Try Hard driver message is code for 'You're only OK if you try hard (but don't actually do it, because if you did it, you wouldn't be trying hard any more')" (p. 53).

This message is the external manifestation of internal psychological and psychobiological systems. Panksepp (1998) identified and mapped seven specific neural circuits and integrated cognition/affect/behaviour patterns that he called "emotional operating systems" (p. 3). These act as "strange attractors" (p. 3) within widespread neural networks, which, Panksepp suggested (p. 3), exert a certain type of "neurogravitational force" on many ongoing activities. Each system is characterised by specific neurotransmitters, is associated with activity in specific subcortical brain areas, and plays a fundamental role in human behaviour. As Panksepp put it:

> Basic emotional states provide efficient ways to mediate categorical types of learned behavioral changes. In other words, emotional feelings not only sustain certain unconditioned behavioral tendencies but also help guide new behaviors by providing simple value coding mechanisms that provide self-referential salience, thereby allowing organisms to categorize world events efficiently so as to control future behaviors ... In addition, arousals of these brain systems are accompanied by subjectively experienced feeling states that may provide efficient ways to guide and sustain behavior patterns, as well as to mediate certain types of learning.
>
> (pp. 14–15)

Some of the systems have to do with individual drive (rage, fear, panic) and some with relationship or relational needs (seeking, lust, care, and play). The "seeking system" is manifested in states of curiosity, excitement, and pursuit. Its chemistry is characterised by dopamine, a neurotransmitter often described as the "power switch" because it turns on and energises the individual in relation to his or her environment and is also linked with the pleasure of discovery and the drive to formulate meaning and causality. While it has these positive features, Panksepp argued that, these days, this system is being overdeveloped and, I suggest from a social perspective, overrewarded. We may think about this in terms of a lack of development of bonding and continuing bonds, which finds expression in a hunger for neurotic control (see Meredith, 2000). There is a separateness and non-relatedness about grabbing that may speak to a struggle with envy and competitiveness. Hargaden (personal communication, 11 March 2007) speculated that these messages come from a macho part of both parents and recalls the story of a client who forced her son to fight another boy and shouted macho things at him as he fought and beat his opponent. In healthy development, the "narcissistic bubble" of infancy is slowly burst by the parents/caretakers in such a way that the child learns that there are other subjectivities in the world – and hence, intersubjectivity. This is usually established through tolerable frustration and, as Little (personal communication, 19 April 2007) observed, "This brings to mind how many folk from the US have difficulty stopping their children eating to obesity". In the United States, the prevalence of overweight among children aged 6 to 11 has more than doubled in the past 20 years, from 7 percent in 1980 to 18.8 percent in 2004; the rate among adolescents aged 12 to 19 has more than tripled, increasing from 5 percent to 17.1 percent (see Ogden *et al.*, 2006).

Following Clarkson's (1992) contribution in reclaiming the aspirational possibilities of driver messages (in praise of speed, experimentation, agreeableness, endurance, and excellence), "Taking it" may be viewed as the appropriate development of mastery with regard to taking in and from the environment in a sustainable way. This illustrates a benign mastery of the environment, which Jahoda (1958) referred to as a concept of positive mental health. The inclusion of and reference to "it" is significant, because I am describing the beginnings of both a mastery of and an alienation from the environment.

Angyal (1965/1973) offered further insight on this in his analysis of the word "possession" with regard to what he considered to be two trends inherent in the human organism: one toward autonomy and the other toward homonomy or a sense of belonging.

> When we possess something we say, "It's mine." But we can mean very different things by these words. We may mean them in the sense of the autonomous orientation: I can do with it what I want; it is under my control ... This is one meaning of possession, but there is another. Consider your relationship to your child or to your wife ... We say "mine" and we say it meaningfully. What do we mean by that? We mean that we identify with the person so that we feel our life extending beyond ourselves and involving those other people.
>
> (p. 22)

Just as Clarkson distinguished "speed" from "hurry", "experimentation" from "trying hard", and so on, the two aspects of "Take it" may be observed and described.

"Take it" – as in "Go for it"

As a driver message, this carries the sense of parental encouragement of a child's contact and active interchange with his or her environment. It describes positive aggression, which Perls *et al.* (1951/1973) defined as including "everything that an organism does to initiate contact with its environment" (pp. 100–101). "Going for it" has a similar sense to the "Get on with" message that Ernst (1971) described as compatible with the "I'm OK, You're OK" quadrant of the OK corral. A simple, everyday activity of picking daisies to make a daisy chain expresses this "both/and" perspective on the organism and its environment. "Can I go and pick the daisies?" a child asks her father. "Of course", he responds with affection. "Just pick enough to make a chain", he says, holding up five fingers. "Oh, but I want to pick more", she responds. "Just pick enough to make a chain", he repeats. The child comes back with five daisies and gives them to her father, who begins to make a daisy chain. It is small. The child goes back and picks some more. The father completes the daisy chain. The daughter looks pleased. "How beautiful!" the father says. She says, "I want to pick more daisies". He responds, "No, you've picked enough daisies for the daisy chain. The other daisies need to grow and to make more daisies". The daughter smiles.

The point here is that there is a relationship in which a child learns to take and to negotiate. This example of taking enough is, in a small way, the foundations of a psychology of sustainable development: taking enough but not too many or too much and being mindful of what the environment needs to be self-sustaining (see Rust, 2004). This mindfulness is more apparent in societies based on the social economics of hunter-gatherers than in the exploitation of labour, land, and resources common in capitalism.

As a driver message, "Take it" (go for it) counters the injunctions Don't, Don't Be Important, Don't Succeed, and Don't Be You. Both the message (external and internal) and its behavioural manifestation can also be experienced as a confrontation in the Bernean sense of disconcerting a person's parent and/or child ego states. I once challenged a trainee as to why, after the completion of her formal training course, she had taken so long to prepare for her certified transactional analyst (CTA) exam, which, for her, was always "around the corner". Having elicited this, I offered a humorous illustration of what I sometimes refer to as a "Slow down" driver (in effect, a "Be perfect" driver), which I observe in some transactions within the transactional analysis community regarding exams. The trainee accepted the confrontation and, within a year, had taken her CTA exam and passed well. Taking in and mastering the environment is an important developmental process and an expression of an integrating Adult that acknowledges being and belonging in a sustainable way (see Angyal, 1965/1973; Jahoda, 1958).

"Take it" – as in "Grab it"

This aspect of the parental (Parental) driver message carries the sense of getting something at someone's expense or "getting one over" them. It gives permission for people to take what they want rather than what they need and thereby encourages greed. As Gordon Gekko, in the film *Wall Street* (Pressman & Stone, 1987), put it:

> Greed, for lack of a better word, is good. Greed is right; greed works. Greed clarifies, cuts through, and captures the essence of the evolutionary spirit. Greed, in all of its forms, greed for life, for money, for love, knowledge – has marked the upward surge of mankind.

Such "taking it" leads to overconsumption, addiction, and alienation. It is associated with a defensive (and aggressive) position of "I'm OK, You're not OK". It describes a pathological position based on a defensive reaction to an early disruption (the withdrawal of the breast or the taking away of the bottle). It explains the behaviour of the playground bully, the ruthless Wall Street trader, and the defensive-aggressive nation state. The neurological view of the seeking system (see

Table 8.1 The Behavioural clues of the "Take it" driver message

Driver	*"Take it"*	*Distinctions and comments*
Words	"It's mine". "I want it NOW". "I'm certain". "There's no doubt".	This driver is often expressed non-verbally, as the drive is fundamentally non-relational.
Tones	Abrupt Certain Low, sharp, growling when bullying High (whiny) when defensive	The high voice of "Please me/others" is squeaky.
Gestures	Pointing with hands open Clenched fists (held out and pointing outward)	The clenched fists of "Try hard" are held defensively, often at the side of the body.
Postures	Square on, one foot in front of the other, leaning forward when threatening Sways slightly forward and back, hunched when defensive	
Facial expressions	Open Eyes look straight ahead but beyond the object Generally show attempts to dominate and/or persuade (e.g. eyes narrowed and piercing, mouth pursed)	

discussion of Panksepp earlier), which acknowledges that we get a chemical "buzz" out of such behaviour, is also an example of the biological advantage of such second and third-degree game playing.

Taking up Kahler's requirement for additional theory and the implicit challenge to distinguish any new driver from his and Capers's original five, Table 8.1 summarises the behavioural clues to "Take it".

Case example

Charles was a successful businessman. He came to therapy as a result of a crisis in his relationship with his wife, who had given him an ultimatum that he should seek help, in particular, as he reported it, "to deal with your feelings".He was confused, resentful, and somewhat remote. In the initial contact on the phone, he was both flattering (the therapist had come highly recommended) and quite demanding in terms of wanting an appointment time to suit his availability. The therapist agreed to meet him. Charles then missed his initial appointment.

The therapist made another appointment, and when they met, commented on this process. Charles picked up on the therapist's use of the word "misunderstanding", claiming that his understanding was correct. He generally spoke in a loud voice and in a rather abrupt and certain manner. Charles spoke rather vaguely about what had brought him to therapy and generally used "you" or "one" to refer to himself. When the therapist expressed or sought to express some understanding of what he did say about himself and his situation, Charles was argumentative. The therapist changed tack and used a more requesting channel of communication (Kahler, 1979). In response, Charles gradually began to relax and open up.

In this first phase of therapy, Charles told the therapist more about his background and life. He had been a "golden boy", brought up by a doting mother and a caring but absent father in comfortable circumstances. When he was 7 years old, he had been sent away to boarding school. He remembered not wanting to go and pleading with his parents to allow him to stay at home and go to the local day school. His parents had refused, telling him what a great opportunity it was. At that point in the story, Charles turned to his therapist and said, "I remember deciding that I would never forgive them and that I would just have to harden my heart". As he said this, his face dropped. Almost immediately he leaned across toward the therapist with his chin jutting forward, looking aggressive. The therapist reflected this, commenting on Charles's vulnerability and the way in which he defended against that. Charles nodded, accepting and responding to, for the first time, the therapist's empathy. This was a turning point in the therapy.

What followed was a second phase, which comprised a combination of and flowing between:

1 History – which uncovered some of what lay behind the façade of comfort and doting, as a result of which Charles and the therapist identified a number of early injunctions, including Don't Be Close (Charles was expected to send large amounts of time on his own), Don't Be Important (although Charles was brought up to think that he and his family were better than others, neither parent accounted for him, especially when he felt vulnerable), and, despite, his parents' apparent ambition for him, Don't Succeed/Make It. During this time, Charles also talked about his career and that he was proud of the fact that he was a "go getter" and even of his reputation at work of being "a mean bastard". It was at this point that the therapist identified "Take it" as a counterinjunction/driver.
2 Relational therapeutic work – which focused on the transactions between Charles and the therapist, with the therapist offering mirroring interpretations (see Hargaden & Sills, 2002; Masterson, 1988).

The end of this phase was marked by Charles leaving therapy. He felt better and did not feel any need to spend further time in therapy. The therapist considered that this ending was premature.

Three months later, Charles rang the therapist, asking him if he knew the name of a therapist who did cognitive-behavioural therapy (CBT). The therapist asked him how he was. Charles responded that things had not gone well, his wife was upset with him, and he wanted some short-term therapy to put things right. He had read about CBT and thought it might help. The therapist suggested that they meet to discuss further what might suit Charles. When they met, Charles was angry with the therapist: "The therapy hadn't worked". However, Charles agreed to spend some sessions working out what he wanted and whether he wanted to continue in therapy with the original therapist.

This was a messy period. Charles came to one session, cancelled the next, then came again and announced that he was going on holiday for 3 weeks. At one point, the therapist said to Charles about therapy: "It seems like you can take it or leave it". Shrugging his shoulders, Charles agreed. In supervision, the therapist reported feeling like he meant nothing to his client. His supervisor reminded him about narcissistic process (as it related to the client) and, specifically, the work of Masterson (1988). When Charles returned from holiday, they had a better session and, soon after, Charles agreed to uninterrupted weekly therapy (which later increased to twice weekly therapy). In response to the therapist working with their present relationship or how they related, Charles began to show more vulnerability and feelings.

In this abridged version of a period in a therapeutic relationship, the "Take it" driver is apparent in the client's behaviour and attitude, which is demanding, abrupt, certain, argumentative, aggressive, disruptive, blaming, and distant. Its relevance for a relational way of working is that, once the therapist gets beyond the client's presenting and surface behaviours, he or she may experience the client as a miserable, alienated soul. It also explains when therapists feel very negative or envied; and, when we work with someone who says all the right things, we may also experience him or her as very needy and greedy, consuming our experiences and time. It explains when we may feel that the therapy, perhaps over a number of years, seems to go down a bottomless pit; when we feel as if we're being taken in and used up and can no longer feel the OKness of the person in front of us. Sometimes our mirroring, empathy and attunement appear wasted because they are not recognised for what they are; the client does not retain his or her experience of therapy and the therapist, while reporting his or her next achievement in the outside world.

As a not OK driver message, "Take it" describes a relational dynamic that expresses and confirms an individual's alienation – from his or her product, productive capacity, other people, species, and the Earth – see Roy (1988), Steiner and Wyckoff (1975), Tudor (1997a) and Steiner (2000). Indeed, alienation is a useful way in which to frame psychopathology because it contextualises pathology as alienation from relationship (see Tudor & Worrall, 2006). Alienation generally leads to individualism and a competitive frame of reference. As Steiner (2003) put it in describing the stroke economy, "Interaction can be divided into competitive and co-operative. Competition is transacted through power plays, co-operation is free of power plays" (p. 180). In this sense, grabbing or taking something for oneself is a power play, whether it is on an individual level, such as bullying, or on an international level, such as war. Grabbing things from others is a highly individualistic (or nationalistic) act that expresses dominance based on and almost beyond competition. Narcissism is the logic of such individualism or, as Kovel (1981) put it with reference to a particular client, "a life led in late-capitalist society, one that chooses a certain kind of sickened narcissism to be its subjective signification" (p. 103).

According to Kohut (1971), the particular affective experiences of narcissistic disorders encompass a spectrum "ranging from anxious grandiosity and excitement on the one hand to mild embarrassment and self-consciousness or severe shame, hypochondria, and depression on the other" (p. 200). This description of two types of narcissism, an "egotistical" type and a "dissociative" type, were confirmed by Broucek (1982) and later described, respectively, by Gabbard (1989, 1990) as "oblivious" and "hypervigilant" and by Masterson (1988) as "exhibitionist" and "closet" (p. 103). This distinction is important because it describes a personal and clinical reality and because the American Psychiatric Association's (2000) *Diagnostic and Statistical Manual of Mental Disorders* (*DSM-IV*) fails to characterise the latter type of narcissism, thereby misrepresenting the range of narcissistic personality process both in type and from trait to adaptation to disorder. However, in my experience, "Take it" drives both types of narcissism. These types are often described as two aspects of one individual or two sides of a vertical split originally identified by Kohut (1971) as developed by Johnson (1994).

Some implications for transactional analysis theory

As noted earlier, and from a systems perspective, one cannot simply introduce something into a system without it having an effect on the other parts of the system, in this case, a body of theory. Following Kuhn's (1962/1996) ideas about the nature of scientific revolutions and the development of theory, any new theory requires some consideration of prior theory and fact. In this case, the addition of a sixth driver message impacts particularly on injunctions, driver messages (Kahler & Capers, 1974), and personality adaptations (Joines & Stewart, 2002; Ware, 1983). In the last section of this article I discuss some of the implications of this addition to transactional analysis theory.

Injunctions

On both personal and social/political levels, the "Take it" driver message is associated with and supported by the following specific injunctions:

- Don't Be Close – to others, especially if they might have different views. This relates to the lack of adequate bonding and lack of development of intersubjectivity, empathy, and interdependence. It includes don't relate, don't be "self and other", and don't negotiate, which, in its positive manifestation, Charlotte Sills (personal communication, 2 April 2007) considers to be "the operationalisation of intimacy and mentalisation".
- Don't Belong – to the family, community, United Nations; don't co-operate (act unilaterally).
- Don't Think – about others or about how others think.
- Don't Feel – this may refer to specific feelings; it also encompasses not being ambivalent.

With regard to mapping these injunctions with personality adaptations (Ware, 1983) and the process model (see Joines & Stewart, 2002), this associates "Take it" more closely with the paranoid, schizoid and antisocial personality adaptations. This, again in part, explains a person's and a nation's defensiveness, alertness, isolation, and unilateral actions.

Driver messages

For each personality adaptation, it is considered that there is a primary or main driver, often accompanied by a secondary driver (and in the cases of the histrionic and schizoid adaptations, two secondary drivers). However, despite the association of the two (or three) drivers with regard to each personality adaptation, there is little in the transactional analysis literature that describes the interrelationship of two particular drivers. So, for instance, with regard to both the obsessive compulsive (responsible workaholic) and paranoid (brilliant sceptic) adaptations, how do the "Be perfect" and "Be strong" messages interrelate and impact each other, and, in this instance, how do they do so differently with regard to the two different adaptations? In her article on personality types, Klein (1985) described what the different combinations of drivers or core elements of the miniscript have in common and how they are opposite. With regard to "Be perfect" and "Be strong", she suggested that what they have in common is rationality and that they are opposite in emotional intensity and detachment. In terms of the impact on another, sixth driver in the theory of drivers, in Table 8.2 I offer some comments on the combination of "Take it" and the other identified driver messages.

These combinations of driver messages describe and confirm the narcissistic picture described earlier with regard to Charles and demonstrate how they can be applied to the social/political world. On a social level, it is significant that one of the most narcissistic nations in the world, the United States, was founded on the forced migration and genocide of the indigenous First Nations peoples and the forced taking or acquisition of the land on which they lived. Similarly, the justification for war on and the subsequent occupation of Iraq made by both US President George Bush and British Prime Minister Tony Blair is well summarised and challenged in Bob Dylan's (1964) ironic anthem "With God on Our Side". It is interesting to contrast these justifications with Thomas Jefferson's assertion (written in a letter dated 28 July 1791 to the American diplomat William Short):

> If there be one principle more deeply rooted than any other in the mind of every American, it is, that we should have nothing to do with conquest. The energies of the nation, as depends on me, shall be reserved for the improvement of the condition of man, not wasted in his destruction.
>
> (Jefferson, 1791/2005: 104)

Personality adaptations and disorders

This suggests that, as a driver message, "Take it" summarises the personal and interpersonal dynamics that underpin narcissism. This is supported by ideas from neuroscience and developmental psychology, as well as from transactional analysis concepts such as human hungers. From a social psychological perspective, the theory of personality adaptations acknowledges the impact of the environment on the individual's personality, precisely because it describes and names various forms of adaptation he or she develops in order to cope with his or her environment (family, culture, society). Ware (1987) suggested that the six personality adaptations can be divided into "surviving" and "performing" adaptations. According to Stewart and Joines (2002), the surviving adaptation "is developed as a means of taking care of oneself when trust of the environment breaks down," whereas the performing adaptation "is developed in order to meet the expectations within the family" (p. 4). Later (Stewart & Joines, 2012), they describe these in terms of Erikson's (1950, 1968) stages of psychosocial development. The surviving adaptations (schizoid, antisocial and paranoid) are responses to the first psychosocial issue, which Erikson characterised as basic trust versus mistrust, and they begin to develop in the first 18 months of life. The performing adaptations (passive-aggressive, obsessive-compulsive and histrionic) develop, presumably (as Stewart and Joines do not comment on this), between 18 months and 6 years in response to the psychosocial crises of autonomy versus shame and doubt (18 months to 3 years) and initiative versus guilt (3 to 7 years).

Table 8.2 The interrelationship of driver messages

"Take it" and "Be strong"	This combination encourages the person receiving them to be bold. As Shakespeare's Lady Macbeth put it when she was encouraging Macbeth to kill Duncan and take the kingdom, "But screw your courage to the sticking-place, And we'll not fail" (Act 1, Scene VII) (Shakespeare, 1623/1997). This combination is supported by the injunction Don't Be You (i.e. don't show if you care what it costs you or others).
"Take it" and "Try hard"	This combination encourages the seeking of any and every opportunity to gain, while extolling the maxim that there is no gain without pain or effort.
"Take it" and "Be perfect"	This combination encourages the justification of accumulation (e.g. money) and possession (e.g. land and/or people), often with reference to self-sealing doctrine or process. Tony Blair's (2005) defence of his decision to invade Iraq has this flavour: "I had to take the decision as prime minister that I thought was right".
"Take it" and "Hurry up"	This combination encourages the person to keep on succeeding. As Gordon Gekko in *Wall Street* (Stone, 1987) puts it, "Lunch is for wimps". This is also supported by the injunctions Don't Be Close and Don't Be You (i.e. don't have other [relational] needs).
"Take it" and "Please me"	This combination has (as with others with regard to the "Pleasing" driver) two implications: (1) to be successful for another (originally a parent) by producing or acquiring something and (2) to please oneself by enjoying the fruits of taking, conquest and acquisition.

In their discussion of narcissism, Stewart and Joines (2002) suggested that in narcissistic personality disorder the individual exhibits a combination of paranoid and antisocial adaptations "on the surviving level" (p. 228). However, they also argued that both narcissistic and borderline structures are "different in kind" (p. 226) from the six adaptations and that, therefore, we cannot think of narcissism (or borderline) as an adaptation. I disagree. Kohut (1971) discussed healthy narcissism. Arguably, most politicians and actors, as well as some eminent psychotherapists, are full-blown narcissists, and, although we may not like their style, ideas, or policies, they are functioning only too well (see Ronningstam, 2005) and could reasonably be described as healthy, if adapted – at least in the same way that an obsessive-compulsive accountant might be healthy.

Other implications for theory

Game theory

"Take it" is associated with the psychological-level Persecutor position on the drama triangle. Of course, at a social level this can come in many guises, with a Victim, for instance, exploiting his vulnerability by perhaps pulling the wool over someone's eyes and then turning Persecutor. Oscar Wilde (1898/1997: 892) summed this up well in *The Ballad of Reading Gaol*:

> Yet each man kills the thing he loves,
> By each let this be heard,
> Some do it with a bitter look,
> Some with a flattering word,
> The coward does it with a kiss,
> The brave man with a sword!

This psychological role theory also accounts for the way in which people and peoples who have been oppressed and victimised may develop a "Take it" driver based on an innate sense of survival and seeking and hunger for control. They may then become grabbing, overly concerned with "rights", and persecutory.

Process scripts

"Take it" reflects a never (type II) script (e.g. "I'll never give in") in which the pattern is looking for the next acquisition, cause, or fight.

Script type

"Take it" reflects a joyless script because there is an open-ended sense to the seeking and no completion or satisfaction.

Conclusion

This article argues that there is – and there is a necessity for – a sixth driver message of "Take it" in order to explain certain seeking and aggressive relational dynamics in and between human beings on personal and wider, social/political levels. The article also argues that we should take theory and the development of theory seriously and that theorists should be able both to argue within an old paradigm in order to expose its deficiencies and to develop new paradigmatic perspectives.

The identification of the "Take it" driver message can help individuals to understand this aspect of and dynamic in their own lives and to distinguish between its assertive and oppressive manifestations. It can also help people resist those who seek to grab rather than to take what they need in a negotiable and sustainable way.

From a social psychological perspective, the "Take it" driver message helps explain why so-called advanced societies take resources from the developing world (minerals, oil, people) and then dump the by-products and waste products of unsustainable development and consumption on those same countries (contraceptives, toxic waste). With its associated injunctions, this driver message accounts for a nation's – and a leader's – defensiveness, isolationism and unilateralism. For example, the US government has refused to sign the United Nations (UN) Convention on the Elimination of All Forms of Discrimination Against Women (1979), the Kyoto Protocol for controlling global warming (1997), and the International Criminal Court Treaty (1998). It has not ratified the United Nations Convention on the

Rights of the Child (1989) and has opposed the International Plan for Cleaner Energy, which has been signed by all the other countries in the G8 group of industrial nations (2001).

At the same time, without UN support but together with the United Kingdom and other countries, the United States has prosecuted an illegal war in Iraq and, to date, still occupies that country. It is important to make this criticism of the United States, both in terms of its own history and development and because of its particular role, influence, and dominance as the world's only superpower. However, while these examples are unique to the United States, the "Take it" attitude in social/political/economic dynamics is not. This driver message equally explains the acquisition of wealth and its uneven distribution, often through corruption, in the leadership of developing and underdeveloped societies, often with divisive and disastrous implications for working people in those societies.

Just as awareness and understanding helps the individual, so too the social psychological analysis of the social, political and economic consequences of the "Take it" driver message may help increase the social awareness of individuals, groups, peoples and even nations so they can better resist oppression and to commit to co-operation.

CHAPTER 9

TRANSACTIONAL ANALYSIS IS RADICAL OR IT IS NOT TRANSACTIONAL ANALYSIS (2008)

Retrospective introduction

This chapter is the English version of an article that was originally published in Italian, in the journal *Neopsiche* (Tudor, 2008b). The published article was an expanded version of a speech I had given in December 2007 at a conference in Turin, Italy, hosted by two Italian associations of transactional analysis (TA): L'Istituto di Analisi Transazionale (the Institute of Transactional Analysis) and L'Associzione Italiana di Analisi Transazionale (The Italian Association of Transactional Analysis). I wrote the original paper in English; it was translated into Italian by Emanuele Milceri and Gaetano Sisali, and revised with the help of Pietro Cardile and Sylvie Rossi, to all of whom I am very grateful. I had lived in Italy in the mid-1980s (see introduction to Chapter 3), and at the conference, I read the paper in Italian, which I have to say, was one of the highlights of my career to date. The conference itself was overshadowed by the death, only a few days before, of Carlo Mosio (1945–2008), a leading Italian transactional analyst and a lovely, generous man. I had been hoping to see him at the conference, was enormously saddened by his premature death, and still miss him. I had met him some 20 years earlier during my training at Metanoia when, at a workshop he was leading, he had challenged me, kindly but firmly about not "trying hard". It was a significant moment in my training, as a result of which he became something of a mentor, and later a colleague and friend, to whom I dedicate this chapter with great affection.

The presentation and original article was – is – part of an ongoing project of mine to review, reclaim, and revitalise the radical psychiatry tradition of transactional analysis (see introduction to Chapter 8), a perspective that continues to influence my work (see Tudor, 2014b, 2016b; Minikin & Tudor, 2016), and a project that extends to the more general field of radical therapy (see Tudor, 2012c; Steiner & Tudor, 2014; Tudor & Begg, 2016). The title of this paper is taken from and inspired by a paper which Peter Schmid, an Austrian person-centred colleague, had delivered the previous year as a keynote speech the 3rd Annual Conference of the British Association for the Person-Centred Approach, with the title: "Psychotherapy is Political or it is not Psychotherapy" (Schmid, 2007), a paper which was published some 5 years later (Schmid, 2012) and again as the lead article in a special issue of *Psychotherapy and Politics International* (which I edit) on the theme of the paper (Tudor, 2012b).

At the time (by late 2008), with regard to transactional analysis in the UK, I was feeling somewhat isolated, even alienated, for a number of reasons:

1 Regarding regulation and registration – despite the extensive critical literature on the subject (for references to which, see Chapter 11) and my own best endeavours (see Tudor, 1999c), most British transactional analysis psychotherapists were supporting increasing professional and statutory regulation. Their obsession with this had already alienated transactional analysts in other fields of application (i.e. counselling, education, and organisations) to the point that a significant number of them had broken away from the then Institute of Transactional Analysis (now the United Kingdom Transactional Analysis Association, http://www.uktransactionalanalysis.co.uk/) to found their own organisation, the Institute of Developmental Transactional Analysis (http://www.instdta.org/). Later, even after the United Kingdom Council for Psychotherapy had turned away from its pursuit of statutory regulation of psychotherapy (in 2009), this view led to the policy of regulating TA training through registered training establishments (Institute of Transactional Analysis, 2013), thereby further restricting practice.
2 Regarding recognition – in 2007, there had been a national TA conference on a theme that was well known as close to my heart, thinking, and work, held in the country in which I lived, yet I had not been approached to be involved in the conference. (In the event, I did put forward a proposal for a workshop, which was accepted.) As a friend and colleague put it at the time (paraphrasing Matthew 13:57, Mark 6:4–6, and Luke 4:24), whilst I was perhaps something of a prophet, it was not in my own country!
3 Regarding personal attacks – earlier in that year (2008), I had been on the receiving end of some pretty unpleasant ad homimem attacks in reaction to the "Take it" article (see introduction to Chapter 8).

All this made the invitation to address the conference in Italy not only a great honour, but also an opportunity for me to speak freely – interestingly enough, in another language.

With regard to the article itself I particularly like the fact that it addresses the radicalism of transactional analysis in terms of its core theory, i.e. ego states, transactions, scripts, and games. Whilst some of this (last) section drew on previously published work, namely Summers and Tudor (2000), in both the keynote and the Italian article, I was able to develop the radical implications of the co-creative approach to transactional analysis. In re-editing the article for this volume, I have retained something of the conversational style of the presentation and deleted some short passages to avoid repetition.

Opening remarks

First, let me thank you for your invitation, which comes as a great honour. I particularly appreciate the recognition you have given me as I have some experience that people who are interested in social and radical psychiatry, and who promote radical forms of psychotherapy and politics, are often not prophets in their own country. As some of you know I lived in Italy for a couple of years, some 20 years ago. In 1987 I attended a TA 101 at the Centro Eric Berne in Milan; and, during my time, in Italy, I studied and obtained my Scuola Media Certificate, one of the qualifications of which I am most proud. When I returned to the UK, unfortunately I did not keep up my Italian, so it is now very rusty. I have prepared this paper in English; and it has been translated by Emanuela Milceri and Gaetano Sisali, to whom I owe my profound thanks; I intend to read it, and ask you to be patient with my Italian. At the end there will be some time for questions to which I will respond via a translator.

Abstract

This paper considers Berne's social psychiatry as the background to radical psychiatry, which the author considers as a "lost tradition" within TA. The paper then offers a reading of radical psychiatry theory and practice as a part of a contemporary development of TA, which not only reclaims this tradition but which also confronts a certain neo-conservatism in psychotherapy in TA and, indeed, in the field of psychotherapy.

Social psychiatry

In 1956 Berne established a series of weekly meetings of mental health professionals under the title The San Francisco Social Psychiatry Seminar (which, in 1960, became an incorporated body which, in turn, led to the establishment of the International Transactional Analysis Association). Berne's seminal work on TA, *Transactional Analysis in Psychotherapy* (Berne, 1961/1975a) is subtitled "*A Systematic Individual and Social Psychiatry*". He defined this as denoting: "the study of the psychiatric aspects of specific transactions or sets of transactions which take place between two or more particular individuals at a given time and place." (p. 12). Despite the apparent importance Berne attached to this concept he only referred to it twice in the rest of the book: once with regard to the maintenance of ego states in relation to the changing flow of sensory stimuli, which observation Berne suggested, "forms the psychobiological basis of social psychiatry" (p. 83); and the other with regard to social intercourse which, he argued, is a form of work or, in terms of his theory of the structuring of time, an *activity*. For Berne, the term "social psychiatry" simply acknowledges the logic of transactional analysis, in terms of the analysis of social level transactions between people; the social diagnosis of ego states; and the social advantages of games.

Berne uses the term "social" to refer to the immediate social environment, and emphasised the "I" and the "You", that is, a person in transaction with another or within a group. Even though Berne originated TA as a group therapy, he worked more with individuals *in* the group, and with individuals *through* the group, than with the group *as* a group. This is very different from radical psychiatry which views groups in themselves as transformative, and organising in groups as a form of social, psychological and, indeed, political action. The original importance given in TA to groups has, in my view, been eroded by decisions within EATA to modify the certifying exam requirements regarding the experience of group therapy, and by trainers who no longer teach much group theory. I think this is significant. As Schmid (2007), a person-centred colleague, put it:

> we do not live in a world of two, [and] the pair is not the ultimate form of living together. There is not only the Other; there is also the Other of the Other. In short: we live in a world of groups … The group is the interface of the

> individual and the society where the person experiences themselves in their substantial and relational dimensions.

In my view, it is this group dimension of TA that makes it political.

Let's just take a moment to remind ourselves what politics is. The word politics derives from the Greek πολις (*polis*) which refers to the city-state. The *polis* originally denoted the castle of a city (the *acropolis*) and the settlement itself; later the city; and, finally, the autarchic political unit, that is, the city and the hinterland and the body of citizens. The equivalent Latin word was *civitas*. The *polis*, including law, culture, education, entertainment and market, were regulated by collective decisions, and provided a beneficial living together for the people inside the community, and activity on the outside, and, therefore, identity and security. For Aristotle:

> the state comes into existence, originating in the bare needs of life, and continuing in existence for the sake of a good life. And therefore, if the earlier forms of society are natural, so is the state...
>
> Hence it is evident that the state is a creation of nature, and that man is by nature a political animal.
>
> (Aristotle, 1946: Book 1, Part 2)

Thus we are social, political beings who actively develop in community. This means that the human being in the community – and only in it – can fully actualise her or his potential, and that only in community can we fully become humans. Politics is the creation of an order that serves this goal. Schmid (2007) reflected that:

> it is interesting that the definition of politics derives from the definition of the human being and vice versa! Politics is the consequence of an image of the human being or the other way round: from a certain image of the human being political action inevitably follows.

Of course, not everyone would agree with Aristotle, Schmid or myself. In a personal (e-mail) communication (22 March 2008), Karpman wrote that: "Well trained [transactional analysts] all know that politics is a CP [Critical Parent] (pseudo NP [Nurturing Parent] Rescue) hard game of I'm OK – You're not OK, and an attempt to exterminate the other 50% of opposite opinion." I think that this perspective is not only wrong but is also very worrying, especially as it comes from someone of Karpman's standing in the TA community. At this point I just want to say "Obama"! Presumably Karpman does not believe his President Elect when in his acceptance speech he promised to listen also to the 46 percent of American voters of the "opposite opinion". I think that one of the great strengths of the ego state model and of Berne's four requirements for ego state diagnosis is that it gives us a specific and structural analysis whereby, for example, politics, and a person's approach to her or his politics, can be analysed and understood as an expression of an integrating Adult neopsychic functioning, or as an expression of Archaic Child or Introjected Parent ego states. Karpman's view is not one based on a transactional analysis but, rather, is one which represents contaminated thinking, based on and revealing a neo-conservative world view.

In an appreciation of Berne's social psychiatry, Moiso (1998) viewed it as "one of the most innovative and useful aspects of Berne's transactional analysis". (p. 1). Moiso continued: "the social dimension of Berne's theory acknowledges that the unit for transactional analysis is not just the stimulus, but the stimulus-plus-response dyad, thus emphasising the reciprocity of cause and effect within the interplay of relationships." (p. 7). I think this is a generous reading of Berne whose focus remained on the individual and, despite his references to the social, on the manifestations of intrapsychic processes. Indeed, after the publication of *Transactional Analysis in Psychotherapy*, Berne only mentioned social psychiatry twice. In *The Structure and Dynamics of Organizations and Groups*, Berne (1963) defined social psychiatry as: "The science which treats of the inner forces motivating specific transactional stimuli and responses" (p. 327), and specifically distinguished this from social dynamics which treat of the "outward effects" of such stimuli and responses. Boulton (1978) has written about this with regard to the origins of an individual's social concerns, which she located within the functional nurturing parent ego state. Later, in *Games People Play*, although Berne (1964/1968) claimed that his (then) present approach was one aspect of social psychiatry, he was clear about his focus: "we are here concerned with *the personal histories* and *psychodynamics* of the individuals involved." (p. 47; my emphasis).

It is clear that Berne made little or no connection "between the consulting room and the larger world" as Jacobs (1996: 207) put it, and neither have many other transactional analysts in the name of social psychiatry. Only 13 out of 1,508 articles in 30 years of the *TAJ* mention the term and, of these, only seven directly address the concept, theory and practice of TA as a social psychiatry. I am not alone in my criticism of Berne's limited use of and reference to the social. Baute (1979) put it succinctly: "TA proposes to be a system of social psychiatry, yet is no more social than almost every other theory of personality and change which are a reflection of our predominant cultural values of individualism, privatism and hedonism." (p. 171). Also Zalcman (1990) argued that the present major divisions of TA – that is, the structural analysis of ego states, transactional analysis proper, script analysis, game analysis and racket analysis (the last two of which she separates) – "*are not sufficient* to establish transactional analysis as a comprehensive theory and method of social psychiatry." (p. 4). Recently Rossi (in Tosi *et al.*, 2008) has pointed out that, from 1984, the *TAJ* dropped from its opening page its reference to and definition of TA as a systematic psychotherapy for *social* change.

Finally and perhaps significantly, given his earlier appreciation of Berne's social psychiatry, in a subsequent article Moiso (1995) argued that ideological and political involvement is crucial for transactional analysts in order to foster Berne's idea of TA as a social psychiatry. In this sense, radical psychiatry, based on an analysis of alienation and oppression, may be viewed as a particular political subset of social psychiatry.

Radical psychiatry

In many ways I think that radical psychiatry is the lost tradition of transactional analysis. Despite its influence, especially in the 1970s, it never had the same impact on TA theory and practice or significantly in the training of transactional analysts as did the other, and original, three "schools" of TA. In their book on *Transactional Analysis* Woollams and Brown (1978) identified radical psychiatry as one of a number of "schools" of TA and offered a brief summary of its treatment emphasis (the stroke economy); aetiology (premature decision in the "Pig Parent"); presenting problems (banal scripts); treatment methods (increase awareness and permissions); tools (organisation against social oppression); and goals (decontaminiation of the "Pig Parent", and autonomy through co-operation). However, since then, it has all but disappeared: in a search of articles in the *TAJ* (1971–2000), [there are only 12 in which there are any references to radical psychiatry (and those are mostly only passing ones). Interestingly, from 2001 to date (2016), 17 articles in or letters to the *TAJ* have mentioned radical psychiatry].

A brief history and context of radical psychiatry

Claude Steiner (2000) reported that he first heard the term "radical psychiatry" in 1968 at the American Psychiatric Association (APA) meeting in Miami, Florida, at which a group of young medical residents, in opposition to the Vietnam War and critical of the psychiatric profession's support for it, called for a radical psychiatry as an alternative to what they saw as a conservative, even reactionary, profession. Prompted by his growing awareness of "psychiatric power abuse", and radicalised by his experiences in Florida, on his return to California, Steiner began to teach a course on radical psychiatry at the Free University at Berkeley. In parallel with other courses on offer, this course dealt with the patterns of power abuse in psychiatry and the oppressiveness of the practice of psychiatry, psychology, psychotherapy and other "helping" professions. A critical analysis of power and oppression was to become a cornerstone of the theory and practice of radical psychiatry.

In September 1969, the APA's conference meeting, held in San Francisco, California, was disrupted by a coalition of women, gay people and others who felt oppressed by reactionary psychiatric practices, and Steiner prepared a "manifesto" (Steiner, 1971b), which was distributed at the conference (and which is reprinted in Steiner *et al.*, 1975; and Steiner, 2000). This coalition of interest groups was also reflected in the theory, practice, and literature of radical psychiatry at that time (see especially the Rough Times Staff, 1973).

During 1969 Steiner joined the Berkeley Free Clinic, an organisation founded by a group of paramedics who had served in Vietnam, together with antiwar medical professionals, and started a psychological counselling section, the Radical Approach to Psychiatry (or RAP Centre). In the course of that year a number of others also joined the centre, notably Hogie Wyckoff and Joy Marcus. At this time Steiner was a clinical psychologist who was also training and working with Berne, and it is interesting to note that many of the pioneers of radical psychiatry were highly influenced by TA. In 1970 Wykoff wrote the first article on radical psychiatry to appear in the *Transactional Analysis Bulletin* on "Radical psychiatry and TA in women's groups".

Radical psychiatry arose, of course, out of a wider social and political context. Roy (1988a) referred to a "melding" of various streams of rebellion, which gave birth to radical psychiatry: the movement for civil rights, especially amongst black people and gay people; the activism in response to the Vietnam war, which led to a "new", if small, political Left in the United States; feminism and the women's movement; the hippie movement; and, as I have already noted, the emergence of organised groups of psychiatric patients and their professional allies challenging the psychiatric establishment in its practice and theory. Many of these contexts, influences and movements were also present outside the US. With regard to radicalising psychiatry, here in Italy, Franco Basaglia was implementing wholesale changes in the running of psychiatric hospitals, beginning in 1971 with a phase of de-institutionalisation (see Basaglia, 1968, 1981). Basaglia was also active politically, and in 1974 *Psichiatria Democratica* was founded. Its activity in this field was highly influential on social policy, and led, some 5 years later to the passing of a new law (180) in 1978, which facilitated community care and the closure of most psychiatric hopsitals (for further details and analysis of which see Tudor, 1990b [Chapter 4]). Basaglia's work was known in radical psychiatry circles in the USA (see Mebane-Francescato & Jones, 1973). At around the same time, in the UK, Aaron Esterson, Joe Berke, David Cooper and R. D. Laing were developing their ideas about the origins and treatment of schizophrenia, and a practice which came to be known as "anti-psychiatry" (see Boyers & Orrill, 1972). This was also influenced by and, in turn, itself influenced the then emerging therapeutic communities (see Windes, 1977; Manning, 1979). This brief history is important in that it illustrates the point that ideas and theories as well as people exist in a social context, and that social and political contexts influence the development of ideas, theory and practice.

Theory and practice

> Radical psychiatry holds that all functional psychiatric difficulties are forms of alienation resulting from the mystifying oppression of people who are isolated from each other. People's alienation is the result of power abuse and is therefore a political matter. Any person in the practice of psychiatry (soul healing) becomes involved in the personal politics of those he or she attempts to help … Radical psychiatry is a political theory of psychiatric disturbance and a political practice of soul healing.
>
> (Steiner, 2000: 578)

From this, we can consider that there are two elements to radical psychiatry:

1 A political theory of psychological disturbance; and
2 A political practice of "therapy" (which is taken to include psychiatry, psychology, psychotherapy and forms of self-help).

We can see these elements in the earliest publications in which Kupers (1971) argued the need for revolutionary theory, and in which Kunnes (1971) wrote about how to be a radical therapist. The key concepts underpinning the theory and practice of radical psychiatry are: alienation; oppression; power; mystification; competition; the stroke economy; the Pig Parent; powerless scripts; autonomy; and co-operation. Here I discuss three of these concepts: autonomy, alienation and the stroke economy.

Autonomy

Despite the reality of groups, western psychology has, in its development and application to the field of therapy over the last hundred years, focused predominantly on understanding the individual, individuality, *self*-actualisation, autonomy, the concept of the *self*, and the importance of *self*-development – and, of course, the goal of autonomy lies at the heart of TA. However, this focus and these concepts are not without their critics: on the individual (e.g. Hillman & Ventura, 1992); on the self (Vitz, 1977; Tudor & Worrall, 2006); on self-actualisation (e.g. Rigney, 1981; Lukas, 1989); on autonomy (e.g. Whitney, 1982; LeVine, 1990); and on self-development and individual *self*-concept (Nobles, 1973).

Autonomy is concerned with self-organisation, whether psychologically or politically. In terms of your political history and organisation as a country, I think Italy and Italians know about autonomy perhaps better than any other European country and peoples. But, from where does autonomy derive? As formulated in his theory of personality and behaviour, Rogers (1951) asserted that the human species, as with other species, has one basic tendency and striving: "to actualize, maintain, and enhance the experiencing organism." (p. 487). It is the human organism's tendency to actualise, the life force that Berne (1947/1971) referred to as *physis*, that gives us the biological and social basis for autonomy. However, Angyal (1941), a Hungarian psychologist on whose work Rogers drew, viewed the organism as having *two* related tendencies: one towards increased *autonomy*, and one towards *homonomy*. He defined the organism as autonomous in the sense that it is "to a large extent, a *self-governing* entity" (p. 23), *and* homonomous in the sense that it longs "to be in harmony with superindividual units, the social group, nature, God, ethical world order, or whatever the person's formulation of it may be." (p. 172). Angyal also acknowledged the notion of *heteronomy*: "The organism lives in a world in which things happen according to laws which are heteronomous from the point of view of the organism." (p. 33). So, human beings live autonomously and homonomously in a world that is heteronomous or other. I think Angyal's concept of homonomy provides us with an important psychological and political counterpoint to the individualism of autonomy, with a biological and conceptual basis for belonging, for relationship, and, as the organism cannot be understood outside its environment, with an understanding of our interdependent relationship with the environment.

Alienation

Autonomy and homonomy, in effect, describe the authentic, experiencing organism/person, in relationship. When we are in some way inauthentic we experience some form of estrangement or alienation also in relationship. As Marx (1832/1975a), the philosopher of alienation, suggested: "Every self-estrangement of man from himself and nature is manifested in the relationship he sets up between other men and himself and nature." (p. 44). Steiner and his colleagues came up with a formula which defined alienation as equal to oppression, plus mystification, plus isolation: Alienation = Oppression + Mystification + Isolation.

Marx talked in terms of relationship and of alienation in four ways:

- man's relation to his or her product
- man's relation to her or his productive capacity
- man's relation to other people
- man's relation to his or her species

– to which Roy (1988) added a fifth:

- man's social relations to the Earth.

Based on a theory of alienation, and an analysis of oppression and power, derived from Marx and influenced by Reich, Marcuse, Fanon and Laing, the tradition of radical psychiatry within TA offers particular co-operative ways of working with individuals and groups to reclaim autonomy (see Steiner *et al.*, 1975) – and, I would add, homonomy or a sense of belonging whether to family, group, tribe, community or an organisation. Echoing Marx's analysis, Steiner (2000) wrote in terms of people:

- being alienated from our hearts, or from love;
- being alienated from our minds, or from the capacity to think;
- being alienated from our bodies, or from our feelings; and
- being alienated from our hands, or from our work

– and, to echo Roy's addition, I would add:

- being alienated from the land, or from our heritage.

Thus, a person who is passive (say, in terms of passive behaviours), who disowns (or discounts) her feelings and behaviour, who blames others "the world" (in terms of their racket or script beliefs) is inauthentic or alienated in some way. In response, a therapy which analyses the transactions by which the client has been oppressed, mystified and isolated, and which invites a client to "own" her impulses and behaviours, and to experience him or herself as a person-in-action in a social world, is a therapy of dis-alienation. This is a process which Bulhan (1980) argued is impossible without a total restructuring of society – and, hence the need to view and understand the individual client/citizen in the context of the *polis* (see, for example, Tudor & Hargaden, 2002).

In these terms, alienation provides us with the core concept of a psychosocial theory of psychopathology (see Tudor & Worrall, 2006). In this context I am interested that in its preparation for the fifth edition of its *Diagnostic and Statistical Manual of Mental Disorders*, the APA is thinking about abandoning its Axis II personality disorders in favour of understanding personality in terms of relational dimensions: extraversion – introversion; antagonism – compliance; constraint – impulsivity; emotional dysregulation – emotional stability; and, interestingly in the context of some of my own experiences within TA, unconventionality – closedness to experience (see Widiger & Simonsen, 2006).

The stroke economy

The stroke economy (Steiner, 1971d) is, in my view, one of the most underrated pieces of TA theory. In his original article Steiner explicitly referred to Reich and Marcuse as writers who have linked "the control of vital human processes and broader economical and political points of view". (p. 10). Drawing on Marcuse's theory of alienation and the concept of surplus repression, Steiner made the point that "This surplus repression forces human beings to live according to the performance principle". (p. 10). Steiner went on to argue that, just as the social order controls people through the economic system – and, of course, this is an argument that is highly topical – so it controls people through the imposition of a stroke economy. You [the audience at the conference] will be familiar with its tenets or injunctions:

- Don't give strokes – when you have them to give, and don't give yourself strokes,
- Don't ask for strokes – when you need them,
- Don't accept strokes – if you want them, and

- Don't reject strokes – when you don't want them.

Whilst I have known about these for the 20 years I have been involved in TA – and have practised their antitheses, i.e.

- Give strokes – when you have them to give, and give yourself strokes,
- Ask for strokes – when you need them,
- Accept strokes – if you want them, and
- Reject strokes – when you don't want them.

– I am always surprised at their power. Earlier this year I invited Claude Steiner to England to run a workshop, and had the pleasure and privilege of working with him and was again reminded of the power of exchanging strokes and of working through the resistance to positive strokes, a practice which is both personal and political.

Having identified and elaborated some aspects of radical psychiatric theory and practice, in the last part of this paper, I turn to some discussion of the radical nature of TA.

The radical nature of TA

I think we need to reclaim the radical project that is psychotherapy, that is, the liberation of the individual from the chains of their past, to be able to live, love and work in the present in authentic relationship with themselves, others, and the world. We may understand this in terms of oppressive scripting, the importance of Adult–Adult transacting, and co-operation based on a sense of belonging, or we may frame this in terms of the slogan, principles and aspirations of the French revolution: liberté, egalité et fraternité. I think the difference of language is important: one is the language of individual psychology, the other is the language of social and psychology and politics. One aspect of our radical project is to reclaim a social language about the individual and about our interconnectedness. I am currently working on a paper which argues that the fundamental life position is not "I'm OK, You're OK", a statement which in my view confuses humanism with existentialism, but which is simply and profoundly: "We are" (see Tudor, 2016b).

I think it is interesting that most of the founding fathers and mothers of psychotherapy, were, in their own time, viewed as radicals, as often they challenged social and cultural norms; and, in their descriptions of psychological processes, they developed a language which was new, challenging, subversive, and sometimes shocking. It is no accident that in the history of psychotherapy there has been a number of practitioners and theorists who were politically minded as well as psychologically minded – Adler and Reich to name but two. However, in the development of ideas, problems often arise in the second generation, which is the one which usually establishes the schools based on the work of the founders, and is often the generation which seeks to conserve rather than to challenge. As Phillips (1995) put it: "Disciples are the people who haven't got the joke." (p. 162). I have experienced this conservatism, for instance, in some of the responses to my article in the *TAJ* earlier this year on a sixth driver (Tudor, 2008f [Chapter 8]), a concept and an article which challenges self-sealing doctrines and closed systems. As far as TA is concerned, I would imagine that most of us here probably represent the third and fourth generations, on whom it falls to reflect on our history and, where necessary, to revise it. So, here, I present four reflections and revisions, which, to take up the challenge implicit in Zalcman's (1990) critique, relate to the foundations of TA: ego states, transactions, scripts and games. All four reflections have implications for the political theory and the political practice of TA.

Ego states

Radical, from the Latin *radix* means root, so in a very real sense, being radical means returning to our roots or "natural" state or process. With regard to the personality, this, in my view, is the *neopsyche*. What this means is that our "roots" are – and our radicalism is – in the present, and an ever-changing present at that. One of the problems we have in TA is that, at the heart of our theory, we have two sets of models about structural ego states – and both these sets of models derive from Berne (1961/1975a). One set comprises those models which represent all three ego states as the "complete" or total personality and the desirable end goal of therapy; the other is the Integrated Adult, or what I have referred to as the "integrating Adult" model (Tudor, 2003), which views the Parent and Child as, respectively, introjected and archaic ego states which need to be integrated into Adult/neopsychic functioning, or abandoned. The integrating Adult is the logic of the co-creative relational approach to TA developed by Graeme Summers and myself (Summers & Tudor, 2000); and the logic of the integrating Adult is a methodology based on empathy and aimed at expanding the client's neopsychic/Adult functioning (see Tudor, 2003, and Figure 9.1).

I think this is radical because it locates the power of change in the experience of the client.

Transactions

Transactional analysis, that is, the analysis of transactions, is radical as it implies a meta-perspective; in other words, we talk with the client about how we talk with each other, so *how* we communicate is on the map or the territory that is therapy. This, together with the principle and method of open communication, means that, again, we do not take away power from the patient. Indeed, at best, TA does not *give* power to the patient or client; it never takes it away in the first place. This, however, depends on the philosophy, attitude and stance of the therapist, trainer, supervisor, facilitator, or consultant, and, in our transactions with clients and trainees I think we need to be particularly careful of subtle "power plays", which, as Steiner (1981) observed "depend on our obedience, which is often mistaken for co-operation. Co-operation very often means going along, not arguing, and doing as others, who know better, tell us." (p. 47). One antidote to acquiescence is disobedience:

> The first step in becoming powerful without using power to control others is to learn to be disobedient ... Refusing to be controlled against your will and judgement frees your own powers for whatever you may decide is good for you. (pp. 50–51)

So, do we as a TA community support this analysis of power and encourage civil and psychological disobedience? I think not.

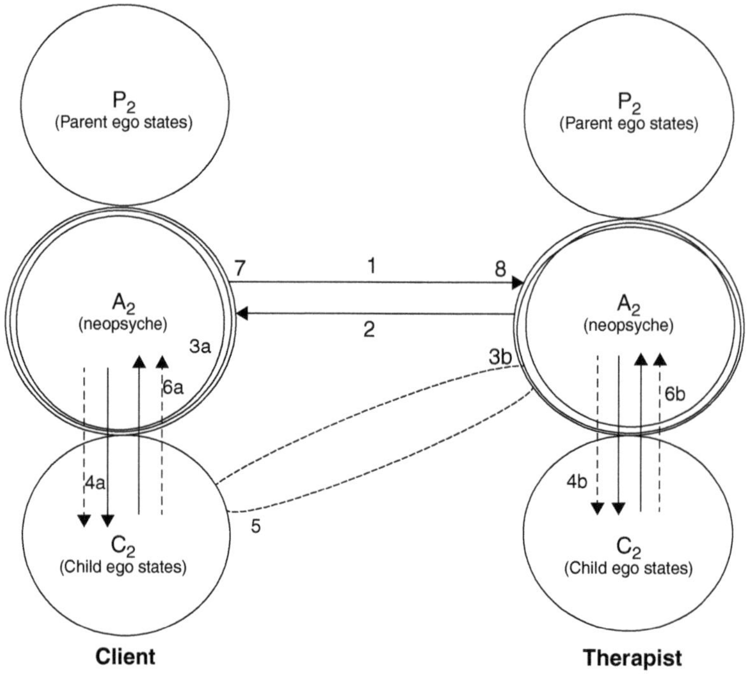

Key

1 The client offers an initial stimulus.	2 The therapist responds.
3a The client resonates with a feeling state in response to the therapist's response ...	3b ... and so may the therapist.
4a ... which, in this case, has an impact on the client's Archaic Child ego state(s),[1] consciously and unconsciously ...	4b ... as it may in the therapist.[3]
5 The client *may* experience the therapist's empathy also at an ulterior level, although it is not the intention of the therapist to "send" an ulterior Adult–Child transaction.[2]	
6a The client abstracts empathic knowledge from the experience of her or his emotional resonance at both social (conscious) and ulterior (unconscious) levels ...	6b ... as may the therapist.
7 ... and integrates this abstracted empathic knowledge into responses that are increasingly acceptant and empathic of self and others ...	8 ...including the therapist who also is affected and expanded by this process.

Notes

1 This transactional process is the same with regard to Introjected Parent ego states (but for reasons of clarity and simplicity is only shown here with regard to the Child ego states).

2 A point and a theme that acknowledges the intersubjective nature of this process.

3 If this is idealised then it would be represented as a Child–Parent and/or Parent–Child idealising ulterior transaction and, as such, offers a representation of how narcissism can be encouraged and perpetuated in therapeutic relating [see Chapter 8].

Figure 9.1 Co-creative empathic transacting

Scripts

As I noted earlier, one element of radical psychiatry is to develop a political theory of psychological disturbance. I think we have this in TA, especially within radical psychiatry, but that we could do more to critique and revise TA theory, not least as a political act in itself. One example of this is script, and specifically, the script matrix (Steiner, 1966). In his critical review of script theory, Cornell (1988) suggested that script, as presented in most TA literature is "overly reductionistic and insufficiently attentive to the formative factors in healthy psychological development" (p. 270) – and I agree with him (see, for instance, Tudor, 2008f). From a philosophical point of view, this is especially ironic given the compatibility of script theory with constructivism (Allen & Allen, 1997). However, if we are to view scripts as constructive narratives which, like memories, are co-created in the present and projected into the past, then we need to reformulate much of our present understanding of script and script theory. Elsewhere, Summers and I have suggested taking the logic of Cornell's (1988) arguments further in developing a narrative map of the influences on co-creative identity (Summers & Tudor, 2000), i.e.

1 We agree with Cornell in drawing the script matrix horizontally, bringing the "parental" influences into a mutual relationship with the "child" or subject; and
2 We extend the mutuality of vectors to include the Parent vector (see Figure 9.2).

Thus, the injunctions, programs [sic] and drivers of the script cut both ways. A child telling her parent to "Go away" may be both receiving and responding to *and* conveying a "Don't Exist" injunction. Of course the relative impact on the parent who, predominantly, has more power than the child, will vary according to her or his own development, history, experiences, pathology and present support, etc. The child who models his parents' various behaviours by, for instance, succeeding at school, also perpetuates the family/cultural "success" story and, again, this impacts on the parents. Similarly, with driver messages: "Pull yourself together, son" (from a father) may be matched by a "Hold me and be there for me always" (from the son) – which may represent mutual drives to "Be Strong".

In addition, and perhaps most significantly and radically,

3 We replace "Mother" and "Father" with any polarity which is significant to the subject, based on their own construction/s of reality (see Figure 9.3).

As well as revising theory we must also apply theory and, I think apply our own theory to ourselves. Thus, for some years I have been interested in analysing TA from a transactional perspective. So, for instance, we might think about what script messages TA trainers, organisations, supervisors and practitioners convey. In a previous paper I have commented on what I see as a certain dogma in TA and identified how this is reinforced through notions of purity, conformity, priesthood, and certainty (see Tudor, 2007d).

Psychological games

Turning finally to games, I think that one game which a number of transactional analysts play is "conformity". Lindner (1953) wrote about what he identified as the eleventh commandment: "Thou shalt comply and conform." He continued:

> And when the child does not (or cannot) adjust, when his rebelliousness that is actually of the essence of his nature appears, he is relegated to the purgatory

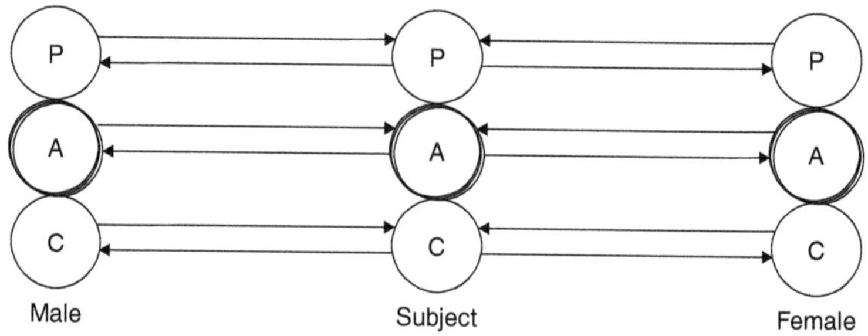

Figure 9.2 Co-creative script matrix (Summers & Tudor, 2000)

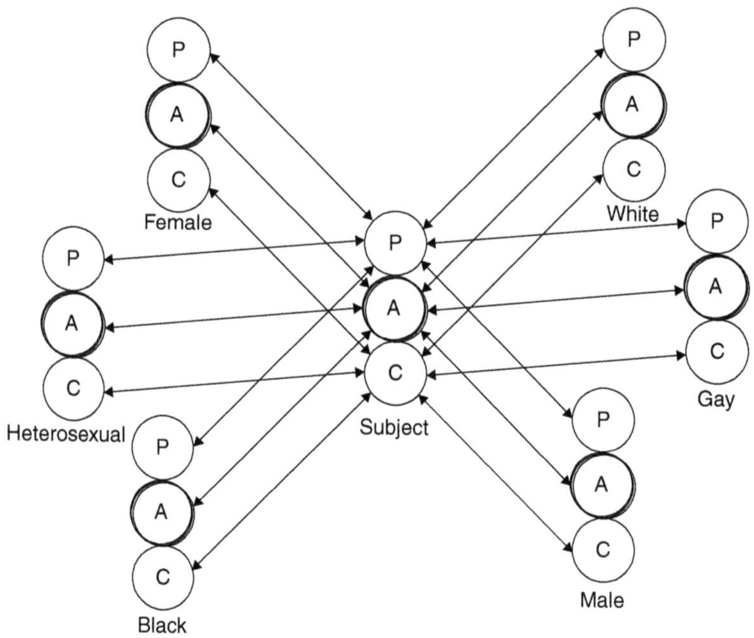

Figure 9.3 A script helix (Summers & Tudor, 2000)

> of parental disapproval, and thereby conditioned to the immediate suppression of his rebellious inclinations.
>
> (p. 73)

This is one reason why I think we need to reclaim concepts of the rebellious Adult and, for that matter, the critical and nurturing Adult (see Tudor, 2003).

One manifestation of conformity is the number of candidates preparing for examinations, especially certifying exams, who are overly concerned about what their examiners might think rather than how they themselves think about and describe their work, their clients, and themselves with reference to the richness and diversity of TA theory. In his keynote speech to the conference of the United Kingdom's Institute of Transactional Analysis in 2000, Cornell expressed his concern that TA candidates were being examined for conformity. In the published version of this speech, referring to EATA oral examinations, Cornell (2000) wrote that: "I finished those exams with the thought that our organization is now teaching doctrine rather than theory and thinking." (p. 270). Of course, this is the end point of a process which begins with the training and supervisory relationship and method. Sadly, I think that too many colleagues operate from a Parental paradigm which schools trainees and supervisees, as distinct from an Adult paradigm which seeks to educate adults (see Lomas, 1987; Tudor, 2007f).

I am not suggesting that these reflections in themselves transform TA into a comprehensive theory and method of social psychiatry, let alone radical psychiatry, but that they begin the task.

Conclusion

So, in conclusion, if TA does not advocate integrating Adult neopsychic functioning; if it does not promote the analysis of transactions, and the meta-theoretical communication of such analysis; if it is not reflexive, that is, it does not reflect critically on its language and its own script messages and organisational games, then it is not TA. If it promotes autonomy at the expense of homonomy; if it trains for conformity rather than critical thinking; if it accepts its neo-conservativism rather than its radicalism, then it is not TA.

Thank you.

PART IV

THE 2010s

Employment, other work, professional qualifications, accreditations/registration and memberships, academic qualifications, and recognitions

Ongoing	Self-employed counsellor, transactional analyst, health care provider, supervisor, researcher, trainer, and consultant
	United Kingdom Council for Psychotherapy, registered psychotherapist
	Auckland University of Technology (AUT), 2009–2010 senior lecturer, 2009–2014 programme leader, from September 2009 certified postgraduate supervisor, 2010–2015 associate professor, 2013–2015 head of department, Department of Psychotherapy & Counselling, from September 2015 professor of psychotherapy, from 2016 head of school, School of Public Health and Psychosocial Studies, and leading researcher
	Ngā Ao e Rua, member
Ongoing–to 2011	European Association of Transactional Analysis, certified transactional analyst, teaching and supervising transactional analyst
From 2010	Waka Oranga, associate member
	New Zealand Transactional Analysis Association (from 2015 Aotearoa New Zealand Transactional Analysis Association), member
2010	PhD in Mental Health Promotion by Public (Published) Works, Middlesex University
	Certificate in Treaty of Waitangi Studies (AUT)
From 2011	New Zealand Association of Psychotherapists, provisional member
From 2012	International Association for Transactional Analysis, teaching member
From 2015	The Critical Institute, honorary fellow
	Univerza na Primorskem (University of Primorska), Slovenia, visiting associate professor
	University of Roehampton, Department of Psychology, London, honorary senior research fellow

CHAPTER 10

THE FIGHT FOR HEALTH

An heuristic enquiry (2010)

Retrospective introduction

This chapter comprises excerpts from my doctoral work, which focus on heurism as a research method. I undertook a PhD by public, i.e. published works, a process which involved presenting three previously published works, in my case, a book (Tudor, 1996b), a chapter (Tudor, 2003), and a chapter (Tudor, 2008e) that had been previously published as an article (Tudor, 2007a), together with a justifying context statement, which ran to some 30,000 words. The final title of the work was "*The Fight for Health: An Heuristic Enquiry into Psychological Well-Being*."

I have had a long interest in research which dates back to 1976 when, as a temporary (trainee) probation officer, I was encouraged to attend a probation service methods development group. My experience of research encompasses the following:

- 1981–1985, my first post-qualification employment as a "counsellor/ researcher" at a youth counselling agency, during which, in addition to offering counselling to clients, I participated in the design and collection of research data, as well as the struggle against an attempt to impose a particular method (see introduction to Chapter 2).
- During the mid-late 1980s, undertaking research into the implications and impact of social policy (see Chapters 3 and 4).
- In 1990, my fellowship at King's College, London, which led to a number of publications on mental health (see Chapter 7), and also research into projects offering programmes to prevent male violence (Tudor, 1993).
- Over some years, researching my own psychotherapy practice: (a) with groups, based on Yalom's (1985) work on the therapeutic factors of groups (see Tudor, 1999a); and (b) with regard to specific, intensive work with clients with serious difficulties, using the Minnesota Multiphasic Personality Inventory (Hathaway & McKinley, 1940/1970) (see Embleton Tudor & Tudor, 1997; Embleton Tudor *et al.*, 2004).
- During the early 2000s, designing as part of the Postgraduate Diploma/MSc course at Temenos, a 12-day module on research methods which, at the time, offered students at Temenos the most input on research of all the psychotherapy training recognised by the Humanistic and Integrative Psychotherapy Section of the United Kingdom Council of Psychotherapy.

- During 2002–2003, being part of a research project into the effectiveness of listening visits conducted by health visitors with women with postnatal depression (see Morrell, Ricketts, Tudor, & Williams, 2011).
- Since 2008, supervising postgraduate students' research and, from 2011 doctoral students' research.

Students of psychotherapy have generally been under-resourced with regard to reading and becoming familiar with research methods and methodology, let alone conducting research. Psychotherapists, and especially those within the humanistic and psychodynamic traditions, are increasingly under attack to "prove" the validity, efficacy and effectiveness of their practice, and more so in the context of the dominance of a particular, "evidence-based" approach to research and evidence (for a critique of the research bias of which, see Tudor, 2008d). In this context, it is important to reclaim, conduct, and promote research methods and methodologies that are more consistent with the science, art and method(s) of psychotherapy and counselling. As McNulty (1997) acknowledged in his review of my book on mental health: "In employing the methodology of critical reflexivity, [the author] provides a worked example of an approach to professional and personal development for people in this field." (p. 119).

With its roots in phenomenology and its explicit links with humanistic therapy, heursistics is a base for and an approach to research that is particularly appropriate to researching psychotherapy and the other "psy" professions. It is also profoundly personal, a perspective which informs the critique in the doctoral statement and this chapter. In this sense I would argue that heuristics is a critical methodology and method, 'though this warrants further elaboration.

The chapter comprises the abstract of and the introduction to the PhD, which gives some overall context to the chapter, including the relationship between the three works presented; a short part on methodology; and two parts on heuristic method, all edited for consistency and coherence as one chapter. In my original context statement, I acknowledged and thanked my wife Louise Embleton Tudor; my colleagues and friends Helena Hargaden, Charlotte Sills, Graeme Summers and Mike Worrall; my supervisor Dr Bernard Burgoyne; my doctoral examiners, Dr John Lees and Dr John Nuttall; and my colleague at Auckland University of Technology, Dr Liz Smythe, who I consulted in and about the last stage of revising my context statement.

In the chapter I refer to myself as a psychotherapist, a title which I claim in most countries in the world – I retain my voluntary registration with the United Kingdom Council for Psychotherapy. In Aotearoa New Zealand I am not a psychotherapist as I am not registered with the Psychotherapists Board of Aotearoa New Zealand, which, as a "responsible authority" under the Health Practitioners Competence Assurance Act 2003, regulates the practice of those practitioners who choose to register as a psychotherapist (for further discussion of which see Tudor, 2011d; and Chapter 11).

Abstract

This statement describes an enquiry into psychological wellbeing by means of a heuristic research process which reflects on three public (published) works, and their cohesive originality. Psychological wellbeing is considered in terms of positive mental health, neopsychic ego state functioning (or ego process), and homonomy.

The thesis reflects the candidate's heuristic process over a number of years in researching and writing these particular works, as well as referencing his work as a whole. The thesis also reflects on the candidate's heuristic process specifically with regard to the examination process, and frames this reflection in terms of the phases, process and key concepts of heurism and heuristic research methodology. Through this reflection a further concept – that of holism – emerges as a cohesive and unifying theme. The statement defends the thesis that the candidate's work, severally and together, has contributed to a shift in the field of psychotherapy, specifically by proposing that the client develops an organismic integrating functioning as a result of the therapeutic method of co-creative empathic transacting.

Keywords: heuristic, mental health, neopsyche, ego states, homonomy, holism

Introduction

...

This extended statement provides the context for the three published works I am submitting for consideration for the award of Doctorate of Philosophy by public (published) works in the field of psychotherapy. The submission comprises: (a) the context statement and (b) my public works, two of which form two of the Appendices to the statement. [The works were: the book *Mental Health Promotion: Paradigms and Practice* (Tudor, 1996b), the chapter "The Neopsyche: The integrating Adult ego state" (Tudor, 2003), and the chapter "Psychological Health: Autonomy and Homonomy" (Tudor, 2008e), which was based on an article published in a Dutch journal (Tudor, 2007a).

I have been studying and practising psychotherapy for over 20 years, and am a widely published author in this field. The three works selected represent my intellectual journey: from an extensive study of mental health; through a re-reading of transactional analysis and a re-writing of a central element of its ego state theory, and the elaboration of the implications for empathic transactions; to a discussion of the significance of the human trend to belonging or homonomy alongside autonomy. This journey has not been an easy one: health is a disputed concept and, in some quarters, is seen as a self-deceptive "flight"; and my own interest in and focus on health, growth and growth models, psycho*sanology* alongside psychopathology and salutogenesis alongside pathogenesis, has, at times, involved struggle and conflict. The "fight" of the title of this submission thus acknowledges both a critical theoretical perspective as well as particular personal, professional and political experiences, and, to a certain extent, my experience of the doctoral *viva voce* (oral examination) process. Specifically, I argue that my work has shifted the field by proposing that the client develops an organismic integrating functioning as a result of the therapeutic method of co-creative empathic transacting....

I see a number of conceptual links between these three public works (see Figure 10.1).

The chapter on the *neopsyche*/integrating Adult is linked with the book on mental health promotion through health psychology; sociopsychology, an *inter*-discipline which draws on both psychology and sociology (see Holland, 1988); and reflexivity, or critical reflection and analysis (see, for instance, Harré, 1983; Holland, 1999). Although ego psychology has its origins in psychopathology and a conception of defence (see Pine, 1990), Hartmann (1939/1958) argued that, as a development of psychoanalysis, ego psychology offers "a *general* theory of mental life". (p. 4). Hartmann (1942) also framed his discussion of the concept of health in

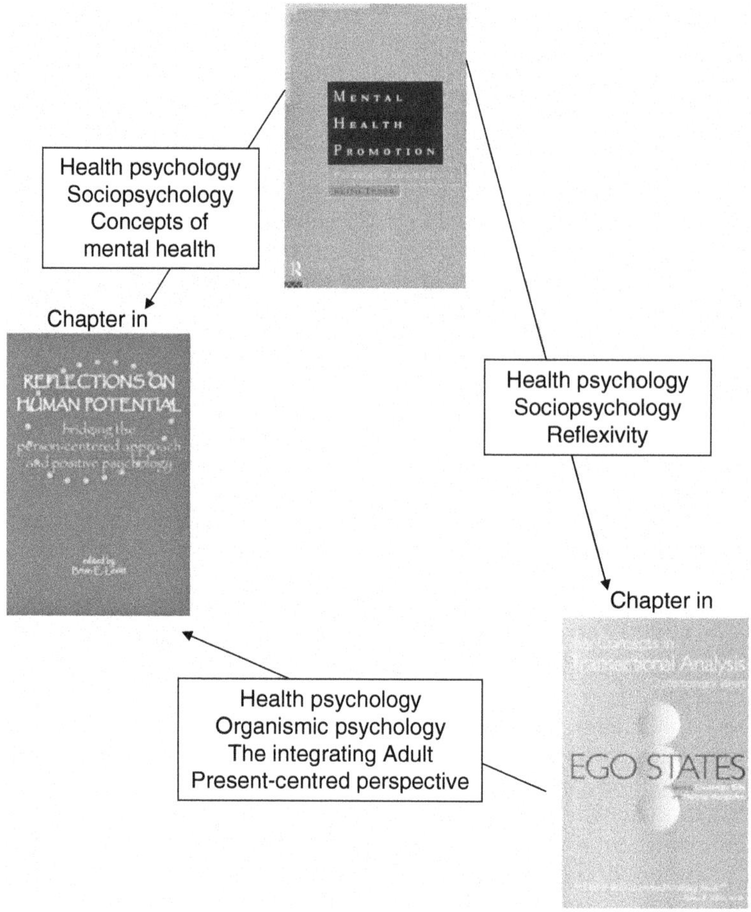

Figure 10.1 Conceptual links between the three public (published) works presented

terms of the ego. My work on the integrating Adult stands in this tradition. There is also an implicit link between the two in that I have also applied paradigm analysis to transactional analysis as an organising framework within which I analysed and located TA theory and method (Tudor, 1996c). In doing so I developed the practice – and potential – of transactional analysis as a social action psychotherapy (Holland, 1988, 1990), and critiqued the notion of integrative psychotherapy (see also Tudor, 2001).

The article/chapter on autonomy and homonomy is linked with the chapter on the *neopsyche* also as a development of health psychology, the common ground of organismic psychology, and an understanding of *neopsychic* functioning as a quality of the organism (also represented by the integrating Adult). This work represents a development of a unitary theory of motivation (Rogers, 1963) to include the trends of autonomy and homonomy (Angyal, 1941), and of a present-centred perspective on the person and his or her psychology (see Mead, 1932/1980; Stern, 2004; Tudor, 2008e). My argument that the present is relatively autonomous from the past is similar to Hartmann's (1939/1958) point about the relative autonomy of an ego which is separate from the conflicts of the past.

The article/chapter (the third public work) also reflects the influence of and, therefore, links with the first public and original work on mental health promotion in terms of health psychology, and a sociopsychological approach to the wider social and cultural aspects and context of mental health, specifically with regard to the elaboration of the human trend to belonging or homonomy. In setting my development of Rogers' (1959) cluster of concepts around congruence as the basis for health in a wider theoretical context, I also draw on Jahoda's (1958) concepts of mental health, to which I referred in the book, and which informed my thinking both about concepts of health and about conceptualisation.

There is, however, a more general and significant link and progression between and across these three works, which is an elaboration of a holistic approach to the person and to the study of the person.

Regarding methodology

With regard to my research into mental health promotion the method I adopted was an empirical–inductive approach. Scientific research is generally divided into discovery and testing. The reductive method of discovery, which has a long history dating back in European thought to the early seventeenth century, is based on the idea of dividing a large problem into several sub-problems that are solved separately by using methods including inductive generalisation. Whereas deductive logic moves from premises to conclusions, such that if the premises are true, then the conclusions must be true, inductive logic involves an inference where the conclusion follows from the premises, not with necessity but with probability. The empirical–inductive approach is a learning model of research whereby the researcher generalises from examples to concepts or models as I did using a paradigm analysis of the field of mental health and its promotion. It is also an approach which examines the theoretical assumptions underlying and the hypotheses of the scientific work under examination.

With regard to both the chapter on the neopsyche and the article/chapter on autonomy and homonomy, I adopted a hermeneutic methodology. Hermeneutics is the art or science of interpretation. In hermeneutic research the activity of research is primarily that of interpretation and the focus, therefore, is on the dialogue with a person or a text. My research into the Adult ego state and into the nature of ego states in general is an example of this in that my writing represents a dialogue with the texts I was rediscovering and reading on the subject. As I did this especially in the chapter on the neopsyche with regard to ego states, I became increasingly interested to clarify definitions of and distinctions between different words and different concepts.

In reading and interpreting texts and presenting an heuristic exegesis (see for example Tudor 2007a), I often find myself adopting a "back to the future" approach in terms of representing texts and focusing on the history of ideas and on what was written by original thinkers, as well as what was not written by them but is attributed to them. One example of this is my consistent representation of Rogers' (1957, 1959) six conditions of therapy and personality change as distinct from the core conditions of Truax and Carkhuff (1967), a concept which is commonly misattributed to Rogers (see Tudor 2000, 2011c). Gillon (2007) has acknowledged this about my work:

> Tudor argues that the way in which the person-centred theory of therapy is so often associated with the three core conditions has become a major problem

> for the approach and part of the reason why the strong psychological basis of the theory is often neglected.
>
> (p. 57)

As I reflect again on these methodologies I think that my use of them was an attempt to develop a certain knowledge, even a knowledge of certainty. Despite my caution against certainty (Tudor 2007d) and my cautiousness in seeking probability and in offering interpretation, there is a sense in which I have been trying to elicit the implicit in search of the explicit. In my original statement I used a quotation from Angyal (1941) as the epigram for the third part on research:

> No scientific work is possible without theoretical assumptions, even if the investigator is not always aware of them. Since hypotheses cannot be eliminated from scientific work, it is certainly more reasonable to admit their presence and consider them critically than to work with implicit unexamined hypotheses.
>
> (p. 9)

However, as Nuttall (2009) pointed out, this quotation contradicted my epistemological position, which, from an heuristic perspective, is more concerned with deriving knowledge, especially tacit knowing, from reflection.

...

At the *viva voce* examination (in July 2009) on my submission and in defence of my thesis, and particularly given that I take a heuristic approach, I was challenged to show more of myself, especially in the process of reflection on these public works. As a result of this challenge and the dialogue with my examiners in the *viva*, I have included in this statement more about heurism and heuristic methodology, and placed this earlier in the statement; an explanatory sub-title; and, throughout, my reflections on this process, including drawing on "data" from the process of the *viva* itself, and the examiners' summaries of the revisions required. These reflections are integrated throughout the statement. Some of the reflections appear[ed] in grey, that is, somewhere between black and white, thereby representing more of a process of discovery, including uncertainty and what Polanyi (1964, 1969, 1983) and Moustakas (1990) refer to as "tacit knowing". Including these refections feels both risky and right.... On the whole I am pleased to be representing my work and thinking in this way and think that this is now a truly creative synthesis (Moustakas, 1990). On the other hand, somewhere less than whole, I am nervous and a little scared. On further reflection, however, [I realise] this is no bad thing and, indeed, represents an aspect of my own journey in health and dis-ease or ill-health, acknowledging an emotional aspect and consequence of a particular journey and fight and more generally of the fight.

Less than a week after my *viva* my family and I emigrated to Aotearoa New Zealand, where I have taken up the post of senior lecturer in the Department of Psychotherapy at Auckland University of Technology (AUT). I – and my family – have been welcomed into the department and into the university by both Māori and non-Māori colleagues. In Māori culture there is a tradition that a person introduces him or herself by offering a mihi or speech of welcome, which includes more or less of her whakapapa or recitation of genealogy or genealogies. One of the meanings of whakapapa means to place in layers, one upon another; the recitation and the layers include spiritual, mythical and human stories that illustrate the person's ancestry, history, and connection – to the sea and the land, ancestors, tribe and subtribe. For a number of years I have been interested in the autobiographical aspect of theory and such questions as: what implicit theory we have as a result of our upbringing and values; why we are drawn to the theories we choose and espouse; and why we develop the theories we do. The elaboration of the autobiographical aspects of theory gave rise to a series of (to date, nine) books published between 1930 and 2007 entitled "A History of Psychology in Autobiography", edited variously by Carl Murchison, Edwin Boring, Gardner Lindzey, Alvin Langfield, Heinz Werner, Robert Yerkes and William Runyan. Thus, observing the Māori protocol of the whakapapa not only makes sense in terms of the bicultural nation that is Aotearoa New Zealand, it also resonates with some sense I have carried of wanting to express myself, personally, theoretically – and autobiographically. I think of this as akin to the self-dialogue and, indeed, dialogue with others, that is essential to heuristic inquiry. I represent this aspect of my experience in the form of a series of what, in acknowledgement of the concept of whakapapa, I refer to as as "layers" [which formed one of the appendices of the final statement].

...

Heuristic methodology: initial reflections

This ... is a prelude in that it comes before the sections which consider the public works presented; and is a postlude in that it is a reflection on research, by definition, written after the publication of these works. Presenting a PhD by public works is, in effect a "post match analysis" of a journey, in this case one covering a period of some 20 years.

In terms of method and methodology, with regard to my research into mental health promotion, the method I adopted at the time was an empirical-inductive approach; with regard to both the chapter on the neopsyche and the article/chapter on autonomy and homonomy, I used a hermeneutic method. However, in terms of my overall development as a researcher, these three public works represent a longitudinal programme of heuristic research. In addition to my reflections on the public works themselves, the further reflection involved in the process of writing this statement entails describing the experience of the discovery, and a further dissecting of or reflecting on the discovery – which is a further heuristic process (see Higgins, 1996).

In [these initial reflections], which set the scene for the rest of this statement, I describe and discuss heuristic research, including my own experiences of and reflections on this process....

The word heuristic, from the Greek *εὑρίσκειν*, means to find, to find out, to discover, to devise, to invent, to procure. Moustakas (1990) stated that: "It refers to a process of internal search through which one discovers the nature and meaning of experience" (p. 9). The focus of heuristic research is, thus, on the researcher, and on the reflexive experience of discovery (see Moustakas, 1961), and the activity of research is primarily that of introspection – which is why it is particularly applicable to psychotherapy (see O'Hara, 1986), to supervision (see Merry, 2004), and to this particular form of PhD by public works. This is not an easy process. As Moustakas (1990) put it:

> The heuristic research process is not one that can be hurried or timed by the clock or calendar. It demands the total presence, honesty, maturity, and integrity of the researcher who not only strongly desires to know and understand but is willing to commit endless hours of sustained immersion and focused concentration on one central question, to risk the opening of wounds and passionate concerns, and to undergo the personal transformation that exists as a possibility in every heuristic journey.
>
> (p. 14)

This chimes with what one of the examiners had written in his comments on the revisions required for my resubmission regarding the rejection of the original manuscript of my work on mental health promotion. He (Lees, 2009) noted that "the early trauma of the rejection of his work in the early 1990s and his subsequent tendency to polarize is not addressed in the text although became apparent as a key issue in the course of the oral examination." I realised, both during the *viva* and with the benefit of further indwelling, how much I had forgotten the hurt of this rejection [see introduction to Chapter 7] and had not dwelt on the connection between that and my subsequent fights with regard to this material. Interestingly, the process of rewriting this statement twice has, to some extent, paralleled this trauma and the fight. Indeed, in his second set of comments (Lees, 2010) speculated whether we [the examiners and I] were getting into a fight over the context statement...

Heurism and heuristic research is based on experience and on the reflection on that experience. In this sense it shares a common epistemology and methodology with person-centred psychology and, indeed, Moustakas (1990) acknowledged Rogers' contribution to his own knowledge and understanding of heuristic discovery. He also referred specifically to Gendlin's (1961) analysis of the meaning of experiencing and his later work (1971) on focusing; to Rogers' (1969) summary of the essential qualities of discovery, including an openness to one's experience; and to Jourard's (1971) investigations into self-disclosure. I find these connections not only interesting but important as I value "philosophical congruence" (Tudor & Worrall, 2006), that is, a fit between one's personal philosophy, the principles of any philosophy or theory that one espouses, and the methodology that follows from or embodies that theory.

Clearly heurism fits with humanism and humanistic psychology. Knight (1961) identified two corollaries of humanism:

1 That virtue is a matter of promoting human wellbeing; and
2 That the mainsprings of moral action are what Darwin called the *social* instincts, that is, those altruistic, co-operative tendencies that are as much a part of our biological equipment as our tendencies towards aggression and cruelty.

These corollaries represent my humanism and are specifically represented in my public works on mental health promotion, and on autonomy and homonomy.

Heuristics is also applied to a system of education in which the student is trained to find things out for her or himself and, is therefore, also consistent with person-centred approaches to education, training, and supervision which encourage a freedom to learn (see Rogers, 1969, 1983; Rogers & Freiberg, 1994), a subject about which I have written a number of papers and edited two books (see Embleton Tudor *et al.*, 2004; Tudor & Worrall, 2004, 2007; Tudor, 2007f).

In addition to the focus, qualities and transparency needed for heuristic discovery, drawing on Polanyi's (1964, 1969, 1983) work, Moustakas (1990) asserted that "Underlying all other concepts in heuristic research, at the base of all heuristic discovery, is the power of revelation in tacit knowing" (p. 20), that is, we know more than we can tell. Such knowing is based on elements of perception that enter into conscious awareness through such skills as focusing and fine observation skills, but also by means of speculative skills such as observing patterns and configurations (gestalt), as well as through intuition, images, and dreams. Moustakas (ibid.) commented that: "Such knowledge is possible through a tacit capacity that allows one to sense the unity or wholeness of something from an understanding of the individual qualities or parts." (pp. 20–21) ... This fits with my interest in the organism, organismic psychology and holism as represented in these present public works (see also Tudor & Worrall, 2006), and, indeed, an alternative title to this thesis could be "*Wholes and Parts*". Significantly, Craig (1978) suggested that the heuristic process moves from whole to part and back to whole again; as he put it: "From the individual to the general and back again ... from the feeling to the word and back to the feeling, from the experience to the concept and back to the experience." (p. 57). This process and tacit capacity is enhanced by what Moustakas (1990) referred to as "indwelling", which refers to: "the heuristic process of turning inward to seek a deeper, more extended comprehension of the nature or meaning of a quality or theme of human experience." (p. 24). He continued: "It involves a willingness to gaze with unwavering attention and concentration into some facet of human experience in order to understand its constituent qualities and its wholeness." (ibid.: 24).

In his book on the subject, Moustakas (1990) identified six phases of heuristic research, an analysis with which I frame my work and development as a researcher. I do this specifically with regard to the writing and examination of this context statement, although I also draw a number of parallels between this process and the process of the original research. ... As these are phases, as distinct from stages, they are not linear ... my own experience of these phases is summarised in Box 10.1 (pp. 156–157). As Moustakas (1990) himself put it, these six phases: "guide unfolding investigations and comprise the basic research design." (p. 27). Here I describe the phases with reference to my reflections, and [in the complete context statement] my autobiographical layers.

Initial engagement

Moustakas (1990) suggested that: "The task of the initial engagement is to discover an intense interest, a passionate concern that calls out to the researcher, one that holds important social meanings and personal, compelling implications." (p. 27). In a sense the "task" of my initial engagement with this study was to undertake and complete the context statement which presented my public works and, whilst I felt passionate about *each* work separately, it took some time for me to engage with the relationship *between* and *of* the three works. As Lees (2009) put it in his comments on my initial context statement: "There needs to be considerable strengthening of the links and progression between the three published works". Whilst I valued – and still value – the supervision I had, it took engagement with the examiners in and, through their comments, after the *viva*, to rediscover the central question: "What are the links and progression between *these* public works?". Moustakas (1990):

> The question lingers within the researcher and awaits the disciplined commitment that will reveal its underlying meanings. The engagement or encountering of a question that holds personal power is a process that requires inner receptiveness, a willingness to enter fully into the theme, and to discover from within the spectrum of life experiences that will clarify and expand knowledge of the topic and illuminate the terms of the question.
>
> (p. 27)

In effect I had three phases of engagement with this process: one at the beginning, and one more recently as I re-engaged with re-writing my second and third [versions of the] context statement.

My initial and subsequent engagement with this present process has some resonance and parallels with the early process of my research into mental health and its promotion. As the senior fellowship post was part-time (2½ days a week) and time-limited (for 1 year), there was a sense in which I "hit the ground running" and so, in the first couple of months of 1990, I also engaged quickly. Similarly, there was a given question and a question which emerged. In that case the central question of that piece of research was given by the remit of the fellowship (Caplan, 1989), that is: "to investigate conceptual issues and implementation of community mental health promotion". However, a further question which soon emerged from my engagement with the material was: "How could the conceptual issues and implementation of community mental health promotion be organised?". Reflecting on this question led me to seek a framework with which to organise and understand the material and, from there, I turned to paradigm analysis.

Following the rejection of the work [on mental health promotion] by the Health Education Authority, I temporarily lost interest in the work. After a while I returned to it, re-engaged with the material, and began to plan a book, some of which would be based on the original material, but which would involve me in doing more research on and developing the subject in my own time.

Since the completion of this initial research I have continued writing, the subject of which has often emerged from initial engagement with an issue or an idea which arises from my practice as a psychotherapist, trainer and supervisor, or from my interest in philosophy and ideas, and, often, in the empirical-inductive approach to enquiry.

Immersion

The second phase of heuristic research is one in which the researcher lives and breathes the question, and this certainly has been my experience, especially in the last stage of re-writing this statement. My experience of the *viva* and, specifically, Lees' (2009) use of the word "trauma" in his comments had a catalytic and crystallising effect on me. From the question "What are the links and progression between *these* public works?" emerged others: "Why is health a fight?", "Why do I (have to) fight?", and "In what ways do I tend to polarise?". These questions held both the "personal power" of the principal question, as well as some of the material with which to address it.

My immersion in this PhD has principally been in three periods: one when I was doing much of the initial writing of my context statement, and the second and third other as I was re-writing – and making more changes to – this statement (see Box 10.1, pp. 156–157).

Again, I experienced something similar also with regard to the investigation into mental health promotion, principally during 1990. Having the part-time fellowship meant that for half the week I could literally immerse myself in the research, reading and writing. At one point in the year, due to a computer crash, I lost some 5,000 words of what I had written. After an initial panic, I decided to stay up late that night and try to recall what I had written – and succeeded. On reflection, I think this demonstrates how much I was immersed in the work and, therefore, could recall from my short-term memory. Since then, when I have been working on other projects, I have often immersed myself in them – and have come to accept that I need to immerse myself, to the exclusion of other things and, at times, other people. When teaching others about writing, I have described this as being – and as having to be – "in the zone". I have found that certain practices help such immersion, for instance, when studying in the local university libraries – and, now, in my own university library: the time spent travelling, even the short walk across the campus, or to the main library in the city; the physical search for books and journals; and being in an atmosphere of concentrated study.

Incubation

This is the process and the phase in which, as Moustakas (1990) described it: "the researcher retreats from the intense, concentrated focus on the question ... [but] on another level expansion of knowledge is taking place ... The period of incubation enables the inner tacit dimension to reach its full possibilities". (p. 28). On reflection I think it is significant that I did not really experience or make time for this phase in the main period of the preparation of my context statement (2008–2009). Lees (2009) picked this up in his comments when he asked for "more clarity about ... the emergent tacit dimension". Having decided to undertake this form of PhD, in the context of applying for a visa to be able to live and work in Aotearoa – New Zealand, I was on a deadline, and needed to take my *viva* before I emigrated. At the time (2007–2008), whilst the process – reading, reflecting, writing and supervision – did not feel rushed, it was intense and relentless. It – I – was also somewhat frustrated as, in the context of a busy professional and personal life, I rarely felt that I could do it – myself – justice. There was no time to pause, which, of course, contradicts what Moustakas (1990) wrote about the heuristic process.

It was only after I submitted the statement and my public works in April 2009 that I had time to pause and, in this sense, the first incubation phase of this heuristic inquiry was between [that] April and the *viva* exam in July 2009. This was an extended period due to various difficulties in convening an exam board and, although a little unsettling in terms of my timeframe with emigration, it was a useful period. The second period of incubation was more intentional. When I and my family arrived in Aotearoa New Zealand, we were in temporary accommodation and, in fact, had three moves in 10 weeks, before finally moving into our home. Even then I could not access all my books. At that stage (October 2009) I asked Middlesex University for an extension of time in which to submit my revised context statement. Not having access to my books initially seemed like a very heavy cloud; the silver lining, however, has been that this has focused me more on my own experience and on reflecting on that experience, rather than looking to external authorities. Perhaps unsurprisingly, this period of incubation and "pause" has been incredibly useful, and has led to a rich period of illumination and explication.

Following the end of my original research fellowship, I have (from 1991 to 2009) been an independent researcher and academic and, as such, have been able to follow my own research interests, which have arisen from engagement with practice and theory and, often, from the writing I have just finished. As a writer I am well organised and keep notes of ideas in files (on my computer) which I constantly update. In this way I allow my intuition – a subject which, interestingly, was the focus of Berne's (1949/1977) early research – as well as my more conscious interests to emerge. Sometimes I make notes on a particular subject over a number of years, one example of which is my work on empathic transactions [see Tudor, 2011a, 2011f] which has come to fruition over a period of some 5 years. In this sense I always have several projects incubating at the same time, and find that each is the richer for it.

Illumination

Moustakas (1990) described this process as "one that occurs naturally when the researcher is open and receptive to tacit knowledge and intuition." (p. 29). As such, it is "a breakthrough into conscious awareness of qualities and a clustering of qualities into themes inherent in the question." (ibid.: 29). Although I had and gained a number of insights during the process of writing my initial context statement, the main breakthrough came, as I have suggested, in the *viva* exam itself, and afterwards, when I received the examiners' comments and requirements, and following further indwelling through incubation, re-engagement, immersion, and explication (see Box 10.1, pp. 156–157). Even then, I do not think I "got it" until I was in the last stage of revisions. I had several moments of revelation – usually in the shower! "Of course", I thought, "It's all about wholes *and* parts". In other words, all three public works are concerned with a holistic approach to the person and to life, and to understanding and integrating "parts" into the particular whole.

A number of writers have described such a breakthrough or turning point as a metanoia or change which represents both the moment of change as well as a continuing process of change. West (1990) described the moment of change and the spiritual quality of metanoia as "repentance, a change of heart, a new direction" (p. 51), whilst Esterson (1970) emphasised the process or dialectical praxis of therapeutic interaction and describes this metanoia as "dialectical rationality, an enterprise of continual and continuing reappraisal and renewal" (p. 240). In my experience as a researcher both aspects of metanoia are important; for further discussion of the concept of metanoia, see Tudor (2001) – and I am grateful to have trained in psychotherapy at the Metanoia Institute in Ealing, west London, UK.

Again, there are parallels with a number of similar moments I experienced in the course of the research on the public works presented:

1 With regard to the research on mental health promotion, that I could – and, indeed, should – describe mental health *qua* health without necessarily referring to mental illness; and that I did not have to come up with *a* definition of mental health.
2 With regard to the chapter on the *neopsyche*, that it was important to describe the neopsyche/Adult ego state as providing an *integrating* function as distinct from being an integrated state.

3 With regard to the paper/article/chapter on autonomy and homonomy, that both are criterial to mental health and the good life.

Explication

The meaning of the noun "explication", from the verb "to explicate", has several elements: (i) unfolding, expanding, and displaying; (ii) disentangling; (iii) bringing out what is implicit; and (iv) explaining. In my experience, this phase of explication is represented in the writing up of research, which, at best, fulfils all four of the above elements. As well as explicating through writing and, importantly, editing my own writing, and getting feedback on it, I also do this through training and teaching – and I have presented and taught courses and workshops on the basis of all three public works. I have experienced that there is nothing like teaching a subject to realise and to learn what I know and, importantly, what I do not know. Moustakas (1990) described the purpose of this phase as one in which "to fully examine what has awakened in consciousness, in order to understand its various layers of meaning." (p. 31). In this context statement, this phase is reflected particularly in the three chapters on heuristic methodology.

In the *viva*, I appreciated being asked to defend my thesis; in other words, to be given the opportunity to explicate, which, for the most part, I did. As Lees (2009) acknowledged: "We had a most interesting and stimulating discussion with the candidate ... [who] was able to engage in a fruitful dialogue". However, as with the example of teaching, there is nothing like a good, rigorous exam to highlight gaps in my thesis, argument, and explication. As Lees (2009) commented: "the viva had a sense of providing debate and input that had not been previously provided". This revised statement reflects my learning from that experience and further self-dialogue, focusing and indwelling. The parallel process to this with regard to other presentations is when I send a completed draft of something I am writing to a friend or colleague. Their comments and critique often draw and require further explication for clarity.

Creative synthesis

This narrative context statement is the creative synthesis of all that I have described – and much more. It represents the weaving together of the single threads of the three public works cited, in a way which acknowledges the link and progression between them and, which, in itself, creates a unified, single thread....

In response to the illumination offered in and by the examination process, this synthesis has involved the deconstruction of the original statement in favour of one which is more heuristic, more reflective, more layered and more creative. This has involved an important period of incubation, as well as re-engagement and further immersion, as well as an intensive period of explication through writing. Moustakas (1990) observed that, in this phase:

> The researcher must move beyond any confined or constricted attention to the data itself and permit an inward life on the question to grow, in such a way that a comprehensive expression of the essences of the phenomenon investigated is realized.
>
> (p. 32)

One of the learning points for me as a researcher and, specifically, an heuristic researcher, has been precisely to move beyond such attention and to be as open to learning in this way as I am in my work as a psychotherapist and educator. In this sense I draw on the phenomenological method in my work as a researcher.

In my experience, this phase often involves and requires a period of immersion in writing and in the actual production of the piece of work, whether book, chapter, article, or statement. When I complete a piece of work, I tend to need to come away from it for a while, and to let it – and myself – settle before returning to it for final editing. At this point I print out the document, read it out aloud, and edit it by hand. In doing this, I often find that, in addition to the usual process of editing involving corrections and changing word order within sentences, I also move or delete passages and even whole sections, some of which may later form the basis for the next piece of research and writing. This process is one of synthesising, and is one which strengthens my argument and thesis, not least in this present work [i.e. the context statement – and also in *this* present work, i.e. this book].

As I have indicated, my heuristic process has not been linear. I have represented the phases of my process with regard to this work and the writing of the statement in Box 10.1, to which I have added a pre-contemplation phase (Prochaska & DiClemente, 1992) as I have been contemplating undertaking a PhD for some time.

Box 10.1. Timeline of the process of heuristic research with regard to PhD by public works

Writing the public works
and
pre-contemplation
(1991–2007)
↓
Initial engagement
in the project of undertaking a PhD by public works
(February 2007–March 2008)
↓
Creative synthesis
with regard to the structure of the context statement
(October 2007–March 2008)
↓
Immersion
in the task of writing my initial context statement
(April 2008–March 2009)
↓
Incubation
whilst waiting for the date of the *viva* exam
(March–June 2009)
↓
Illumination
in the *viva* examination
(7 July 2009)
↓

Incubation
following the examination and emigration/immigration
(July–October 2009)
↓
Re-engagement, immersion, explication, and further creative synthesis
in rewriting and completing the second context statement
(October–November 2009)
↓
Further incubation
Whilst waiting for the result of the revised submission
(November 2009–January 2010)
↓
Crisis, incubation, and immersion
In response to the examiners's second reports
(January–March 2010)
↓
Re-engagement, immersion, illumination, explication and further creative synthesis
in making a fresh start and writing two new sections and completing the third version of the context statement
(March–April 2010)
...

An ongoing heuristic response to the examination process

Heuristic enquiry is a process that begins with a question or problem which the researcher seeks to illuminate or answer. The question is one that has been a personal challenge and puzzlement in the search to understand one's self and the world in which one lives. The heuristic process is autobiographic, yet with virtually every question that matters personally there is also a social – and perhaps universal – significance (Moustakas, 1990).

This [chapter in the PhD] forms the third and final reflection on the heuristic methodology used in this research and context statement and, as a key aspect of that process, reflects an ongoing heuristic response to the examination process and, specifically, to the external examiners' reports (Lees, 2010; Nuttall, 2010) on my second context statement (submitted November 2009).

In heuristic methodology Moustakas (1990) wrote that: "one seeks to obtain qualitative depictions that are at the heart and depths of a person's experience." (p. 38). He went on to cite depictions of situations, events, conversations, relationships, feelings, thoughts, values and beliefs, as well as passages from documents and correspondence as examples of experience essential to the heuristic quest. Thus, heuristic research is based on experience and on reflection on that experience. In this it shares a common epistemology and methodology with person-centred psychology and, indeed, Moustakas (1990) acknowledged Rogers' contribution to his own knowledge and understanding of heuristic discovery and cited Rogers (1969b) own heuristic process. Etherington (2004) went further and stated that heuristic process developed out of humanistic psychology. Heurism and heuristic method then fits or is congruent with my philosophy of life and practice as a humanistic psychotherapist. According to Moustakas (1990) in a heuristic quest "the focus is on recreation of the lived experience and full and complete depictions of the experience from the frame of reference of the experiencing person" (p. 39), in this case me. All enquiry and all heuristic enquiry begins with a question. In the case of presenting work which has already been published the question shifts somewhat and in my experience has been at times somewhat elusive, a process which I now understand as to do with a certain compartmentalising of the three works presented (see following section). As a result of some "concentrated gazing" (Moustakas, 1990) and focusing, especially through the examination process, I have clarified the question as "What is the cohesive originality of my work?". Clarifying this question this has helped me to shift my focus, albeit belatedly, on the whole rather than the parts.

... [Finally], as a further and final reflection or turning back on my heuristic experience and process in writing and presenting my public works, this chapter comprises my ongoing response to the examination process framed in terms of [the seven] key concepts and processes of heuristic research (Moustakas, 1990).

Identifying with the focus of enquiry – parts and wholes, and homonomy

With regard to my revised submission, Lees (2010) asked the question: "Why does the narrative still seem to be about parts rather than wholes?". When I read this question, I, too, was puzzled. "Why was I (still) compartmentalising?", I asked myself. What was I missing? What part was missing? What whole was missing? In many ways I feel whole and holistic. I have, as Grof (1993) expressed it in the title of one of her books, "*A thirst for wholeness*", and yet I was having trouble expressing myself holistically. In the revised submission this was manifested in a number of ways with regard to the title and a structure that included an interlude which had done a disservice to my argument about the links between and the levels of the public works (see Nuttall, 2010).

Reflecting on my writing through this lens, I think that much of my writing represents a tension between wholes and parts: attempting to describe the whole and yet and perhaps inevitably focusing on parts, for example, my work on mental health. Whilst much of my work is an attempt to reclaim a positive association of "health" from the term "mental health" (which generally is more associated with mental illness) [see Chapter 10], I realise that, to a certain extent, arguing for positive mental health has become a fight over a term and a territory which has led to polarisation rather than to differentiation and integration. Moreover, even using the adjective "mental" to describe an aspect of health, carries the danger of compartmentalising a more holistic vision of health, as one which encompasses the mental/affective/behavioural/cognitive/somatic/spiritual and more. This perspective resonates with indigenous experiences and views of health, see, for instance, Durie (1998), and I am increasingly coming round to using the term "wellbeing" instead of mental health. Similarly, my work on ego states and specifically the neopsychic integrating Adult is an attempt to clarify a healthy aspect of the personality distinct from Introjected Parent and Archaic Child ego states, which thus makes a more integrated or integrating whole – and, interestingly, at least one colleague has suggested that the integrating Adult might encompass the Parent and Child ego state material. Similarly, my work on homonomy represents an attempt to challenge a one dimensional and predominantly western view of self-determination at the expense of a determination which includes others. In this sense my work represents and reflects a progression from polarisation to integration or at least to a "both..., and..." approach.

When I first wrote the previous sentence I noticed that I had used the singular word "work"; as I reflected on why I had noticed this, I realised that it was the first time that I had considered the significance of the plural term "public works". The three pieces of writing for which I have written this context statement are three *works* (plural), yet my task and statement concerns them as *a* body of *work* (singular) and in this sense they are – or it is – more of a whole than separate parts. This is also reflected in the changing title of the context statement from "The Fight for Health" (original submission, March 2009) to "The Fight for Health: A Heuristic Enquiry into Mental Health, Neopsychic Functioning, and Homonomy (revised submission, November 2009) to the present title: "The Fight for Health: A Heuristic Enquiry into Psychological WellBeing" [final submission, April 2010], a subtitle which is both more unified and more unifying (see Nuttall, 2010).

As Moustakas (1990) observed, heuristic process is autobiographical and social. The changes in the title represent my developing process with regard to my identification with the focus of this enquiry, which has shifted from the three separate works to this body of work as a whole, a focus and an identification which represents a coherent line of research and enquiry about health and holism. As below so above: my struggle with parts and wholes reflects a broader struggle about wholes and holism. As Smuts (1926/1987) put it:

> What is not generally recognised is that the conception of wholes covers a much wider field than that of life that its beginnings are traceable already in the inorganic order of Nature and that beyond the ordinary domain of biology it applies in a sense to human associations like the State and to the creations of the human spirit in all its greatest and most significant activities.
>
> (p. 98)

As I have struggled with identifying the focus on the whole work so, too, I have struggled with homonomy. In both his sets of comments (Nuttall, 2009, 2010) picked up on the disproportionate coverage in Chapter 2 [of the original context statements] of the three respective public works whereby I devote less text to the article/chapter on homonomy. In part, this was due to the fact that, as the most recent of the three public works (which were published in 1996, 2003 and 2008, respectively), it may be less mature, developed or integrated in my thinking and presentation. It is also the shortest. In the [first] revised context statement, whilst I integrated some references to the work of Horney, Lewin, and Fromm, the discussion of homonomy was still less and less integrated. It is, ironically, as if the concept of belonging itself did not belong here as much as the other concepts discussed and integrated; and, especially following Nuttall's (2010) second comment about this, I am curious about this, again in terms of both autobiographical and social processes.

On a personal level, whilst I have a strong sense of my family, of the philosophical and cultural roots of my identity, and of the collective and of community, I also have a sense of not belonging, of being on the edge of things, of opposing and, at times, of being oppositional. To a certain extent this explains the tangle, fight and polarisation to which Lees (2010) referred. As I turn this back on itself once again, I realise that I had not accounted for the fact that I have been writing this context statement in the context of having made a decision in February 2007 to emigrate: to pull up my roots, and to relocate to the other side of the world. Not surprisingly, I am experiencing the tension between belonging, being welcomed, making friends, etc., and not belonging, not knowing, and not being known. On reflection I think that, just as I have felt somewhat dislocated and disintegrated, I did not sufficiently locate or develop the material on homonomy. Whilst I was – and am – engaged with the material at a philosophical and intellectual level, there is a sense in which I was not fully engaged with the focus of this aspect of the enquiry. In terms of this as a representation of a wider social process, it is clear that western – and northern – psychology gives greater value to autonomy than it does to homonomy. In a recent search on Google Scholar (April 2010), the entry "autonomy" produced 1,180,000 hits, whilst one on "homonomy" produced only 661 hits, a mere 0.06 percent of the total number of hits on these two related subjects.

Self-dialogue – reflexivity, and relationship with theories

According to Etherington (2004) reflexivity is "the capacity of the researcher to acknowledge how their experiences and contexts (which might be fluid and changing) inform the process and outcomes of inquiry." (pp. 31–32). In the context of this research and this context statement, reflexivity is the primary methodological vehicle for the enquiry – and yet, whilst I have been reflective and have referred to self-dialogue in previous chapters of this PhD, I have not specifically referred to reflexivity.

In my book on mental health promotion, and drawing on a number of authors such as Buss (1979), Ray Holland (1981, 1987), Harré (1983), and Schon (1983), I discussed and employed reflexivity as critical reflection. As McNulty (1997) acknowledged in his review of the book, "In employing the methodology of critical reflexivity, [the author] provides a worked example of an approach to professional and personal development for people in this field". (p. 119). I had quoted Ray Holland (1981), who linked reflexivity and sociopsychology:

> Discriminating between various transformations and kinds of emphasis is part of the effort to become aware of what we are making of the theory – to become reflexively aware of our activity by means of sociopsychological analysis. And since it is a theoretically guided empirical investigation of theory construction – a theory about theories – it is well described as metatheory.
>
> (p. 25)

Then I had framed reflexivity then as more of an intellectual, abstract and abstracting activity – which had served me well in developing a paradigm analysis of the field of community mental health (Tudor, 1996b), but it had also taken me away from myself and my reflections on what I was making of the theory and theories. Schon (1983) observed that: "practitioners themselves often reveal a capacity for reflection on their intuitive knowing in the midst of action and sometimes use this capacity to cope with the unique, uncertain, and conflicted situations of practice." (pp. viii–ix). In the process leading up to the *viva*, I had not sufficiently exercised this capacity with regard to my intuitive knowing (see section below for the consistent discipline involved in reflecting or turning back on reflections).

As a result of the examination process I have more of a personal sense of reflexivity and that this relies on a constant turning back like turning over a leaf and another and another and on self-dialogue and self-disclosure. In some ways I am or have been reluctant to make myself manifest, as Jourard (1971) put it: "showing yourself so that others can perceive you" (p. 17). Also, writing about self-disclosure in the context of reflexivity, Douglass and Moustakas (1985) stated that: "At the heart of heuristics lies an emphasis on disclosing the self as a way of facilitating disclosure from others – a response to the tacit dimension within oneself sparks a similar call from others" (p. 50).

My adoption and valuing of reflexivity – or reflexivities, as Etherington (2004) acknowledged, has a number of roots:

- Philosophical critique – influenced by my non-conformist family background, and my own study of philosophy and theology.
- Social critique – also influenced by my family background, as well as training and working as a social worker, and being drawn to radical and critical thinking about social work and society.
- The concept of "prefigurative politics" – from my involvement in the political group *Big Flame* (see http://bigflameuk.wordpress.com/), and 10 years of collective living.
- Being a reflective practitioner – as a result of my experience of being a client, training and working as a psychotherapist, and continuing training, personal therapy, supervision, and professional and personal development.

Tacit knowing

In his comments on my original submission and the *viva* examination and specifically with regard to my account of heuristic methodology, Lees (2009) had referred to the need for more on the "emergent tacit dimension". In my revised statement I had attempted to address this by the inclusion of a number of text boxes, which included both reflections on the process as well as layers of biography and personal story. However, these appeared more as recollections than illuminations and, in his second set of comments, Lees (2010) challenged me: "What about really being bold, letting go of the limitations of the intellect and rational linear thinking?". In his comments he included a reference to the "Johari window", a cognitive psychological tool created by Joseph (Jo) Luft and Harry (Hari) Ingham (whence Johari) in 1955, in order to help people develop awareness of themselves, their interpersonal communication, and consequent relationships (see Figure 10.2). I had taught this model on a number of counselling courses in the early and mid-1990s but had not used it much since, and had not remembered it as a heuristic exercise.

Reflecting on my experience with regard to this present work and using this model as a way of mapping this experience, I think that the *viva* examination and both sets of comments from the external examiners have been encouraging me to explore the unknown (see Figure 10.3). This echoes a point Etherington (2004) made: "By using reflexivity in research we close the illusory gap between researcher and researched and between the knower and what is known." (p. 32). It is this second gap which I have been closing in this heuristic process. In Figure 10.3 the vertical arrow represents the effect of feedback, and the horizontal arrow represents the effect of self-disclosure and greater reflexivity.

As Polanyi (1983) put it, we should start from the fact that "we can know more than we can tell" (p. 4). He termed this pre-logical phase of knowing as "tacit knowledge". Of course, it is difficult to know what is unknown and so we

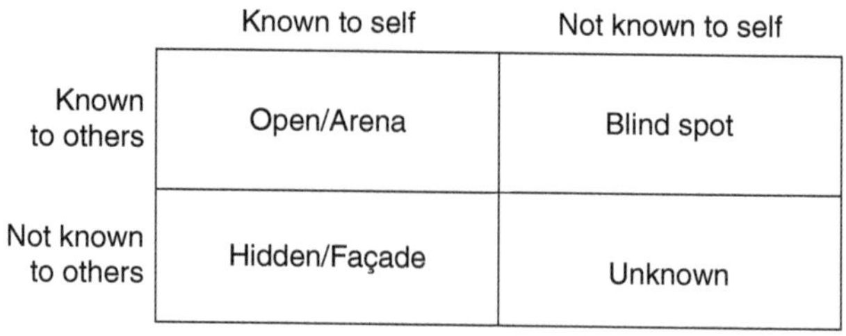

Figure 10.2 The Johari window (Luft & Ingham, 1955)

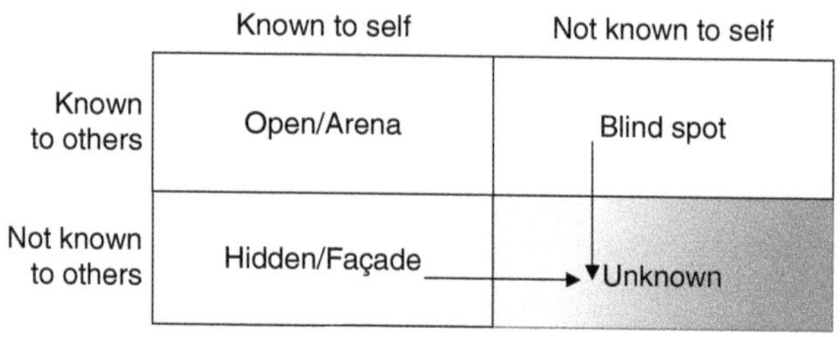

Figure 10.3 The Johari window (Luft & Ingham, 1955) showing the movement and impact of feedback and self-disclosure

have to access it in creative, even bold ways. I realised that during the more recent period of writing my second context statement and further revision, I had also been doing other writing. I decided to examine these for what they might "tell" (see Figure 10.4), in which the arrows represents what becomes known to self and/or others.

With regard to making the tacit more explicit, I am especially interested in the poems I wrote during this period. The poem "When I saw her, I said hello" was a poem I had written in response to Bob Dylan's (1974) song "When you see her, say hello", which completes an implicit dialogue about a lost love. "Calvados" was a poem I had written during a visit to the beaches and war graves in Normandy. During the Second World War my father had been a conscientious objector, one consequence of which was that I had had an ambivalent relationship to commemorations of war, and had somewhat polarised war and peace. As an adult, as a result of my experience on a men's workshop with Robert Bly and Michael Meade [in the 1980s], I had decided that I wanted to visit the beaches and cemeteries, a project enhanced by meeting and getting to know my father-in-law who had fought in the war. In 2008 I had fulfilled this when I went with a friend to Normandy where I wrote this poem, and started another, "Leslie and Albert", about my father and father-in-law. Last year, just I was saying goodbye to my father-in-law for what I knew to be the last time, and leaving the UK, I returned to and revised the poem.

As I was in the last stages of writing this statement I wrote the following poem:

The mint

I remember the fresh white taste of the mint
And its smooth hardness,
Feeling its shine, and
Tracing its name with my language.

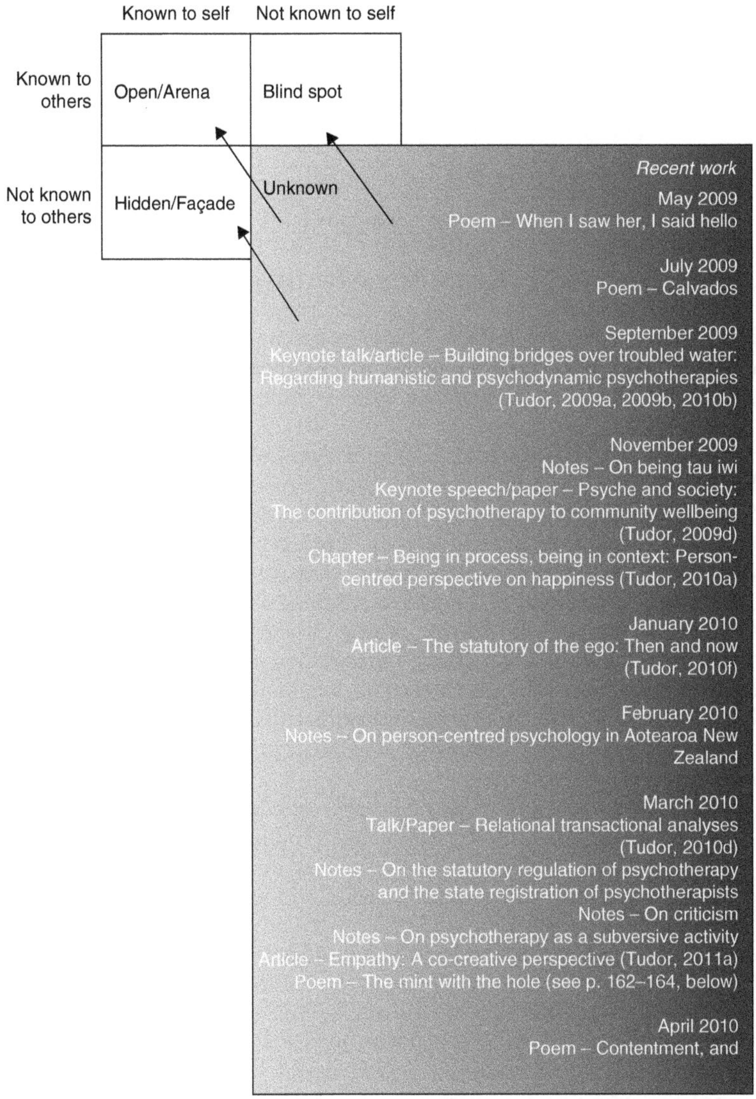

Figure 10.4 The Johari window (Luft & Ingham, 1955) applied to my [then] recent writing

I remember the hole in the middle, of course,
And, pushing the tip of my tongue into the hole,
Marvelling that it didn't break.

I remember cradling the round gently in my mouth,
Willing it to last, and to last longer.
Sometimes it broke,
Then I snapped and crunched it, useless.
But, on other days I nurtured it to champion thinness,
And sometimes showed it proudly.
'Though invariably it did not survive this exposure.

Now I remember the whole:
The whole mint round
And its outside edge,
And running it with the groove of my tongue
Like a drunken penny rolling down a hill

And which, like a coin,
Holds obverse and reverse two faces
By means of a third side.
Tamaki Makaurau | Auckland, March–April 2010

The theme that emerges from these poems and from some of my other writing in this period is one of difference and dialogue, and balance and wholeness, a theme which is also reflected in my recent academic writing:

- The keynote talk and article, "Building Bridges Over Troubled Water: Regarding Humanistic and Psychodynamic Psychotherapies" (which I delivered both in the UK [Tudor, 2009a] and in Aotearoa New Zealand [Tudor, 2009b]) is a personal reflection on the similarities between these different traditions and, given that I am the programme leader of a psychodynamic training course, something of a personal dialogue and manifesto for bridge-building.
- My notes on the subject of being tau iwi, literally, the "other" tribe, i.e. non-Māori, form the basis of an article I am writing about my identity as an immigrant specifically in relation to tangata whenua, the first people of Aotearoa New Zealand, and thus it represents another dialogue which involves historical, social, philosophical and psychological arguments in favour of embracing biculturalism in this country.
- The keynote speech and paper, "Psyche and Society: The Contribution of Psychotherapy to Community Wellbeing" (Tudor, 2009d) was concerned with shifting the conceptualisation of therapy as an individual and individualistic enterprise to one which is more social and which encompasses a sense of community.
- The article "The State of the Ego: Then and Now" (Tudor, 2010f) is a clarification of the two different sets of ego state models – and, whilst it takes issue with some TA authors, interestingly and significantly, the current draft reflects a more reflective, dialogic and inclusive stance and tone.
- The talk and paper on relational transactional analyses (plural) represents an attempt to outline two principal contributions, represented by Summers and Tudor (2000) and Tudor (2003), and by Hargaden and Sills (2002), to the development of a relational tradition in TA, and, again, their similarities as well as their differences (Tudor, 2010d).

Intuition

Intuition, for Moustakas (1990), is "a kind of bridge ... between the implicit knowledge inherent in the tacit and the explicit knowledge which is observable and describable. [It] is the realm of the between, or the intuitive". (p. 23). When Lees (2010) challenged me to be bold and to let go of "the limitations of the intellect and rational linear thinking", I took this as a challenge to rely more on the intuitive and the not-so-rational, and even the irrational. Just as I was finishing this chapter, a second verse to a poem I had written some 5 years earlier came to me, again in the shower, where I seem to have had most of my recent illuminative moments!

Contentment, and

Said slowly
Contentment
Harbours its promise.

In turn, the harbour contains
Its own promise of ebb, flow, and storm:
Of rocking boats, and upsetting contents.

Sheffield, June 2005; Tamaki Makaurau |
Auckland, April 2010

To me, this speaks of necessary balance: content(ment) with discontent and, more broadly, of health and illness, of parts and wholes, of single-mindedness and group-mindedness. As Moustakas (1990) reflected: "Intuition makes possible the perceiving of things as wholes". (p. 23).

Indwelling – verification, and interpretation

I discuss indwelling in Chapter 1 [of the PhD]. Here I address this process of turning inward with regard to the issues of verification and interpretations.

In order to establish the trustworthiness of qualitative research, and specifically with regard to verification, Lincoln and Guba (1985) used terms such as: credibility, transferability, dependability, and confirmability; and, in order to operationalise these, they propose assessments and techniques such as prolonged engagement, persistent observation, and the triangulation of data of sources, methods and investigators. Applying this to my own enquiry, I would claim that my work on positive mental health over some 20 years demonstrates both a prolonged engagement, as well as a certain persistence in my observation of and engagement with and in the field. The "triangulation" of data included in all three works and this work as a whole has involved a huge amount of sources from literature, legislation and social policy, which has been subjected to paradigm analysis, and, more recently, heuristic methodology, under supervision. Regarding credibility, Lincoln and Guba (1985) proposed the use of general concepts such as trustworthiness and authenticity to establish credibility, concepts which form a background to the demands of heuristic research and, in particular, reflexivity (see pp. 160–161 above). Eisner (1991) also discussed the credibility of qualitative research in terms of seeking "a confluence of evidence that breeds credibility, that allows us to feel confident about our observations, interpretations, and conclusions" (p. 110) and, interestingly in the light of my interest in holism, the formulation of a "compelling whole" (ibid.: 110). Eisner proposed three standards by which qualitative research should be verified: structural corroboration, consensual validation, and referential adequacy.

Structural corroboration involves the use of different types of data to support or contradict the interpretation. With regard to this submission, the data which is different from the original data of literature is that generated by my own reflections and processing, stimulated initially by my supervisor and then in and since the *viva* exam by the external examiners. I have felt both stimulated and challenged in this process to be and bring more of myself and to be bold, and hence my drawing on other types of data such as poetry.

Consensual validation refers to the researcher seeking the opinion of others, in this case my various academic (and clinical) supervisors from Ray Holland in 1990 onwards; the peer reviewers of the journals to which I have submitted articles; the editors of the journals and the book to which I contributed these works; the external examiners; and, most recently, my colleague [Liz Smythe] at AUT. Writing about reflective practice, Bolton (2001) argued that an examination of our personal practice: "needs to be undertaken alongside open discussions with peers on the issues raised, an examination of texts from the larger field of work and politics, and discussions with colleagues from outside the practitioners' own milieu." (p. 29). She also viewed this way of reflecting as "becoming politically, socially, as well as psychologically useful." (p. 29).

Referential adequacy refers to the importance of criticism which illuminates the subject matter, this statement and the process of rewriting is a case in point. Despite my initial resistance to some of the criticism and comments from the external examiners, I have felt illuminated and educated – in the sense of being "drawn out". I have felt encouraged and even pushed or pulled to explore and examine the tacit dimension (see Figures 10.3 and 10.4). This process began in the *viva* when the examiners questioned the methodology of the original statement (see Lees, 2009; Nuttall, 2009); continued in my subsequent reflections on the *viva* and my initial context statement; and was furthered in my continued dialogue with the examiners, by means of their comments (Lees, 2009, 2010; Nuttall, 2009, 2010), and in my rewriting of this context statement. Both examiners offered alternative interpretations: the significance of the "trauma" of the rejection of my work on mental health by the HEA; my tendency to polarise and "fight"; and the incommensurable positions of ontology and methodology taken in the first statement. These interpretations and criticisms not only gave me pause for thought and reflection, but generated further reflections about my process and positionality with regard to health and holism.

Creswell (2007) viewed dependability as equivalent to the "reliability" demanded by quantitative research; the qualitative researcher, however, as Creswell put it, "seeks dependability that the results will be subject to change and instability". (p. 198). This certainly fits with my experience of the process which, I think, overall, has made this whole statement more authentic, trustworthy, and reliable.

Focusing – fight, and focus

Moustakas (1990) acknowledged the influence of Gendlin (1978) on the heuristic process of focusing which involves:

1. clearing an inner space in order to tap into thoughts and feelings;
2. getting a handle on the question;
3. elucidating its constituents;
4. making contact with core themes; and
5. explicating the themes.

One of the difficulties I have had in the process of researching and writing this statement is a lack of inner space, and perhaps a lack of clearance. As a result I have had some difficulty in getting a handle on the question of what the link was between the works and in the work. One of Lees' (2009) comments on the original submission was that the context statement was merely a draft still in the process of making and, although I did not appreciate it at the time, I think he was right. In many ways the processing of writing the resubmission and doing further work on this version has been the process of clearing space, including the text and getting a handle on the question of the enquiry. The continuing dialogue has enabled me to elucidate the constituents specifically regarding the methodology and to explicate the emergent of holism.

Another process and theme that has emerged in the ongoing examination process is that of the fight. I have explored this to a certain extent in terms of polarities, and polarised and polarising positions. However, as ever, there is another layer! My intellectual journey from Unitarianism and non-conformism, through libertarian socialism, to humanistic psychology (gestalt therapy, transactional analysis, and the person-centred approach) appears coherent, consistent and, in terms of values, method, and practice, congruent. Reflecting further on this, what I realised is that they have in common a sense of opposition to the dominant ideology: Unitarianism to Trinitarianism, socialism to capitalism, libertarian socialism to the traditional extra-parliamentary Leninist and Trotskyist Left, and humanistic psychology to behaviourism and psychoanalysis. Due to this heritage I am comfortable with taking and holding a position because I think it is the right one, 'though at times I have been less aware of the impact that taking a position has on the other. Sometimes I have promoted a view – on mental health, on the integrating Adult, or homonomy – in order to reclaim a position or territory without necessarily appreciating the impact of that claim or reclamation on the other. This can be experienced as polarising, which, ironically, has the opposite effect to the one I want – which is dialogue. Moreover, as I am constituted in the social context which I seek to transform, I am inscribed with that against which I struggle (see Lather, 1993), that is, my ill-health or dis-ease, my introjects and fixated archaic experiences, and my independence and self-sufficiency autonomy.

In many ways the ongoing heuristic process and journey represented in this statement is one from a polarised conception and epistemology to one which embraces more than polarities (see Tudor, 2007c). In order to maintain this, my challenge is to focus or make time and space for focusing.

Internal frame of reference – a continuing inquiry

As Moustakas (1990) put it: "Heuristic processes relate back to the internal frame of reference." (p. 26). Rogers wrote about this frame of reference in the context of empathic understanding: when we experience empathic understanding of our own view of the world or internal frame of reference, it is then that we can grow and change.

In heuristic research when the researcher is both object (my public work) and subject (me and I) of the enquiry, then we (I, me, supervisors and examiners) need to pay attention to tacit knowing, intuitions, images and felt sense – and this has been, and is still an emerging process. As Stern (1985) put it, when describing the emergent sense of self: "It is a sense of organization in the process of formation

... it is coming into being." (p. 38). I think that in some ways I have only recently come to appreciate another layer to the coherence of this continuing enquiry which is that of holism, alongside health or psychological wellbeing. Particular moments of emergence have included:

- In Autumn 2008, when preparing for supervision, I decided to change my third public work from a chapter on verbal being and present-centred language (Tudor, 2008h) to the present article/chapter on autonomy and homonomy.
- In [northen hemisphere] winter 2008/2009, when writing the section on links, I saw the progression and development of ideas *between* the works, including, perhaps most significantly, between the first and third works, concerning health psychology and sociopsychology.
- On 7 July 2009, in the *viva* examination, when I was asked to outline and defend my thesis, and, specifically, to describe the links between the works.
- On 4 March 2010, when I remembered that I sometimes feel only a part of a whole – I have a sense of losing a twin when myself *in utero* – and that I had omitted this from the autobiographical layers of my second context statement.
- In March 2010, when writing the poem "The mint with the whole", I realised the significance of the personal connection with my enquiry into health and holism.
- In March 2010, when writing an earlier draft of this section, I realised that I was describing a unifying enquiry or work (singular), as distinct from three separate works.
- On 8 April, when a second verse of the poem "Contentment" (see p. 165) came to me, and I realised (again) that in my desire for health and contentment, I can lose the importance of discontent or dis-ease – and the sense of balance that a "both ... and" perspective brings.

Moustakas (1990) suggested that: "One completes the quest when one has had an opportunity to tell one's story to a point of natural closing". (p. 39). As I reflect on my writing, on the dialogue with myself and others, and as I write and edit, I experience my responses and self-analysis as an ongoing process of turning back layer after layer. It is therefore an ongoing enquiry. The reflexivity of heuristic research, the constant turning back, the uncovering and discovering, opens up space for layered and multiple meanings – and for further reflection and exploration. In my end is my beginning ... It is, therefore, an incomplete enquiry. At the same time, as is the case with most writing which is public or published, I am writing to a final deadline, so this ending is both a closure and a continuation.

CHAPTER 11

THERE AIN'T NO LICENCE THAT PROTECTS

Bowen theory and the regulation of psychotherapy (2011)

Retrospective introduction

The article reproduced in this chapter is a discussant paper, that is, a paper/article which discusses another one. The editors of the *Transactional Analysis Journal* (*TAJ*) were planning a special issue of the journal on "Dialogues in Ethics" and invited me to contribute an article which was to discuss an article on the licensing of psychotherapists by Smith (2011), which had been accepted for the issue (Cornell & Eusden, 2011). The broader background to this, which was known to the editors of the *TAJ*, was my interest in and research into professional regulation over (then) some 15 years, and my critique of increasing moves towards the statutory regulation of psychotherapy and the state registration of psychotherapists. I had first presented on this in 1999, and earlier in 2011 had published an edited book on the subject (Tudor, 2011e).

I was delighted to be invited and enjoyed the discipline of writing a discussant paper, especially as it involved me in some background reading on Bowen family systems therapy, with which I had not been familiar before reading Smith's paper. I have chosen to include this article in this selection: (a) because of the subject matter; (b) as it demonstrates the continuity of my critical thinking; (c) for its form, which demonstrates my ability to take on a task with a specific brief and to undertake the necessary background research in a timely fashion; and (d) as it shows the development of my style of writing in the specific context of an invited paper. Given the brief and the word limit, there's not a lot I would change, 'though I would be interested to read more about Bowen and family systems theory and to apply his – and its – theoretical concepts to other aspects of psychotherapy and the social/political world.

Abstract

The author discusses Smith's (2011) article and draws further on the example and criticisms of moves toward the statutory regulation of psychotherapy and the state registration of psychotherapists as an example of societal – and professional – regression.

Smith's paper

"Licensing of Psychotherapists in the United States: Evidence of Societal Regression?" by James B. Smith (2011) is an interesting and stimulating introduction to the work of Murray Bowen (1913–1990) and his psychosocial concepts (see Bowen, 1978). Smith reflects poignantly and critically on the pressure on psychologists and other mental health professionals to be licensed and on courses training such professionals to be accredited. For some 20 years, I have been an advocate of free association and voluntary professional membership and registration, and more recently, have been heavily involved in debates about and criticism of moves to the statutory regulation of psychotherapy and the state registration of psychotherapists in a postregulation society (see Tudor, 2010c, 2011e). As such I found Bowen's concepts both interesting and pertinent and Smith's application of them accessible and relevant, if not always thorough. I wish Smith had analysed licensing more directly in terms of Bowen's theory and, in this sense, found the two halves of his article a little disjointed. In this discussant paper, I offer some further elaboration of Smith's application of Bowen's theory, specifically to the issue of regulation of psychotherapy and the licensing or registration of psychotherapists, and some further application of Bowen's original analysis.

Despite my reservations about the structure and some of the style of Smith's article, I agree with much of his analysis, and in my discussion here review and briefly elaborate his argument with reference to three of Bowen's concepts: natural systems and family systems (Bowen's nuclear family emotional system); emotional processes in society (Bowen's societal emotional process), specifically, those of regression and progression; and the differentiation of self.

Natural systems, family systems, and emotional systems

From Bowen's view that human beings are part of all life, it follows that practitioners and professionals are part of all life. This is consistent with holism (Smuts, 1926/1987), organismic psychology (Goldstein, 1934/1995; Murray, 1938) (for a discussion of which with regard to transactional analysis, see Hagehülsmann, 1984 and Tudor, 2003), and most indigenous wisdom traditions. This perspective questions the distinctions and divisions between human being and professional, practitioner and client, personal/private and public, person/family and social systems, the clinic and society, and the clinical and the social.

Drawing on systems thinking, Bowen based his theory and concepts on a core assumption that an emotional system, which has evolved over several billion years, governs human relationships. Bowen proposed that this system affects most human activity and is the principal driving force in the development of both interdependence as well as clinical problems or, more accurately, systemic psychosocial problems that are presented in the clinic. Knowledge of how this emotional system operates personally, in the family, at work, and in social systems reveals both the old systems as well as new and more effective options for co-creating new ways of relating (see Summers & Tudor, 2000) and reflecting and taking action (see Tudor & Hargaden, 2002). It is the nature of the family and of other groups that its members are connected emotionally.

> Family members so profoundly affect each other's thoughts, feelings, and actions that it often seems as if people are living under the same "emotional skin." People solicit each other's attention, approval, and support and react to each other's needs, expectations, and distress. The connectedness and reactivity make the functioning of family members interdependent. A change in one person's functioning is predictably followed by reciprocal changes in the

> functioning of others. Families differ somewhat in the degree of interdependence, but it is always present to some degree.
>
> (Bowen Center, 2010)

This idea of an *emotional skin* or *emotional membrane* makes sense both in terms of a literal family and a professional "family" system or association. Members of an association or an organisation are, more or less, part of and connected to others in the association – freely or otherwise (see Kirsner, 2000). They – we – connect with, disconnect from, respond to, react to and against, support, stroke/recognise, honour, approve of, disapprove of, complain, and gossip about each other. While associations differ in the degree of interdependence, which is somewhat affected by the size of a particular association, it is always present to some degree. I write "more or less" because people can be inactive, distant, or reluctant members of an association, in which case the membrane may be stretched. In this context, it is interesting to note that the Code of Ethics of the New Zealand Association of Psychotherapists (NZAP) (2008) has, as part of psychotherapists' responsibilities to self, colleagues, and the profession, to "maintain participation in the profession" (Section 2.6).

Bowen's concept of emotional systems in human systems and family systems is a useful one in understanding the emotional interdependence of association members. In other words, professional associations are themselves an expression of a human need to affiliate (Allport, 1955/1983) and belong: to associate and promote a certain aspect of and activity in our lives. We join because we are political or social animals, however much we may then rail against the rules, regulations, and responsibilities of associations. And, of course, all this (joining, railing, being responsible or irresponsible, and so on) causes anxiety, and, according to Bowen, as anxiety increases, so the emotional connectedness of members becomes more stressful than comforting. Current tensions within the NZAP and other associations, including the New Zealand Transactional Analysis Association, regarding the statutory regulation of psychotherapy and the state registration of psychotherapists, and between some registered members and non-registered members, is a case in point.

Emotional process in society: regression and progression

Bowen's interest in emotional process/es in society is in the tradition of, among others, Wundt (social psychology), Adler (social interest), Reich (the mass psychology of fascism), Adorno and others (on aggression), and transactional analysis as a social psychology. Despite the fact that TA is a social psychology (see International Transactional Analysis Association, 2010), there are few specific discussions of transactional analysis as a social psychology, two exceptions being articles by Price (1978) and Massey (1996). There are a number of articles that describe applications of transactional analysis to social systems on topics such as the dependency cycle (Symor, 1977), modern racism (Batts, 1982), and notably, the work of Jacobs on autocratic power (1987, 1990, 1991, 1997). Smith's article, then, is a useful prompt for us to consider Bowen's concepts – and perhaps other transactional analysis concepts such as emotional literacy (Steiner, 1984) – and their application to the social/political sphere (see Antidote, 2010).

Bowen's concept of societal emotional process describes how the emotional system governs behaviour on a societal level. Working in the 1960s, Bowen identified certain parallels between the permissiveness of families (specifically the parents of juvenile delinquents) and that of the courts, with the result being a certain downward spiral or cycle that Bowen viewed as an anxiety-driven regression. Smith presents Bowen's ideas clearly and cites Comella's (2009) summary of some of the characteristics of societal regression, as well as progression. However, Smith is not so specific in his own application of Bowen's ideas and, specifically, these characteristics, to his own concern about the licensing of psychotherapists.

If we apply Bowen's analysis to our global society (population explosion, shortage of new habitable land, depletion of raw materials, etc.), it is clear that we are in a regressive phase. Regarding the specific issue of regulation and licensing (registration), the question is whether Bowen's characteristics are applicable to this issue and, if so, what they suggest. For a response to this question and an application of Bowen's characteristics of societal regression to the regulation of psychotherapy and the registration of psychotherapists see Table 11.1.

Much of the argument for licensing (registration) and regulation is based on the largely unexamined assumption that it protects the public, and Smith is correct when he reports that there is little evidence to support this. Indeed, there are 11 books (and many more papers) that have rebutted this assumption (for references see Table 11.1). Smith goes on to make a second point: that the licensing of professionals has more to do with protecting or enhancing the professional and the profession rather than the public, an analysis that, again, is reflected in the literature that is critical of the professionalisation of the activity of psychology and psychotherapy (see House, 2003).

Differentiation of self

Families and groups have a tremendous effect on how people act, feel, and think, and they vary in the amount of pressure they exert for conformity. For their part, individuals vary as to their susceptibility to "groupthink" (Janis, 1972), a process whereby people make faulty decisions because group pressures lead to a deterioration of "mental efficiency, reality testing, and moral judgment" (p. 9), with the result that the group ignores alternatives and tends to take irrational actions that, ultimately, can dehumanise other groups. According to Bowen's theory, people with a poorly differentiated self depend heavily on the acceptance and approval of others (in transactional analysis terms, in response to the Parental "Please me" driver) to the point that they overadapt to groupthink. A person with a well-differentiated self recognises her or his realistic dependence on others – or, better, interdependence.

In his discussion of this, Smith (2011) suggests that the individual needs to ask how she or he can become more of a defined self. With reference to regulation, he suggests that "the only thing I have any chance of doing is to better regulate me. Can I be – and let others be themselves?" (p. 145). This appears a somewhat individualistic and laissez faire response to taking constructive action and to regulation or co-regulation. In contrast, in a contribution that develops a politics of professional regulation based on the neuroscience of regulation, Embleton Tudor (2011) has argued for "a regulatory process which reflects human development" (p. 169). Also, and given the emphasis in Bowen theory on systems, surprisingly, Smith does not apply this concept to different systems or models of regulation (see Figure 11.1).

The taxonomy shown in Figure 11.1 is also useful in that the distinctions and differentiations between the various models may be seen clearly, as can the conflation

Table 11.1 Characteristics of societal regression as applied to the regulation of psychotherapy and the registration of psychotherapists

Characteristics of societal regression (based on Bowen, 1978; Comella, 2009)	*Examples and responses with regard to statutory regulation and state registration or licensing*
Emotionally driven choices to allay anxiety	The drive on the part of psychotherapy associations to seek state regulation of the profession has often been an emotionally driven choice in response to increasing moves to professionalisation (for a history of which in Aotearoa New Zealand see, for example, Manning, 2006; Bailey & Tudor, 2011; Dillon, 2011).
Automatic, instinctual responses to a sustained, underlying, and unknown, unacknowledged, or unrecognised societal-level threat	"I hope that it [registration] encourages recognition of Psychotherapy." (Hemmingson, cited in Manning, 2006: 27); "I think we should go for registration as all the other health providers will be. If we don't, we lose credibility" (Smith cited in Manning, 2006: 28).
Intellect more cut off from knowledge of the underlying threat	In moves to regulation and state registration, there is a distinct lack of analysis or meta-analysis of the threat or apparent threat posed to the profession or the public by unregistered practitioners, a lack reflected in the dearth of literature in favour of regulation and registration.
Vague awareness of the anxiety elicited by the underlying threat	Similarly, there has been a lack of analysis from those in favour of regulation and licensing regarding any anxiety elicited by the perceived threat posed by existing models of professional and self-regulation (for commentary on and critiques of which see Mowbray, 1995; Parker & Revelli, 2008).
Felt anxiety expressed in action, usually directed at resolving some issue, especially one perceived as threatening and around which societal conflict has erupted	Moves to regulation on the part of a profession predominantly have been based on seeking greater professional authority and credibility, usually in the eyes of the state and other professions, and justified with reference to particular examples of exploitative and unethical practitioners and to the "fact" that regulation and registration protects the public, for rebuttals and critiques of which see Gross (1978), Hogan (1979), Koocher (1979), Alberding, Lauver, & Patnoe (1993), Dawes (1994), Mowbray (1995), House & Totton (1997, 2011), Wampold (2001), Postle (2007); House (2009, 2010), Postle & House (2009), and Tudor (2011e).

(*continued*)

Table 11.1 (*cont.*)

Characteristics of societal regression (based on Bowen, 1978; Comella, 2009)	*Examples and responses with regard to statutory regulation and state registration or licensing*
Threatening issue inaccurately perceived at the intellectual level as causing the underlying anxiety	The threatening issue is seen as the unlicensed practitioner and not, for example, the increased professionalisation, medicalisation, and bureaucratisation of and the increased "audit culture" in psychotherapy (see, for example, King & Moutsou, 2010).

Least restrictive

Self-regulation
(also known as peer regulation)
For example, through voluntary membership in a professional organisation or group
(see, for instance, Heron, 1997; Totton, 1997)

Negative licensing
For example, being allowed to practise unless listed on a
register of practitioners ineligible to practise

Co-regulation
Whereby members of a professional association are regulated by that association
in conjunction with government
(such as currently being considered by the New Zealand Association of
Counsellors, 2010)

Reservation of title
Whereby a statutory registration authority reserves a professional title
(e.g. "psychotherapist") only for those eligible and approved to be registered
(the system currently administered by the
Psychotherapists Board of Aotearoa New Zealand)

Reservation of title and certain core practices
Which restricts both title and some activities or practice,
usually designated as "restricted activities"

Reservation of title and wholesale practice restriction
Which restricts both title and an entire scope of practice to only members
of the registered profession and other specified registered health professions

Most restrictive

Figure 11.1 Models of regulation (based on Macleod & McSherry, 2007)

of or any slippage or creep between different models. Thus, for example, in Aotearoa New Zealand, the regulation of psychotherapy under the Health Practitioners Competence Assurance Act 2003 (the Act) and administered by a regulatory authority, the Psychotherapists Board of Aotearoa New Zealand (PBANZ), appointed by the Minister of Health, is an example of the "reservation of title" model of regulation. However, in some of its policies, PBANZ has reflected a more restrictive model (for an analysis of which, see Tudor, 2011d), although, at times, it appears to accept a more pluralistic model as is embodied in a number of publications from the Ministry of Health (2010a, 2010b). Bowen's concept of differentiation of self is useful in reminding us of the importance of person-to-person relationships; interdependence; resisting unilateral models of regulation and licensing; and supporting the theory and practice of differentiation, options, and pluralism in the licensing or registration of practitioners. As the Director-General of Health (2009) in New Zealand has stated, "The Act is largely based on certification of title rather than licensing of activity.... *The Act does not prohibit unregistered people from performing activities that registered health practitioners perform*" (p. 2; emphasis added).

The representation of the various models in Table 11.2 along a continuum from least restrictive to most restrictive is also interesting socially and politically in that, with regard to social legislation, conservative governments tend to be less restrictive, while labour and socialist governments tend to be more willing and even keen to legislate. One example of this with regard to the regulation of psychotherapy and counselling has been in the United Kingdom, where, for a number of years, a Labour government had been promoting regulation under a Health Professions' Council and a medical model of competence and regulation (Health Professions Council, 2009). After much campaigning by the profession and, perhaps significantly, a change of government, the new Conservative–Liberal coalition government decided not to pursue such regulation, stating that,

> by freeing society from unnecessary laws, the Government aims to create a better balance of responsibilities between the state, business, civil society and individuals, and to encourage people to take greater personal responsibility for their actions. The Government therefore believes that the approach to professional regulation must be proportionate and effective, imposing the least cost and complexity consistent with securing safety and confidence for patients, service users, carers and the wider public.... Effective regulation of healthcare workers and social workers can support and develop the notion of professionalism by promoting self-regulation at an individual level.
>
> (Department of Health, 2011: 3–4)

Bowen's theory of differentiation of self is useful in thinking about group and organisational pressure with regard to licensing: how governments and their regulatory authorities may seek to impose conformity; how professions without sufficient differentiation may overadapt to such pressure; and how professions and professionals may express homonomy *and* autonomy, interdependence *and* independence.

Further analysis and application

In his article, Smith focuses on three of Bowen's eight principal concepts. I would have been interested in his application of some of Bowen's other concepts to the subject of regulation and licensing. For example, Bowen's concept of a "family projection process" (Bowen Center, 2010), which describes the primary way parents transmit their emotional problems to a child, appears a potentially useful way to understand the motivation and process behind some government policies in this area and the hierarchical organisation and transmission of professional culture (see Embleton Tudor, 2011). Similarly, Bowen's concept of "multigenerational transmission process" (Bowen Center, 2010), whereby small differences in one generation lead to marked differences in subsequent generations, appears a useful way to understand some of the history of concerns and debates about licensing from Freud (1926/1959) onward.

Conclusion

The licensing or registration of psychotherapists may enhance the professional and even the profession itself, at least from a certain perspective. It does not enhance the client by guaranteeing good practice, understanding, love, cure, or change; neither does it protect the client by guaranteeing safe or ethical practitioners, an argument that is based on unexamined assumptions and that has been discredited by some 11 books on the subject. Moreover, it is arguable that licensing actually lulls the public into a false sense of security about professionals and professions and fosters an institutionalising of the transference (see Mowbray, 1995). Members of the public are not protected by professionals who have a tick-box approach to membership and accountability or who register as a passive behaviour (i.e. as a result of doing nothing or of an overadaptation to groupthink and conformity). Moreover, it is hard to reconcile the transactional analysis values of dignity, self-determination (autonomy), and mutuality, as well as principles of respect, empowerment, protection, responsibility, and commitment in relationship (see European Association for Transactional Analysis, 2008), with any closed or unilateral system of licensing and any extension of regulatory authority or scope without consultation. The responsibility of the practitioner to the public is better discharged by professionals who are mature, well-trained, reflective, supervised, active, and engaged members of relevant associations, autonomous – and homonomous, and who have a sense of civic accountability. These are all qualities we might claim as the basis of genuinely transactional, analytic and relational ethics.

CHAPTER 12

SOUTHERN PSYCHOTHERAPIES (2012)

Retrospective introduction

Shortly after emigrating to Aotearoa New Zealand, I came across the book *Southern Theory: The Global Dynamics of Knowledge in Social Sciences*, written by Raewyn Connell, an Australian sociologist. It was one of those books that I read almost at one sitting and then for a while carried around with me, re-read, and kept making connections with what I was thinking and experiencing. Apart from learning a lot from the content of the book, which is fascinating, and the argument, which is extremely well made, the book has been an important part of finding my intellectual place in a new country and, indeed a new hemisphere. Looking back, I think it has also given voice to – and some analysis of – some disquiet I have had at times when I have travelled abroad when colleagues, both visiting and resident, have taken theory for granted or as given, one of the implications of which is that theory is somehow "neutral" and/or acontextual. For some years I have been aware of and drawn on the concept and practice of "cultural intentionality" (Shweder, 1990; see also Singh & Tudor, 1997); *Southern Theory* has helped me extend this to theory, and specifically, the cultural origins, assumptions, and biases of theory.

In the original paper, I acknowledged that it was a revised and expanded version of one presented at the World Council for Psychotherapy 6th International Congress, Sydney, Australia, on 25 August 2011. At the conference I attended a number of interesting and stimulating presentations. When I returned home, I decided, as editor of *Psychotherapy and Politics International*, to make a special, themed issue of what I referred to as "The Political Papers" from the World Conference (Tudor, 2012b). I expanded my speech and submitted it through the usual peer-review process and, as the editor of the journal in which the original article appeared, was especially grateful for the single-blind reviewers' comments on the first draft of the paper. Apart from editing the article for consistency, the only change I have made to the original is that I have updated my Pēpehā.

I have included the article in this selection as I like the analysis it advances, and as I think there is more in the critique that could be developed – certainly by me and hopefully by others. At the end of the article I refer to the East, which, as it transpired, was somewhat prescient as I was subsequently invited to give a keynote speech to the Japanese Association for Clinical Psychology at its 2014 conference in Yokohama, Japan. In speaking about "Alienation, Aliens, and Alienists: A Critical and Cross-Cultural Perspective on Psychopathology" (Tudor, 2014b), I used the critique offered by *Southern Theory* to acknowledge "eastern" theory and the need for a continuing critique of the dominant "western" – and "northern" – intellectual tradition, a perspective that continues to stand me in good stead as I engage in more cross cultural dialogues (e.g. Komiya & Tudor, 2016; Ioane & Tudor, 2016).

I have two critiques of the article. The first, a general one is that I would like to have used some more specific examples: whilst I made some important points about context and theory (pp. 180–181), and offered general principles that outline the counterpoints of a southern psychotherapy, I would have liked – and still would like – to take this to another level of practice (for a good example of which, see Fay, 2016). My second critique is a more specific one in that, over the 3 years since this publication, my knowledge about bilcultural issues and, specificially Te Tiriti o Waitangi, has developed. I have moved away from referring to what have become known as the *principles* of the English version of the treaty to referring to the articles of *Te Tiiriti*, i.e. the version signed by Māori chiefs. The principles – of partnership, participation, and protection – were identified in the Education Act 1981 and by the Royal Commission on Social Policy (1988) following judgements in the courts and findings and recommendations of the Waitangi Tribunal. They are, however, principles that have been identified by politicians, and, predominantly, white, Pākehā politicans at that, whereas the original articles – which acknowledge kāwanatanga (governorship), tino rangatiratanga (sovereignty), ōritetanga (equitable outcomes), and wairuatanga (spiritual freedom) – reflect the te reo Māori version of Te Tiriti. I am particularly grateful to my colleague and friend, Dr Heather Came, for advising me on this; see also Tudor and Grinter (2014) for an application of these Articles to client consent regarding publication.

Abstract

Drawing on Connell's ground-breaking and ground-affirming work, *Southern Theory*, published in 2008, this paper explores the concept and possibility of "southern psychotherapy" – or, more accurately, as the author advocates pluralism in psychotherapy, "southern psychotherapies". The paper first discusses the significance of context, personally and in theory, and the relationship between culture and theory. From this, it then addresses the hegemony of western theory, the arguments by which this is maintained, and the "northernness" of general theory. The second half of the paper responds to the "characteristic textual moves" of northern theory, identified by Connell, and offers four "textual" counterpoints as defining the theory and practice of southern psychotherapies.

Pēpehā (2016)

Tēnā koutou, tēnā koutou, tēnā koutou katoa.	Greetings to you all.
Ko Helvellyn te maunga.	My mountain is Helvellyn (in the English Lake District).
Ko Don te awa.	My river is the Don (which flows through Sheffield).
Ko Waka Oranga te waka.	My waka is Waka Oranga (see Hall, Morice, & Wilson, 2012)
Ko Ingārangi raua ko Werehi oku iwi.	I have English and Welsh ancestry.
Ko Tudor te hapū.	My family name is Tudor.

Ko John Tudor te tangata.	My oldest ancestor (that I have traced, back to the early 18th century) is John Tudor.
He tangata Tiriti ahau.	I am a person of te Tiriti | the Treaty (see Waitangi Tribunal, 2011)
Ko Ngā Wai o Horitiu te marae. Nō Sheffield, kei Ingārangi ahau. Kei Titirangi, kei Waitakere ahau e noho ana.	My marae is Ngā Wai o Horitiu (the marae of Auckland University of Technology). I am from Sheffield in England. I live in Titirangi, in the Waitakere (west Auckland).
Ko Leslie Charles Tudor taku papa. Ko Joan Cherwell Philipson taku mama. Ko Louise taku hoa rangatira. Ko Saul raua ko Esther aku tamariki. Ko Keith Tudor taku ingoa.	My father was Leslie Charles Tudor. My mother was Joan Cherwell Philipson. My wife is Louise. My children are Saul and Esther. My name is Keith Tudor.
Tēnā koutou, tēnā koutou, tēnā tatou katoa.	Greetings to all, greetings to us all.

Introduction

Two years ago I emigrated from the United Kingdom to Aotearoa New Zealand: from the Northern Hemisphere to the Southern Hemisphere, where things are, at least from a northern perspective, a little different: the flora and fauna are different, although there are imports of both that are familiar, but which, in many cases, also have a history of having colonised native plants and animals, some to extinction. There is different food, and certain food (such as Marmite, a childhood favourite) which looks the same but tastes different. Some of the (English) language is different; and, of course, there is a different, and second, official language: teo reo Māori. I have moved from being "at home" and indigenous (at least as far back as I know and have researched) or, in te reo māori, "tangata whenua" (people of the land), to being "tau iwi" or of the "other tribe": an immigrant settler in my new homeland, a permanent resident but not yet a citizen. Furthermore, I moved from a western (and northern) intellectual tradition to a southern land in which law, social policy, thinking and attitudes are hugely influenced by the West (and North), but often at the expense of indigenous wisdom and traditions. Whilst the outcomes of this influence are strangely familiar, they are not comfortable, as there are daily examples of colonial, colonising, and racist attitudes, behaviour, assumptions, and thinking.

I come to this land, and a new position, situating myself in new ground, as a cultural being: both in the sense of being cultured (as in educated), and of having a culture and being "culturally intentional" (Shweder, 1990). I was brought up in a liberal household, influenced by non-conformist religious beliefs, with strong parental and family values of social service and social justice, and of internationalism, and benefitted from a liberal education. I have always had a sense of being English, though more in the liberal and radical tradition of culture then patriotism (see Bragg, 2006), and, partly as a result of living in Italy for 2 years in my thirties, have a strong sense both of my own Englishness and of this as a part of European culture.

In the late 1970s and '80s I was actively involved in community politics, was part of a group which founded a housing co-operative and for 10 years lived in collective houses. These political and personal activities and commitments were influenced by the politics of movement (as distinct from party), and both feminism and the politics of *autonomia* (autonomy) in Italy (see Lotringer & Marazzi, 1980), and by a libertarian socialism (see Howell, 1981), which aspired to reflect a "prefigurative politics", i.e. ways of being, relating, and organising that articulated and reflected personal and social liberation – before the revolution. I took this interest in and concern about the state of the social/political world, culture, and context to my training as a psychotherapist in the United Kingdom (1987–1994), and found some resonance for it in the radical psychiatry tradition of transactional analysis (the Radical Therapist Collective, 1971; see Tudor, 2011g). Whilst an interest in the social/political world and the context of people's lives is, of course, not confined to liberals or socialists, it is generally those on the Left who tend to interrogate and articulate more about the social/political world than the conservative Right, some of whom are even sceptical about the concept of society – epitomised by Margaret Thatcher's infamous comment that "There's no such thing as society" (Keay, 1987). Significantly, some research in psychotherapy suggests that 40 percent of improvement in clients as a function of therapeutic factors is due to client variables and extra-therapeutic events (Asay & Lambert, 1999), which suggests that psychotherapists across the political spectrum should, at least, be interested in the society that surrounds their client(s). As the systemic family therapist, Virginia Satir put it: "I count, you count, context counts." (see Tudor & Hobbes, 2007).

Context and theory

If – or, rather, as – we need to count or account for context with regard to clients and their lives, so too we need psychotherapeutic practice and theory which account for and, indeed, is embedded in context.

There are, of course, a number of approaches to and forms of western and northern psychology and psychotherapy which account for the context outside the consulting room, and are more psychosocial than others, e.g. the therapeutic community movement (Main, 1946); radical therapy (the Radical Therapist Collective, 1971; Wyckoff, 1976); feminist therapy (Chaplin, 1988; Mitchell, 1975); radical psychiatry (Steiner *et al.*, 1975; Steiner, 2000); sociodrama (Moreno, 1978); social action psychotherapy (Holland, 1988, 1990 [see also Chapter 4]); pink therapy (Davies & Neal, 1996, 2000; Neal & Davies, 2000); and psychodynamic social relations (Clarke, Hahn, & Hoggett, 2009). Nevertheless, these forms of and perspectives on therapy are the exception rather than the rule, and the rule – and those that rule and regulate – tend to be more conservative, conformist, and even reactionary, than liberal or radical (see Fay, 2008).

A number of the founding fathers and mothers of psychotherapy were themselves either overtly political and, therefore, interested in the social/political world and context, and/or interested in culture and in different cultures, including:

- Alfred Adler (1870–1937), an early psychoanalyst and, later, psychotherapist, who was also a socialist, and emphasised in his theory and practice the understanding of power dynamics and the importance of equality; and espoused the development of "social interest" and democratic family structures, especially in raising children.
- Carl Jung (1875–1961), the founder of analytic psychology, who travelled widely, encountered different cultural perspectives, and made efforts to value

and include indigenous wisdom traditions into his version of psychoanalysis, a project which has been continued by analytic psychologists and post-Jungians (see, for example, Petchkovsky, San Roque, & Beskow, 2003).

- Karen Horney (1885–1952), one of the first women to enter a German university as a medical student, and an early feminist and psychoanalyst, who instigated research into female sexual development, and wrote, contrary to Freud, that the source of penis envy was in the way that female children were treated by the parents. Her work was influenced by her studies of sociology and anthropology and, in 1941, she founded the Association for the Advancement of Psychoanalysis, which focused on the importance of culture in shaping personality.
- Wilhelm Reich (1897–1957), a psychoanalyst and a Marxist, who argued that neurosis is rooted in the physical, sexual, economic, and social conditions of the patient, and wrote *The Mass Psychology of Fascism* (Reich, 1933/1970); he also promoted adolescent sexuality, and the availability of contraceptives and abortion, establishing the first sexual hygiene clinics in Europe; and argued the importance for women of economic independence.
- Eric Berne (1910–1970), the founder of transactional analysis, who, like Jung, also travelled widely, and was highly influenced by his anthropological studies.
- Paul Goodman (1911–1972), an anarchist and early gestalt therapist, who brought his particular social perspectives to influence the theory and practice of gestalt therapy (see Aylward, 1999).

Nevertheless, the extent to which such political, social and cultural influences and interests have impacted on psychotherapeutic theory and practice is arguable, as psychotherapy is not generally viewed by its proponents, let alone its clients, as revolutionary, anarchic, subversive, kinky, queer, or genuinely cross-cultural. It follows that we should not assume that a theory which has been developed and grounded in one culture is necessarily transferable to another. Indeed, I tend to assume that theory is not transferable until proved otherwise; in other words: a theory is guilty, or at least suspect, until proved innocent! There are two specific arguments which support this critique, regarding the myth of universality, which leads to universalism; and the magnification of error; as well as political analysis of the impact of colonialism.

The myth of universality

Universality refers to the notion that a (one) theory provides a complete understanding of everything, in this case, the field of human personality including behaviour, human relations, health and illness, healing and cure, and so on. Universalism refers to the view that a theory is applicable everywhere. Universality – and universalism – has been a popular notion in western philosophy and theology, and the subject of recent debates in the fields of linguistics, geography and human rights – more so than in the field of psychotherapy. There are a number of theories and aspects of psychological theory which are based on universality. One example is the notion that there is a set number of personality disorders (American Psychiatric Association, 2000) or personality adaptations (see Ware, 1983), for a critique of which see Tudor and Widdowson (2008). This kind of universal explanation is based on essentialism, i.e. that there are unchanging universal qualities, attributes or, in this instance, categories of personality, which pre-date existence; and on an assumption of cultural neutrality, i.e. the (supposed) neutrality of theory across culture(s) and, therefore, the (universal) applicability of theory. The assumption of universality (again, in both senses) is challenged by the reality of different views in different cultures and different wisdom and intellectual traditions about human beings; about being, personality, self, and o/Other; about knowledge and understanding; and about the principles of practice. Such differences about human nature, ontology, epistemology, and methodology, respectively, reflect different and differing paradigms (see Kuhn, 1962/1996; Burrell & Morgan, 1979).

The magnification of error

This refers to a philosophical argument about the development and application of theory which Rogers summarised well:

> when the theory is projected to explain more remote phenomena [an] error may be magnified. ... Thus every theory deserves the greatest respect in the area from which it was drawn from the facts and a decreasing amount of respect as it makes predictions in areas more and more remote from its origin.
> (Rogers, 1959: 193)

Rogers was writing in the context of a discussion about the application of theory that originates in the clinic, e.g. the theory of therapeutic conditions, to other fields of application such as supervision, education or training, or the nature, structure and dynamics of organisations. I suggest that the same caution could – and should – be extended on a geographical basis; i.e. that what is founded in one country and culture is more tested (rather than disrespected) the further it travels from its geographical origins. Akhtar and Tummala-Narra (2005) have discussed this (although without reference to the concept of the magnification of error) with regard to the translation, development and questioning of certain Freudian concepts in psychoanalysis in India – and the independent development of psychoanalysis in the subcontinent through the work of Girindrashekhar Bose (1887–1953). As Connell (2008) put it: "Since the ground is different, the form of theorising is often different too" (p. xii). Thus, the further we are, geographically, culturally, and intellectually from the source and the ground of a particular theory, the more we need to question and test its application and applicability. In this sense, this argument about the magnification of error follows on from the myth of universality – and both need to be considered in the context of colonisation.

The impact of colonisation

Theory only exists in context and, as far as some geographical areas or countries are concerned, their context involves colonisation. The word "colony" comes from the Latin *colonia* meaning settled land, farm, or landed estate, and was a translation of the Ancient Greek word *apoikia*, which referred to "people from home" so, originally, colonisation referred to the settlement of a place by emigrants. Whilst the Greek association of colony is benevolent, the development of colonies in Roman history became associated with the settlement of a community, usually as a garrison, in a conquered territory. Thus colonisation has come to mean the appropriation and exploitation of a geopolitical territory by an external power, through conquest and, often, spurious claims, consolidated by the coloniser's law, policy, and the imposition of language – and, as Stewart-Harawira (2005) put it, "the marginalization of indigenous sovereignty and self-determination within the structural framework of world order" (p. 24). This process also applies to theory, whereby a dominant theory, such as the western medical model, is imposed on a non-western society or culture, whilst indigenous wisdom and theory are discounted and/or outlawed. As Nandy summarised it:

> This colonialism colonizes minds in addition to bodies and it releases forces within the colonized societies to alter their cultural priorities once for all. In the process it helps to generalize the concept of the modern West from a geographical and temporal entity to a psychological category.
>
> (Nandy, 1983: xi)

Also, theory itself may be colonial, such as those theories which "justified" racism; and other theories, however "universal", may be used to reinforce colonial and colonising attitudes. In a letter to Bose, written in response to having received a birthday present from him (an ivory statuette of Vishnu, for his 75th birthday), Freud (1930/1961) wrote: "As long as I can enjoy life it will recall to my mind the progress of psychoanalysis and the proud conquests it has made in foreign countries" (p. 128). We may well speculate about Freud's conscious or unconscious use of the word "conquest". Although some take this reference to "conquest" as referring to the challenge posed by psychoanalysis to conventional psychology and psychiatry, dominant in western/northern countries, others offer a different reading. Commenting on aspects of this correspondence and, specifically, on Freud's use of the word "conquest", Akhtar and Tummala-Narra (2005) decried "an unfortunate tendency of psychoanalysis to colonize other idioms of thought rather than enter into a mutually enhancing, dialectical relationship with them." (p. 8, n1).

Culture and theory

There are many ways to describe the relationship between one culture and another, and between culture and theory. Some view cross-cultural psychology as holding the promise of a movement and a trade across and between cultures; however, as with cross-cultural studies in other disciplines, cross-cultural psychology – and psychotherapy – generally ignores colonisation, and the effects of colonisation on the colonised. Taking account of the three arguments articulated in the previous section, it is important to ask, first, "Whence the theory?" and, second, "Is it relevant here?".

For example, Akhtar (2004) has noted that there are at least four separate and distinct concepts implied in psychoanalysis and, one might say, more broadly, psychotherapy: a theory of mental functioning; models of development (which vary, depending on the school or modality of psychotherapy); concepts of psychopathology; and the technique and practice of analysis or therapy. Of these, however, for Akhtar, only the theory of mental functioning, including conscious and unconscious forces, projection, internalisation, regression, and so on, is universally applicable across cultures and ethnic groups. He considered – and considers – that the other aspects of psychoanalysis and psychotherapy are profoundly culture bound and, from a cautious or critical perspective, that they are not necessarily or easily transferable across cultural, ethnic, and geopolitical boundaries. However, for others, including myself, the logic of Akhtar's argument includes a critique of the universal "nature" of mental functioning. Akhtar himself is particularly critical of "western" developmental models, which have been all been uniformly developed from empirical observation in western settings and, often, within specific settings within western culture. For example, the developmental model of separation and individuation espoused by Mahler, Pine, and Bergman (1973) was derived largely from observation of white, upper-class children in Manhattan, New York. Moreover, formulations about what constitutes normal or abnormal behaviour, and concepts such as regression or the need for transitional objects are very different from one culture to the other. The imposition of such concepts (ideas, models, idioms, theories, etc.); the assumption that they are "universal" or "neutral"; and their uncritical application in other areas, whether conceptual or geographical: all support a "top-down" approach to the relationship between "western" and "non-western" cultures and theories.

Assuming, however, that those bringing together different theories founded in different cultures are interested in a genuine and respectful engagement and dialogue, the issue becomes one of whether there is necessary and sufficient cross, trans or bi-cultural knowledge between the parties, as well as knowledge, comprehension, application, analysis, synthesis, evaluation, and agreement about meta-theoretical constructs (e.g. regarding ontology, epistemology, methodology and method) – and, crucially, an equality between the parties to the "dialectical relationship" that discuss such integration. Given the history of colonialism, power imbalance between certain cultures, knowledge and paradigms, this is problematic, and so I now turn to a more radical relationship between culture and theory: that of comparing theories from the "bottom-up", subordinate, subaltern or peripheral position.

Southern theory

In her book *Southern Theory: The Global Dynamics of Knowledge*, the Australian sociologist, Raewyn Connell advanced the thesis that "modern social science embeds the viewpoints, perspectives and problems of metropolitan society, while presenting itself as universal knowledge" (pp. vii–viii). The global "metropole" refers to the "northern" capital exporting countries of Europe and North America. Connell uses the word "southern" for several reasons: first, to highlight relations in knowledge between "centre" and "periphery"; second, to acknowledge that theory emerges from the social experience of the periphery; and, third, to draw attention to the fact that social thought occurs in particular places such as Australia or "the south land" – and that the land (ground and context) situates the social theory of the people who inhabit it. She has defined southern theory as informed by the view: "that colonised and peripheral societies produce social thought *about the modern world* which has as much intellectual power as metropolitan social thought, and more political relevance" (p. xii). Thus "southern" is used not so much to describe or represent a geographical location – indeed, many Southern Hemisphere countries are, in terms of culture and theory, predominantly "western" or "northern" – but, rather, to indicate a particular analysis and attitude, and one which seeks to challenge the assumption and colonising influence of the West (see Nandy, 1983).

Connell has argued that the northernness of general theory is expressed in four, related "characteristic textual moves" (p. 44):

- the claim of universality;
- reading from the centre, e.g. sociology *in* Australia or *in* New Zealand, a move or manoeuvre which presupposes that sociology or psychology has a centre and that this centre is "neutral";

- gestures of exclusion, i.e. the exclusion of ideas from the "periphery" such as Aboriginal or Māori concepts of health and healing;
- "grand erasure", i.e. the erasure of key experiences such as colonisation.

In order to counter these textual and political "moves", we need, from a southern perspective:

1 theories that are specific and contextual;
2 theories that are generated from and that reflect readings from the periphery, the edge and the margins;
3 theories that are inclusive and specifically inclusive of ideas from the periphery; and
4 theories that present and represent experiences from the periphery and, therefore, that reclaim erased wisdom, knowledge, and experience.

Southern psychotherapies

The final part of this paper considers these counterpoints and advances some ideas as to and examples of what southern psychotherapies would represent. I use the plural first because I acknowledge and, indeed, advocate that there are many forms or modalities of psychotherapy, counselling, psychology, and psychiatry or "soul healing" (Steiner, 1971b: 3); and, second, because pluralism (see Samuels, 1997) is an inclusive concept which challenges a certain trend in psychotherapy to unilateralism as manifested, for example, in the statutory and unilateral regulation of the profession (in some countries) (see Tudor, 2011e), and in governments' obsession about so-called "evidence-based practice".

Specificity and context

Southern psychotherapies challenge theories and practices which claim universality and universal relevance, as well as the theory, language and methodology of, as Connell (2008) put it, "talking in universals" (p. 44). This involves making the origins of these universal and dominant theories explicit; challenging the rewriting (and colonisation) of indigenous wisdom in the conceptual language of the dominant paradigm, e.g. the western – and northern – intellectual tradition, without the experiential and contextual knowledge and appreciation of such wisdom; and drawing on theories and practice that are specific to local conditions.

The counterpoint here is to develop theory and practice which are specific and contextual and that name and promote the periphery as the beginning of its analysis and/or understanding. An important example of this is kaupapa Māori research theory (KMRT) which, as Woodard (2008) has commented:

> is an attempt by indigenous researchers to develop their own methodology in order to take ownership of research. KM[R]T draws from an indigenous knowledge base to construct meaning (Pihama, 1993) and includes rectifying the damage of oppressive practices and promoting a social change agenda.
> (p. 11)

Woodard identified and summarised seven key principles which guide indigenous research:

1. The principle of the Treaty of Waitangi: Te Tiriti o Waitangi provides a basis through which Māori may critically analyse relationships, challenge the status quo, and affirm Māori rights (Pihama, 2001).
2. The principle of collective philosophy: the kaupapa refers to the collective vision, aspiration and purpose of Māori communities.
3. The principle of emancipation: Tino rangatiratanga relates to sovereignty, autonomy, control, self-determination and independence.
4. The principle of socio-economic mediation: this principle asserts a need for kaupapa Māori research to be of positive benefit to Māori communities.
5. The principle of cultural aspiration: within a kaupapa Māori paradigm, Māori ways of knowing, doing and understanding the world are considered valid in their own right.
6. The principle of growing respectful relationships: the principle of āta [respectful thoroughness] (Pohatu, 2005) relates specifically to building, nurturing and maintaining wellbeing in relationships with Māori.
7. The principle of extended family structure: the principle of whānau acknowledges the relationship that Māori have with the world around them and to one another. It also identifies the intrinsic connection between the researcher, the researched and the research (p. 12).

One example of this counterpoint would be to develop a psychotherapy education/training programme that reflects "local conditions" such as the extended family structure, and promotes psychotherapeutic work with clients in the context of whanau (extended family), rather than one that focuses on the individual and, at worst, an individualising psychoanalysis of the individual client. Another example would be to include KMRT as a research methodology in courses or papers on research, most obviously in "southern" universities and psychotherapy training institutes.

Reading from the periphery

As with southern social science, southern psychotherapies (would) register the different situations of metropole and periphery as a requirement for psychological science to work on both a local and a world scale and, therefore, they embrace wisdom from the periphery or margins – and reposition it as central. As Connell (2008) acknowledged:

> white Australians often think of themselves as living at the end of the earth, and their distance from the metropole produces odd effects in social science. But Australia also has an Indigenous population for whom this is not the end of the earth, but the centre. Australian Aboriginal civilization is the oldest continuously existing culture in the world.
>
> (p. ix)

This counterpoint both plays with notions of periphery and centre, and "reads" (interprets, understands) the centre from the periphery – and, perhaps somewhat mischievously, subverts notions of centrality, neutrality and universality by offering its own universalism. As Nandy (1983) put it:

> The aim is not to adjust, alter or refurbish Indian experiences to fit the existing psychological and social theories – to make a better case for cultural relativism or for a more cross cultural psychology. The aim is to make sense of some of the relevant categories of contemporary knowledge in Indian terms and put them in a competing theory of universalism.
>
> (p. 17)

One example of this is – or would be – the promotion of the principles of Te Tiriti o Waitangi | The Treaty of Waitangi, which is often referred to as the founding document of Aotearoa New Zealand, i.e. the principles of partnership, protection, and participation, to contexts outside or beyond Aotearoa New Zealand. Although these principles are upheld in many (though not all) settings within the public sector in Aotearoa New Zealand, including, for example, at universities in the country, there also appears to be a certain trend to downgrade or even remove (erase) references to these principles [let alone the articles – see introduction to this chapter]. I was party to an interesting discussion at a university faculty board of studies in which an argument was made to remove these principles from papers (courses) aimed at international students as they (the principles) were viewed as too local and too specific. I and others argued (successfully) to retain them precisely because they were – are – both specific (to Aotearoa New Zealand) *and* universal, in that they could form the basis or the basis of discussions about bi-cultural relationships elsewhere. Nevertheless, the discussion revealed and represented a worrying trend towards an imagined, neutral and neutralised "centre", and, at times, a certain lack of confidence at the periphery, which, on the whole, is not shared by the more confident western and northern centre/periphery.

The "reading" that is southern psychotherapies recognises and embraces the impact of diversity with regard to the (plural) essence of things (ontologies) (see, for example, Stewart-Harawira, 2005); to multiple theories of knowledge (epistemologies), including oral traditions; and to the principles of investigation of experience (methodologies), e.g. kaupapa Māori research theory (see Smith, 1997; Smith, 1999) – and to respectful engagement with this diversity and, in the context of Aotearoa New Zealand, to bi-cultural relationships (and hence the opening to this paper).

Gestures of inclusion

Connell (2008) referred to "gestures of exclusion" (p. 46) as the third of the four geopolitical assumption of the northernness of general theory, and one which is maintained (or gestured) through the exclusion of anything that is not northern (or western) and, therefore, "metropole" or mainstream. Connell cited the example of reading lists which rarely include theorists from the colonised world. By contrast, southern psychotherapies counterpoint this assumption by consciously including such theorists in reading lists, and, importantly, as Connell emphasised, *ideas* from the periphery.

Another example of this counterpoint would be to apply ideas and concepts from indigenous wisdom traditions to critique the western epistemology that informs taxonomies such as the APA's *Diagnostic and Statistical Manual of Mental Disorders* (American Psychiatric Association, 2000) ([then] in its fourth edition). For example, thinking about "depression" as despair or even as a form of alienation positions both the practitioner and the patient differently:

> Māori have always struggled to accept the division of illness into physical and mental disorders. The demarcation is never that clear in experience or in language. Pukiriri, the word for fury or hostility, locates feelings of anger in the stomach (puku) rather than the head. Manawa-pa, apprehension, and manawa-pouri, a term for sadness, link anxiety and depression not with the mind, or with free floating emotions but with the heart – manawa.
>
> (Durie, 2001, p. 115)

There is a striking parallel between this exclusion and the marginalisation in mainstream psychotherapy of ideas from voices that are most often excluded, i.e. clients and patients. It is only relatively recently (in the last 20 years) that psychotherapy clients – in some cases, psychotherapy survivors – have found their published voices on the(ir) experiences of therapy (e.g. Heyward, 1993; Alexander, 1995); and that researchers have become interested in the view from the couch or the other chair in the consulting room. This discounting of the client may be traced back to the earliest days of psychoanalysis when Anna O's comment about the value of "the listening cure", i.e. what the analyst/therapist needed to do, was reinterpreted and reframed as "the talking cure", i.e. what the patient/client needed to do.

Other important gestures of inclusion that psychotherapy, at least from a southern perspective, could and should include are: naming the client's experience of being peripheral and marginalised; undoing the erasure, denial and distortion of experience, especially of colonisation; acknowledging the experience of oppression and of dominant narratives; and, of course, acknowledging the experience of trauma, dispossession, and loss (see Durie, 2011).

Grand "rasure"

In *Southern Theory*, Connell (2008) referred to "grand erasure", a concept which refers to the effect of assumptions of "northernness":

> When ... empirical knowledge derives wholly or mainly from the metropole, and where the theorist's concerns arise from the problems of metropolitan society, the effect is the erasure of the experience of the majority of human kind from the foundation of social thought.
>
> (p. 46)

Such theoretical erasure and insensitivity, and the lack of reflexivity about certain geopolitical and geopsychological assumptions, often intersect with similar social and legal assumptions. Perhaps the most devastating example of this in Australia was the legal notion – and fiction – of "terra nullius", meaning no one's land or empty land, a term applied by early settlers to Australia, a fiction which was overturned by the Australian High Court only as recently as 1992 in the Mabo judgement, which found that "native title" to land had existed in 1788! Reflecting on this notion, Connell commented: "*Terra nullius*, the coloniser's dream, is a sinister presupposition for social science. It is invoked every time we try to theorise the formation of social institutions and systems from scratch, in a blank space". She then added: "Whenever we see the words 'building block' in a treatise of social theory, we should be asking who used to occupy the land" (p. 47).

Just as we recognise the psychopolitical concepts and realities of internalised sexism, racism and homophobia, so we must recognise internalised colonialism whereby the oppressed (individuals and/or groups), to a greater or lesser extent, also "erase" themselves: their history, connection to land, family, tribe, culture, etc. Montero (1984) described this as altercentricism, whereby external, foreign (alter) figures are viewed as having and holding positive qualities, in contrast to the indigenous subject who views themselves as negative (see also Montero, 2007).

If erasure means the rubbing out and obliteration of what has gone before, I suggest that the neologism "rasure" can stand for the careful scraping away, in an archaeological sense, to reveal what was before. After all, one nation's national holiday is another people's "Invasion Day" (see Westergren, 2011).

At best, of course, psychotherapy, both southern and northern, is a process of rasure: of uncovering and reclaiming previously "erased" and forgotten trauma, memory, oppression, mystification, isolation, disconnection, and so on. Southern – and, indeed, radical northern or western – psychotherapies acknowledge local inequalities of wealth and health and power, and their impact on psychological as well as social indicators; and are informed by local configurations of social forces, whether poverty, class struggle, or indigenous land rights' movements. Southern psychotherapies, then, clearly represent a political psychology and praxis of liberation (see Fanon, 1961/1963; Nandy, 1983; Montero, 2007).

On the day of the presentation at the World Congress of Psychotherapy on which this article is based, an article in *The Sydney Morning Herald* reported that incidences of indigenous imprisonment, child abuse and chronic disease continue to rise 2 years after Kevin Rudd, the then Australian Prime Minister, announced the ambitious programme to "close the gap" (Martin, 2011). Similarly, in New Zealand, the gap in health indicators for Māori and non-Māori continues to grow rather than narrow. An important part of this "rasure" is stating these realities in order to acknowledge and textualise the experience of the oppressed, and especially those omitted from, as Connell (2008) has put it, "the hegemonic narratives of history and modernity" (p. 214).

Southern, eastern, northern, and western

When we think about things on a global basis, we may conjure up the image of the Earth as a round planet. It is, however, somewhat symbolic that the Earth, our world, is not perfectly round; it is, in fact, an oblate spheroid: the distance between the North and South Pole being shorter than the distance between the opposite sides of the world at the Equator. This unevenness, this unequalness, stands as a useful geographical metaphor for the geopolitical and psychopolitical realities of inequality, hegemony, and colonisation.

As I acknowledged in the earlier discussion of context and theory, there are a number of approaches and forms of western and northern therapy which are more psychosocial and psychopolitical than others. However, neither the critical tradition in western thinking, nor the radical therapy tradition in western psychology and psychotherapy, emphasises the relationship between people and land in quite the same way that indigenous wisdom traditions or "southern theory" do. From this perspective, those of us trained in the western and northern tradition need southern – and eastern – wisdom and theory to inform and enhance our practice in a colonial or post-colonial landscape (bearing in mind that post-colonial does not mean that "they" have gone).

Southern theory and southern psychotherapies do not stand against northern or western social or psychological sciences; they do stand against the assumption that northern/western social and psychological thought is a universal knowledge; and they stand for "southern" knowledge and method – and, for that matter and by similar argument, "eastern" knowledge (see Watts, 1961/1971). Similarly, southern theory and southern psychotherapies do not discount the problems and perspectives of metropolitan centres (indeed, there are significant metropolitan centres in the "South", with significant problems); they do stand against the notion that the metropole is the only place that produces social and psychological thought about the modern or postmodern world; and they stand for the wisdom that comes from the periphery.

It is my contention that the four counterpoints identified in the previous section constitute the basis of southern psychotherapies which, whatever their local variations, theorise in and on different ground from the western and northern intellectual tradition; are informed by indigenous wisdom and healing traditions; share a critical and radical analysis of the world from the periphery; and (re)present an anti-oppressive, post-colonial psychosocial therapeutic practice which is predominantly concerned with alienation and, therefore, dis-alienation, and with altercentricism and, therefore, the reclaiming of the subject and their social relations.

CHAPTER 13

THE RELATIONAL, THE VERTICAL, AND THE HORIZONTAL

A critique of "relational depth" (2014)

Retrospective introduction

Like the article that forms Chapter 9, this chapter reproduces an article that was originally published in a non-English publication, this time, in the German journal, *Person* [The International Journal for Person-Centered and Experiential Psychotherapy and Counselling], and was also an invited publication. Also like the other chapter, it has a certain history! I had originally submitted an earlier version of the article to a person-centred journal; the reviews were mixed: two reviewers liked it; two did not, and more strongly so; overall it was rejected, with the suggestion that I would need to make certain substantive revisions. Whilst I was disappointed with the decision, I felt fine about the process as I am supportive of the peer-review process (as, in my experience, it always makes the final version so much better). Accordingly, I revised the article, addressing all the points the reviewers had made and resubmitted it. It was rejected again, and, after another round of revisions, yet again. At this point I began to wonder if at least one or two of the reviewers and, indeed, the journal editor(s) were enacting something as the article itself was critiquing a dominant model within person-centred psychology with which many associated with the journal were closely identified. (I knew of another article, similarly critical of this particular model, which had also been rejected from the same journal.) In the end I decided to let it go. Shortly after I had done so, Gerhard Stumm, a valued colleague, who I had met at a number of international person-centred conferences (and who knew about the article), wrote to me to ask if I would be interested in submitting the article to *Person*, a German language international journal. I was delighted. I updated it, and submitted it; the peer reviews were positive; I made some minor revisions, and it was published.

The article is a development of the work that I and Mike Worrall had done and published in 2006, a significant aspect of which was to reclaim the roots of person-centred therapy in organismic psychology (Goldstein, 1934/1995; Murray, 1938; Angyal, 1941). Although I was disappointed that it hadn't been published in the English language journal, I do think that the article has matured with age and benefitted from my more recent work on two-person-plus psychology (Tudor, 2011f) and my reading of Foulkes (1975). In undertaking the final version for *Person*, I came up with the metaphors of the vertical and the horizontal which, I think, helps to hold and contain the critique. I have included the English version of the article in this selection as I wanted to (re)present my more recent work within person-centred psychology, with which I still identify, despite the fact that it is not particularly influential or grounded in Aotearoa New Zealand. As for my own critique of the work, I have to say, that, having gone through more revisions of this article than any others I have had published, I am pretty pleased with it as it stands.

Abstract

Within person-centred psychology, "relational depth" appears to be *the* predominant contemporary conceptualisation of the therapeutic relationship and of working in this relationship. This article offers a number of critiques of the theory and practice of "relational depth" and of "working *at*" relational depth. In doing so, the article is based on and argues for a shift in thinking: from "relationship" to "relating"; from a relational perspective based on the self to one based on the organism; and from a perspective which privileges the vertical to one which encompasses the horizontal, not only between people but also beyond people.

Keywords: relational depth; relationship; relational, relating; vertical; horizontal

Relational depth

The term "relational depth" was first coined by Mearns in an article published in 1996 in which, in relation to what he refers to as the contact spectrum, he defined relational depth as "relating with the client at very high levels of psychological contact" (p. 306). This concept, and Mearns' subsequent collaborative book, *Working at Relational Depth in Counselling and Psychotherapy* (Mearns & Cooper, 2005), has been generally well received both within and outside the person-centred and experiential approach. The book was the subject of an enthusiastic review by Schmid (2006a) who referred to it as "a great, most important and ... groundbreaking book" (p. 149). Both Mearns and Cooper have written further articles based on their book (for example, see Cooper, 2005b). Relational depth has been the subject of a special issue of the world journal *Person-Centered & Experiential Psychotherapies* (edited by Cooper, 2006); has become the basis of research (see for instance, Cooper, 2005a; McMillan & McLeod, 2006; Knox, 2008; Knox & Cooper, 2010; Wiggins, Eliott, & Cooper, 2012); and has been the subject of a number of other articles (see, for instance, Cox, 2009; Lambers, 2006; Cooper & Ikemi, 2012). The theory and practice of relational depth may be considered both as a one-and-a-half and a two-person psychology, as these are proposed and described by Stark (1999). In his article, Cooper (2005b) described relational depth as serving a "corrective relational experience" (p. 18), which represents a one-and-a-half person psychology, and that it could be thought of as "co-presence" (p. 18), which represents a two-person psychology.

However, although relational depth appears to be the predominant way of conceptualising working in the therapeutic relationship in contemporary person-centred psychology, it is not without its critics. Here, I present a critique of relational depth, focusing particularly on the language used to describe and claim relational depth as language is significant in representing meaning and the underlying philosophy of theory and practice (see Tudor & Worrall, 2006).

Critiques of relational depth

In her article on the subject Wilders (2007) expounded a number of criticisms of relational depth which here I summarise:

1 That the theory and practice of "relational depth" is inconsistent with fundamental ideas of the person-centred approach and its therapy, in particular, the principle of non directivity. In support of this argument Wilders (2007) cited a number of instances in which Mearns and Cooper advocated a view of the therapist as expert, directing and leading the client and, worse, "a variety of idiosyncratic behaviours on the part of the therapist, which may at times be erratic, confrontative, and controlling" (pp. 2–3). Another example of this theoretical incongruence is that their approach implies therapist judgement of the client's functioning in selectively implementing confrontative "depth" responding.
2 That, in proposing the theory of relational depth, Mearns and Cooper have isolated and elevated emotional distancing as the most significant response to conditions of worth, and, therefore, the most significant of psychological problems. Moreover, this is at odds with the phenomenological method of equality or horizontalisation whereby therapists give equal consideration to all experience, and do not give any aspect of a client's presentation a differential or hierarchical significance.
3 That in promoting "relational depth" as a new development, Mearns and Cooper tended to caricature person-centred therapy as a narrow set of skills, and failed to recognise how fundamentally relational person-centred therapy is and, specifically, that the concept of engaging equally with different parts of the client is not new and, indeed, is integral to person-centred therapy. Also, in his article, Cooper (2005b) claimed that he and Mearns introduced the term "holistic listening" when, in fact, Rowan wrote an article on this concept in 1985. I would also add to this point that some claims of the effectiveness of relational depth have been exaggerated, for instance, in his article Cooper (2005b) simply asserted that "Experiencing the therapist at relational depth can give the client a sense of safety that far exceeds the norm for therapeutic relationships" (p. 19).
4 That in their book, Mearns and Cooper (2005) have a tendency "apparent throughout the book, to contradict themselves" (Wilders, 2007: 2). Thus, whilst on the one hand Mearns and Cooper reject any objectifying view of clients in order to diagnose, assess, and hypothesise, on the other hand they apply exactly such considerations in their concrete therapeutic actions and interventions. This, in part, may be due to the fact that, as they acknowledged in their preface, the two authors took the lead on different chapters in the book. This would explain, for example, the inconsistency in the capitalisation and view of "the Self" (for further discussion of the significance of which, see below, pp. 198–199).

In an unpublished paper Hilton and Canavan (2008) have also offered a critique of relational depth in which:

1 They express concern about the gendered and even sexualised associations of the metaphor and the language of depth, and argue that, with some clients, the metaphor, with its associations of penetration, would be misdirected and inappropriate. Cooper (2005) continued this association in his article with his reference to co-presence involving an "interpenetrative" cycle (p. 18). Instead of an approach which is based on some notion of being "inside" the other, they favour the kind of relational approaches which advocate being "alongside" the other, such as those developed by the Stone Centre in Boston (see Jordan,

Kaplan, Baker Miller, Stiver, & Surrey, 1991; Jordan, Walker, & Harling, 2004).

2 They discuss the implications of the therapist's language of depth in terms of the dynamics of power in the therapeutic relationship.

3 They discuss the sufficiency if not the necessity of being met at the surface, "for in the space between the external world and our surfaces we can co-construct the narrative of our lives in the presence of another." This echoes Rogers' (1953/1967b) image of the end point of the process of therapy as one in which "the client discovers that he can *be* his experience, with all of its variety and *surface* contradiction" (p. 80; my latter emphasis).

4 They argue that most of the writing on relational depth is therapist-centred in that it privileges the therapist's perspective regarding the therapeutic relationship and encounter, as distinct from the client's perspective or frame of reference.

I agree with the points that both Wilders, and Hilton and Canavan have made, and have some further criticisms of the concept of relational depth.

Further critiques of relational depth

In their original publication Mearns and Cooper (2005) wrote about "relational depth" in terms of:

1 "[R]eal meeting and connection" (p. xi); and
2 that it is: "A state of profound contact and engagement between two people in which each person is fully real with the Other, and able to understand and value the Other's experiences at a high level." (p. xii);

They also stated that it encompasses:

3 a particular *quality* of relationship or "an *enduring* sense of contact and interconnectedness between two people" (p. xii).

Here I discuss and critique these different aspects of the concept, especially the second.

Realness

There is a problem with claiming and qualifying some things as "real" as it implies that other things are in some way unreal. All meeting and connection is "real" both in terms of being actual, and from the phenomenological perspective which informs and underpins person-centred psychology. In their work on therapeutic relationships, Gelso and Carter (1985) made the same mistake in referring to the transferential relationship as "unreal". Mearns and Cooper compound this when they used the adverb "fully", in effect, to describe degrees of realness. Used in this way, "real" and, worse, "fully real", carry implicit value judgements, as in the vernacular "Get real!" (an admonition which also implies a double-bind). In response I suggest that, in this context, adjectives such as "genuine", "open", and/or "immediate" each and all have a clearer, richer, and more accurate meaning than "real". This point is significant in that it lays the ground for the critique of "depth" in relational depth (see pp. 196–197 below).

Meeting and connection

Given that the concept and practice of encounter has been well elaborated within the person-centred approach by Rogers himself (Rogers, 1970/1973a) and, more recently by Schmid (1998), I think that "encounter" would have been a more appropriate and significant word than "meeting". Indeed, Mearns and Cooper (2005) themselves referred to encounter, when they advocated – and I agree with them – that:

> A therapeutic approach in which dialogue and interaction take more centre stage: one in which it is the *encounter* between the therapist and client, rather than the *provision* of a particular set of conditions *for* the client, that is conceptualised as being key to the healing process.
>
> (p. 9)

This suggests a focus on a relational perspective as distinct from an emphasis on the individual: the person *and* person as distinct from the person *to* person. Of course, these are not "either ... or ..." positions, but, rather, ones of different emphasis.

Contact

One problem with extolling "profound contact" is that there are different readings within the approach regarding contact. Rogers (1957) defined psychological contact as a binary phenomenon, by which he means that two people are either in psychological contact or they are not. In his 1959 paper he stated specifically that the other five conditions "exist on continua" (p. 215), implying that psychological contact, at least as he understood it, does not. Others disagree. Mearns (1996), for instance, has asserted that "the phenomenological reality of psychological contact to both clients and counsellors is that there are *degrees* of contact" (p. 306) – although it is unclear how anyone can assert another person's phenomenological reality as if it were an uncontested fact. Elsewhere, Mike Worrall and I have argued that it is simpler, more elegant, and more parsimonious to leave the concept of (psychological) contact as Rogers defined it, and to agree instead degrees of acceptance, empathic understanding, communication, and perception (Tudor & Worrall, 2006) and that, as Rogers (1959) put it: "If more than this simple contact between two persons is intended, then the additional characteristics of that contact are specified in the theory" (p. 207). We think that this is unambiguous and that Rogers viewed psychological contact as a binary pre-condition. One practical and theoretical benefit of our reading of Rogers is that the kind of work described as pre-therapy (Prouty, 1994; Prouty, Pörtner, & Van Werde, 2002) is better conceptualised as an aspect of acceptance and empathy rather than viewed as pre-therapy and, therefore, somehow not part of therapy.

There is a certain irony in Mearns and Cooper's emphasis on "profound contact" as, in consistently referring to "the core conditions" (of congruence, unconditional positive regard, and empathy), rather than the six necessary and sufficient conditions, they omit any consideration of "contact" or "psychological contact" from the therapist's experience or way of being, as Cooper (2005b) put it. On this basis, the single phrase that Cooper suggested as a way of thinking about the core conditions as a single way of being should at least and more accurately be "genuinely *contactful* empathic acceptance". Moreover, the focus on the core conditions – or, including contact, the therapist's conditions – also omits the client and the client's conditions (contact, incongruence, and perception of unconditional positive regard and empathy) from this encounter, for further discussion of which see Tudor (2011c). Indeed, one way that therapists can enhance their receptivity which, I agree with Cooper, is important, is, theoretically, to acknowledge and understand the significance of what Rogers (1958/1967a) referred to as the sixth, and "assumed condition" (p. 130).

Depth

The use of the adjective "profound" (in "profound contact") brings us to the issue and question of depth. In their formulation, Mearns and Cooper were clearly advocating both profound contact and high levels of valuing. Both images and strategies are problematic.

Whilst Mearns and Cooper (2005) have claimed that they do not attach any value judgement to the term "depth", it is clear that they do. The emphasis of the term "relational depth" is on *depth* and, as the noun, it is the substantive concept. It would be different if, for instance, they had advocated "depth relating". In their very next sentence Mearns and Cooper stated that "*some* depth of relating is essential for optimal human functioning" (p. xii), and elsewhere Mearns (2005) referred to the therapeutic alliance as a superficial level of relationship. There is, of course, no issue with Mearns and Cooper or anyone else suggesting that "depth" is a value; indeed, "depth psychology" is based on this view; one can simply agree or disagree with it. There is a problem, however, when people (practitioners or theoreticians) state that they do not attach a value judgement to a view, in this case depth, when their whole theory is based on it. By contrast, Rogers was very clear about the value/s which underlie psychotherapy: for instance, in his paper on "A process conception of psychotherapy" (Rogers, 1958/1967a), he acknowledged that he valued fluidity as a desirable state of being – and that not everyone would agree with this.

A further problem with extolling depth is that anything less is viewed as less, shallow or surface. Indeed Mearns and Cooper (2005) have referred to "relational engagement at a surface level … [as a] presentational level of self' (p. 58) – and that "transferential phenomena belong to a much more superficial level of relating where people are still being symbols for each other" (p. 53). By proposing depth and referring to the presentational level as surface, Mearns and Cooper not only sound judgemental, but also are in danger of not accepting self-protective defences, distancing, and avoidance, and the fact that the organism tends to actualise in terms of maintenance as well as enhancement – which contradicts Mearns' (1996) emphasis, when referring to configurations of self, on the equality of and valuing different aspects of self.

In his early article Mearns (1996) referred to the client deciding what is depth; in the book (with Cooper), this becomes "working *at* relational depth" (my emphasis). This reflects a clear shift from a person-centred perspective that "depth" is in the eye of the beholder, that is, the experience of the client, to a therapist-centred perspective whereby the therapist is focusing on depth and deepening – and concerned if she or he is not achieving this. Mearns and Cooper appear ambivalent about this enterprise: on the one hand they clearly promote working at relational depth; on the other hand, in their writing, they put in a number of caveats about both the term and the activity, at one point cautioning that "for a truly deep relational encounter to happen ... the therapist must let go of her 'aims', 'anticipations' and 'lusts' ... and this includes a 'lust' for relational depth" (Mearns & Cooper, 2005: 113). Nevertheless, whilst Mearns and Cooper have clearly stated that they do not intend that therapists lust after relational depth, the language and metaphors they use consistently, including talk of thrust, lust and flirting, imply precisely this.

Whilst the concept and practice of "relational depth" focuses on relationship, in the field of psychology "depth" refers also to personality. The metaphor of depth applied to personality implies a topographical and even an archaeological view of the psyche, which has a particular psychoanalytic provenance and, in this sense, relational "depth" echoes and inaccurately links person-centred psychology with psychodynamic and analytic "depth psychology" with its views of the unconscious and the importance of transference in relationship (for a critique of which, see Tudor & Worrall, 2006; Tudor & Summers, 2014). Schmid (2006b) has dismissed this criticism of the depth metaphor by simply asserting that it does not represent a topographical category. I think that, in this, Schmid has underestimated the power of language and of the metaphor, and the power and influence of "depth psychology", for a critical history of which see Wyss (1966). Hilton and Canavan (2008) were also critical of what they referred to as "the growing imperative towards 'depth' in person-centred writing". Rogers (1942) himself was critical of "deep" therapy by which he referred to interpretive therapy, psychoanalysis (of children), and the encouragement of dependence. In his discussion of the three main dimensions of personality structure – progression, i.e. means-end relations, depth, and breadth, i.e. channels for expression – Angyal (1941) offered a different view of depth whereby "the person grows from a median position toward both the depth and the surface." (p. 356). He continued:

> A well-organized person has to develop also toward the surface ... In our terminology this means the development of greater facility and perfection in expressing in actual behaviour that which is in the depth of the personality. The development in this direction is a struggle for self-expression.

Height

There is a similar problem in Mearns and Cooper's writing with the metaphor of height, as in "high levels" of understanding and valuing. Putting it this way, Mearns and Cooper were, in effect, aligning themselves with the skills-based approach of Carkhuff and Truax (Carkhuff, 1967; Truax & Carkhuff, 1967) and their "levels" of empathy, and promotion, and reification of "accurate empathy".

Transference

In terms of the kind of relationship that "working at relational depth" promotes, it is interesting that researchers into the client's experience of relational depth (McMillan & McLeod, 2006) report that: "all but one of the informants who reported deeply facilitative relationships described the therapist in terms of a parent, with many of them characterizing the therapist as being *like a good or ideal mother*." (p. 285). At the same time Mearns and Cooper (2005) stated that, as a consequence of the degree of mutuality in the therapeutic relationship as they conceptualise it, "there are absolutely no transference phenomena" (p. 53) and, later, "there are absolutely no transference phenomena at this level of continuing connection" (p. 58). This is an extraordinary claim which not only, as Bazzano (2013) observed, dismisses over 100 years of psychotherapeutic work and theory, but also again makes assumptions about the client's experience, perception, and construction of reality – and, moreover, assumptions which are also contradicted by McMillan and McLeod's research. Furthermore, Mearns and Cooper's concern about transference – and, presumably, countertransference – appears at odds with Rogers who acknowledged "transferential attitudes" (Rogers, 1951), or, I prefer, "co-transferential relating" (see Summers & Tudor, 2000; Tudor & Summers, 2014; and p. 200 below).

Hierarchy

The practice of "working at relational depth" is implicitly hierarchical in that it is viewed as an "advanced" skill and only achieved through advanced or post-graduate training or through the therapist's continued professional development; and indeed, Mearns and Thorne (2000) view this as the "developmental agenda" of the therapist. Elsewhere, they put it thus: "The essential challenge for the person-centred counsellor ... [is to] be able to offer an encounter at relational depth not just to some clients but to *every client who comes to her door*", and emphasise that: "*This is not achieved in initial training*" (Mearns & Thorne, 2007: 145), although this view is contradicted by the emphasis on some diploma/undergraduate person-centred training courses on relational depth and its practice.

The other/Other

Another issue in the theory of relational depth is the reification of the (capitalised) "Other". In the introduction to their book, Mearns and Cooper (2005) stated that in using the term "depth" they "are not wanting to imply an object-like model of the 'self' in which a person is seen as having some deep 'inner core'" (p. xii), and that what they mean by "deeper" is those things which are "truer" and more "real" for a person. However, while saying that they do not want to imply such things, the language they use, along with the capitalisation of "Self" and "Other" does precisely imply an object-like and, indeed, object-relations view of self and other. This is no slip of the pen or the finger, or oversight of the author/editor, but is a consistent reference to a reified "Self". Whilst some take the self (whether, in the English language, lowercase or uppercase), represented by the pronoun "I" (interestingly enough, in English, always capitalised), as representing an existential understanding of the person as agent, I think that there are important distinctions between the concepts of "person", "self", and organism (see Tudor & Worrall, 2006). This is significant in that the same authors are, and especially Mearns, specifically associated with self theory and "configurations of self" (Mearns, 1998, 1999), although it should be acknowledged that it was Zimring (1988) who first coined the term "self-configuration". Whilst the capitalisation of the other may be common in original writings on dialogical philosophy and therapy, it is significant and should not simply be ignored.

The broader problem here is that Mearns and Cooper based their theory of relational depth on a self-relational theory without acknowledging it, and without locating self, selves, and self theory within the context of the organism and organismic theory, as Rogers does. As the self is a differentiated part of the organism, the organism is logically and developmentally prior to the self; as Matthews (1991) has put it: "The paradigm instance of the self is, of course, indisputably, the organism – from primitive amoeba to highest mammal" (p. 129).

Enduring

As noted above, Mearns and Cooper (2005) described relational depth as also encompassing "an *enduring* sense of contact and interconnectedness between two people" (p. xii). Whilst it is clear that their conceptualisation of the relational encompasses contact and interconnectedness, "enduring", which implies longevity and a certain sense of survival during hard times, appears somewhat different to "depth" and is, therefore, in their formulation as it stands, not sufficiently elaborated. Also, as "enduring" implies a relatively long-term relationship, such a quality or necessity seems to contradict Rogers' (1942) challenge to the assumption in psychoanalysis and psychodynamic psychotherapy that therapy is necessarily long term; and to be something of a luxury in the context of concerns to offer brief, short-term, or time-limited versions of therapy (see Tudor, 2008a).

The relational, the vertical, and the horizontal

Having offered some specific critiques of relational depth, I briefly offer some links between these critiques and wider discussions in and beyond person-centred and experiential psychotherapy and counselling.

The relational: from relationship to relating

Person-centred therapy is the original "relationship therapy". It is well documented that Rogers took the term, with due acknowledgement, from Jessie Taft (1882–1960) who wrote about it in her influential book on *The Dynamics of Therapy in a Controlled Relationship* (Taft, 1933), which thus predates the more recent interest in what has been referred to as "the relational turn" (see Greenberg & Mitchell, 1983) by half a century. Taft, who was a pupil (and later biographer) of Otto Rank (1884–1939) was, with Frederick Allen, Elizabeth Davis and Virginia Robinson, very influential in Rogers' development of a "newer psychotherapy" (Rogers, 1942). In many ways, I wish that Rogers had maintained the term "relationship therapy" rather than renaming it "non-directive therapy" (Rogers, 1942), as this began a shift away from an emphasis in person-centred psychology on the therapeutic relationship, for a detailed argument about which see Ellingham (2011).

In my work with Mike Worrall (2006), we reclaimed the logic of Rogers' relational theory and approach and did so by articulating his organismic theory and the organism as the root metaphor of relational person-centred therapy. The human organism tends to actualise. This sentence is both simple and rich with meaning. The human organism has a number of qualities – holistic, experiential, relational, dialogic, interdependent, directional, needs driven, goal-directed – all of which imply action: experiencing, construing reality, differentiating, being in dialogue, being in a constant process of becoming, regulating, behaving according to need, valuing, aggressing, and, of course, relating. As humans we are beings in process, and thus it is helpful to use the language of process to describe this experience. Elsewhere (Tudor, 2008g, 2008h), I advocated the use of process language and, in particular, verbs, to reflect and emphasise human activity and process; and I am particularly interested to shift our current focus on "*the* therapeutic relationship" (noun) to "therapeutic relating" (verb, present participle) which, thereby, emphasises the present, active, and dialogical quality of this particular human encounter (see also Summers & Tudor, 2000). By now, the reader will be aware of my interest in and attention to language; indeed, "languaging" represents an activity which Maturana (1995) argued is a biological phenomenon or process which "takes place in our relational domain as a manner of living in recurrent interactions". (p. 154). It is my contention that the concept of the organism is more useful in promoting such languaging and relating than the concept of the self, not least as relationship therapy seeks to provide – or co-create – a therapeutic environment which, as Taft (1933) put it: "permits a realization of wholeness" (p. 290).

In this sense, the phenomena described by Mearns and Cooper as "relational depth" is not new and it does not add anything to our understanding or experience of therapeutic relating; and, as I hope to have demonstrated, as a concept it is problematic. Furthermore, I have come across a number of practitioners, and especially students, for whom the hegemony of relational depth has become oppressive and even dogmatic – which was not the intention of the original authors. Whilst it is clear that there are keen advocates of the concept and its practice, perhaps especially in the United Kingdom, it is not the only person-centred theory of relationship/relating and the relational; and, as person-centred approaches to therapy are both non-dogmatic and anti-dogmatic, we need to be wary of any creeping orthodoxy (see Tudor, 2007d, 2007e). Furthermore, from an organismic and experiential perspective, I think that we should be less concerned with depth and the therapist's communication, and more concerned with the relational and the client's experience and perception (Rogers' sixth or "assumed" condition), as well as with how both therapist and client engage and work with this and with each other.

The vertical and the horizontal

Given the emphasis in person-centred psychology on mutuality, which describes a horizontal relationship between client and therapist, there is something strangely vertical about the promotion of relational depth and of working "at" relational depth. This is problematic for a number of reasons.

- It encourages the client to think of their ability to be contactful, aware, real, authentic, respectful, regarding, loving, empathic, fully functioning, and so on as "deep" down within them, rather than as aspects of an intersubjective and inter-relational encounter, supported by certain co-created conditions.
- It perpetuates an archaeological, "depth psychology" image of the person and their psyche which contradicts person-centred personality theory.
- It subtly elevates the therapist as a figure who, if not above – or behind – the client (as represented in the "one-person" psychology of the classical analytic stance), is at least in a higher degree or angle of asymmetry (see Aron, 1996) with regard to the client than would be expected of the classical or relational person-centred therapist. In this sense, I would argue that the therapist working at relational depth is not only being directive but also

> subtly promoting rather than dissolving the transference or transferential attitudes. This is particularly ironic both given Mearns and Cooper's view of transference, and as, in the wider psychotherapy world, including psychoanalysis and psychodynamic psychotherapy, there has been more interest in the significance and importance of "symmetrical and horizontal relationships" as Foulkes (1975: 3) referred to them, and, more recently in "horizontal transferences".

In response, I would argue for more discussion and praxis of horizontal relating, not only between therapist and client but also between clients, one example of which was research that demonstrated the benefit and efficacy of clients' empathic understanding *of each other* in group therapy (Giesekus & Mente, 1986). Beyond this, I would advocate for a greater appreciation of the impact of horizontal relationships and relating on the client from family, friends, partners, the workplace, and the environment (see Tudor, 2013c).

Conclusion

In order to further a relational approach which (I think) is more consistent with Rogers' initial conceptualisation and promotion of "relationship therapy", I suggest three propositions to represent both present strengths of and future challenges for person-centred and experiential therapies:

1. That, as the organism is at the heart of the person-centred approach and its theory of therapy (Rogers, 1959), the organism is – or should be – at the centre of the theory and practice of person-centred and experiential therapies, and logically prior to theories of (the) self.
2. That the principles and features of organismic psychology provide the most appropriate and consistent base for person-centred therapy, its practice and theory and, specifically, its theory of relationship or, more accurately, (therapeutic) relating (see Tudor & Worrall, 2006).
3. That an organismic perspective transforms our view of life and of therapy from an analytic and individualistic "one-person" and even "one-and-a-half-person" psychology (Stark, 1999) to a relational "two-person" psychology and, indeed, further, to a contextual, social, environmental/biospheric "two-person-plus" psychology (see Tudor, 2011f).

LEGAL STATUTES

England and Wales

Disabled Persons (Employment) Act 1944. 7 & 8 Geo. 6. Ch 10. London, UK: His Majesty's Stationery Office.
Mental Health Act 1959. 7 & 8 Eliz. 2. Ch 72. London, UK: Her Majesty's Stationery Office.
Mental Health Act 1983. 1983 Ch 20. London, UK: Her Majesty's Stationery Office.

Italy

Legge 17 luglio 1890 n. 6972 (Legge Crispi) Sulle istituzioni pubbliche di beneficenza [Regarding public charitable institutions]. Rome, Italy: Gazzetta Ufficiale.
Legge 14 febbraio 1904, n. 36 Legge sui manicomi e sugli alienate, disposizioni e cura degli alienate [Law regarding the mentally ill and the insane, their provision and cure]. Rome, Italy: Gazzetta Ufficiale.
Legge 2 aprile 1968, n. 482 Disciplina generale delle assunzioni obbligatorie presso le pubbliche amministrazioni e le aziende private [General regulations regarding the obligations of public services and private agencies]. Rome, Italy: Gazzetta Ufficiale.
Legge 30 marzo 1971, n. 118 Conversione in legge del decreto-legge 30 gennaio 1971, n. 5, e nuove norme in favore dei mutilati ed invalidi civili [The conversion into law of the decree-law 30 January 1971 no. 5 and new norms in favour of maimed and disabled civilians]. Rome, Italy: Gazzetta Ufficiale.
Legge 4 agosto 1977, n. 517 Norme sulla valutazione degli alunni e sull'abolizione degli esami di riparazione nonche' altre norme di modifica dell'ordinamento scolastico [Norms regarding the evaluation of pupils, the abolition of remedial examinations and other modifications to the education system]. Rome, Italy: Gazzetta Ufficiale.
Legge 13 maggio 1978 n. 180 Accertamenti e trattamenti sanitari volontari e obbligatori [Voluntary and statutory health investigations and treatment]. Rome, Italy: Gazzetta Ufficiale.

Legge 23 dicembre 1978, n. 833 Istituzione del servizio sanitario nazionale [The establishment of the national health service]. Rome, Italy: Gazzetta Ufficiale.
Legge 11 febbraio 1980, n. 18 Indennita' di accompagnamento agli invalidi civili totalmente inabili [Attendance allowance for completely disabled civilian invalids]. Rome, Italy: Gazzetta Ufficiale.

New Zealand

Education Act 1981. Wellington, Aotearoa New Zealand.
Education Amendment Act 1990. 1990 No. 60. Wellington, Aotearoa New Zealand.
Health Practitioners Competence Assurance Act 2003. Wellington, Aotearoa New Zealand.

REFERENCES

Akhtar, S. (2004, October). *Psychoanalysis and Eastern cultures: Adversaries or allies?* Paper presented at the American Psychiatric Association's Institute on Psychiatric Services, Atlanta, Georgia, USA.

Akhtar, S. & Tummala-Narra, P. (2005). Psychoanalysis in India. In S. Akhtar (Ed.), *Freud along the Ganges: Psychoanalytic reflections on the people and culture of India* (pp. 3–25). New York, NY: Other Press.

Alberding, B., Lauver, P., & Patnoe, J. (1993). Counselor awareness of the consequences of certification and licensure. *Journal of Counseling & Development*, 72, 33–38. DOI: 10.1002/j.1556–6676.1993.tb02273.x

Alexander, R. (1995). *Folie à deux: An experience of one to one therapy*. London, UK: Free Association Books.

Allen, J. R. & Allen, B. A. (1997). A new type of transactional analysis and one version of script work with a constructivist sensibility. *Transactional Analysis Journal*, 27(1), 89–98.

Allport, G. W. (1983). *Becoming: Basic considerations for a psychology of personality*. New Haven, NJ: Yale University Press. (Original work published 1955)

American Psychiatric Association (2000). *Diagnostic and Statistical Manual of Mental Disorders* (4th ed., text revision). Washington, DC: APA.

Angyal, A. (1941). *Foundations for a science of personality*. New York, NY: Commonwealth Fund.

Angyal, A. (1973). *Neurosis and treatment: A holistic theory*. New York, NY: Wiley. (Original work published 1965)

Antidote (2010). *About Antidote*. Retrieved from www.antidote.org.uk/about-us/our-history/

Antonovsky, A. (1979). *Health, stress and coping: New perspectives on mental and physical well-being*. San Francisco, CA: Jossey-Bass.

Antonovsky, A. (1987). The salutogenetic perspective: Toward a new view of health and illness. *Advances*, 4, 47.

Antonovsky, A. (1993). The structure and properties of the sense of coherence scale. *Social Science and Medicine*, 36, 725–733.

Argent, I. (2009). [Letter to the Editors]. *Transactional Analysis Journal*, 39(3), 262–263.

Aristotle. (1946). *Politica* (B. Jowett, Trans.; rev. ed.). Oxford, UK: Oxford University Press.

Aron, (1996). *A meeting of minds: Mutuality in psychoanalysis*. New York, NY: The Analytic Press.

Asay, T. P. & Lambert, M. J. (1999). The empirical case for the common factors in therapy: qualitative findings. In M. A. Hubble, B. L. Duncan & S. D. Miller (Eds.), *The heart and soul of change: What works in therapy* (pp. 33–36). Washington, DC: American Psychological Association.

Ascoli, U. (Ed.) (1984). *Welfare state all'Italiana* [The Italian welfare state]. Bari, Italy: Editori Laterza.

Audit Commission (1986). *Making a reality of community care*. London, UK: HMSO.

Aylward, J. (1999). The contributions of Paul Goodman to the clinical, social, and political implications of boundary disturbances. *Gestalt Review*, 3(2), 107–118.

Bachman, J. E. & O'Malley. P. M. (1977) Self-esteem in young men: A longitudinal analysis of the impact of educational and occupational attainment. *Journal of Personality and Social Psychology*, 35, 385–380.

Bailey, P. & Tudor, K. (2011). Letters across "the ditch": A trans Tasman correspondence about regulation and registration. In K. Tudor (Ed.), *The turning tide: Pluralism and partnership in psychotherapy in Aotearoa New Zealand* (pp. 77–95). Auckland, Aotearoa New Zealand: LC Publications.

Banton, R., Clifford, P., Frosh, S., Lousada, J., & Rosenthal, J. (1985). *The politics of mental health*. Basingstoke, UK: Macmillan.

Barclay, P. M. (1982). *Social workers: Their role and tasks*. London, UK: Bedford Square Press/National Council of Voluntary Organisations.

Barrett, M. (1980). *Women's oppression today*. London, UK: Verso.

Basaglia, F. (1968). *L'istituzione negata* [The denied institution]. Torino, Italy: Einaudi.

Basaglia, F. (1981). Breaking the circuit of control. In D. Ingleby (Ed.), *Critical psychiatry* (pp. 184–192). Harmondsworth, UK: Penguin.

Batts, V. (1982). Modern racism. *Transactional Analysis Journal*, 12(3), 207–209. DOI: 10.1177/036215378201200309

Baute, P. (1979). Intimacy and autonomy are not enough. (Is TA a middle-class tranquilizer?) *Transactional Analysis Journal*, 9(3), 170–173.

Bazzano, M. (2013). Togetherness: Intersubjectivity revisited. *Person-Centered & Experiential Psychotherapies*, 13(3), 203–216. DOI: 10.1080/14779757.2013.852613

Becker, T. (1985). Psychiatric reform in Italy: How does it work in Piedmont? *British Journal of Psychiatry*, 147, 254–260.

Benigni, B., Ciappi, F., Germano, G., & Martini, P. (1980). *Il Nuovo Servizio Psichiatrico*. [The New Psychiatric Service]. Rome, Italy: La Nuova Italia Scientifica.

Berne, E. (1963). *The structure and dynamics of organizations and groups*. New York, NY: Grove Press.

Berne, E. (1968). *Games people play: The psychology of human relationships*. Harmondsworth, UK: Penguin. (Original work published 1964)

Berne, E. (1971). *The mind in action*. New York, NY: Simon & Schuster. (Original work published 1947)

Berne, E. (1975a). *Transactional analysis in psychotherapy: A systematic individual and social psychiatry*. London, UK: Souvenir Press. (Original work published 1961)

Berne, E. (1975b). *What do you say after you say hello: The psychology of human destiny*. New York, NY: Grove Press. (Original work published 1972)

Berne, E. (1977). The nature of intuition. In *Intuition and ego states* (pp. 1–31). San Francisco, CA: TA Press. (Original work published 1949)

Bhugra, D. (1998). [Review of *Mental health promotion* by K. Tudor] *Behaviour Research and Therapy*, 36(2), 248–249.

Birtchnell, J. (1993). *How humans relate: A new interpersonal theory*. Westport, CT: Praeger.

Blair, T. (2005, 20 April). *The Paxman interviews* [Interview]. London, UK: British Broadcasting Company.

Boadella, D. (1985). *Wilhelm Reich*. London, UK: Arcana. (Original work published 1973)

Boal, A. (1979). *Theatre of the oppressed* (C. A. & M. L. McBride, Trans.). New York, NY: Urizen Books.

Bolton, G. (2001). *Reflective practice: Writing for professional development*. London, UK: Sage.

Boulton, M. (1978). The Nurturing Parent and social issues. *Transactional Analysis Journal*, 8(2), 117–120.

Bowen Center (2010). *Bowen theory*. Retrieved from www.thebowencenter.org/pages/theory.html.

Bowen, M. (1978). *Family therapy in clinical practice*. New York, NY: Jason Aronson.

Boyers, R. & Orrill, R. (Eds.) (1972). *Laing and anti-psychiatry*. Harmondsworth, UK: Penguin.

Bragg, B. (2006). *The progressive patriot: A search for belonging*. London, UK: Bantam Press.

Briggs, M. J. (2001). *Building on strengths: An innovative approach to developing a mental health promotion strategy for New Zealand*. Unpublished Master's thesis, University of East London, London, UK.

British Association for Counselling (1992). *Code of ethics and practice for counsellors*. Rugby, UK: BAC.

Broucek, F. J. (1982). Shame and its relationship to early narcissistic developments. *International Journal of Psycho-Analysis*. 63, 369–378.

Brown, K. (1979). *Towards a Marxist theory of personality*. Unpublished MA dissertation, University of Kent at Canterbury, Canterbury, UK.

Brown, K. & Tudor, K. (1981). Social work education and practice: Reform and revolution – a theory for change. *Contemporary Social Work Education*, 4, 101–112.

Bulhan, H. A. (1980). Fritz Fanon: The revolutionary psychiatrist. *Race and Class*, 21, 251–270.

Burrell, G. & Morgan, G. (1979). *Sociological paradigms and organisational analysis*. London, UK: Heinemann.

Buss, A. R. (1979). *A dialectical psychology*. Irvington, NY: Halstead Press.

Butler, D. & Butler, G. (2010). *Twentieth century British political facts*. Basingstoke, UK: Palgrave Macmillan.

Caldwell, L. (1986). Reproducers of the nation: Women and the family in fascist policy. In D. Forgacs (Ed.), *Rethinking Italian fascism*. London, UK: Lawrence & Wishart.

Came, H. & Tudor, K. (2016). Bicultural praxis: The relevance of Te Tiriti o Waitangi to health promotion internationally. *International Journal of Health Promotion and Education*, 54(2). DOI: 10.1080/14635240.2016.1156009

Cameron, R. (1997). The personal is political: Re-reading Rogers. *Person-Centred Practice*, 5(2), 16–20.

Campbell, P. (2000). Surviving social inclusion. In C. Newnes, G. Holmes & C. Dunn (Eds.), *This is madness too* (pp. 93–102). Ross-on-Wye: PCCS Books.

Caplan, R. (1986). *The implications of socio-theoretical constructs for the evaluation of health education theory*. Unpublished MSc dissertation, Kings College, University of London, London, UK.

Caplan, R. (1989). *Proposal for the establishment of a fellowship to investigate conceptual issues and implementation of community health promotion*. Paper available from the Health Education Authority, London, UK.

Carkhuff, R. R. (1967). *Beyond counseling and therapy*. New York, NY: Holt, Rinehart & Winston.

Cariapa, A. (2009). [Letter to the Editors]. *Transactional Analysis Journal*, 39(3), 263–264.

Carper, B. (1978). Fundamental ways of knowing in nursing. *Advances in Nursing Science*, 1(1), 13–23.

Carver, T. (1975). *Marx: Texts on method*. Oxford, UK: Blackwell.

Caspary, W. R. (1991). Carl Rogers – Values, persons, and politics: The dialectic of individual and community. *Journal of Humanistic Psychology*, 31(4), 8–31.

Cervi, B. (1990, 26 July). Election pandering. *Community Care*, p. 9.

Chaplin, J. (1988). *Feminist counselling in action*. London, UK: Sage.

Clare, S. & Tudor, K. (2016a). *Eco-friendly psychotherapy: Obstacles and solutions to practice*. Manuscript submitted for publication.

Clare, S. & Tudor, K. (2016b). *Interpreting the environment: A literature review and a contribution to pluralist research*. Manuscript submitted for publication.

Clarke, S., Hahn, H., & Hoggett, P. (2009). *Object relations and social relations*. London, UK: Karnac.

Clarkson, P. (1989). *Gestalt counselling in action*. London: Sage.

Clarkson, P. (1990). A multiplicity of psychotherapeutic relationships. *British Journal of Psychotherapy*, 7, 148163. DOI: 10.1111/j.1752-0118.1990.tb01329.x

Clarkson, P. (1992). In praise of speed, experimentation, agreeableness, endurance, and excellence: Counterscript drivers and aspiration. *Transactional Analysis Journal*, 22(1), 16–20. DOI: 10.1177/036215379202200103

Cohen, S. (1972). *Folk devils and moral panics: The creation of the Mods and Rockers*. London, UK: Routledge.

Collingwood, N. (1991). People and politics. *Self & Society*, 19(5), 2–6.

Comella, P. (2009 18–19 April). *Bowen's concept of societal emotional process*. Paper presented at the New England Seminar on Bowen Theory, Conference on Emotional Process in Society, Wooster, MA.

Connell, R. (2008). *Southern theory: The global dynamics of knowledge in social sciences*. Crows Nest, Australia: Allen & Unwin.

Cooper, M. (2005a). Therapists' experiences of relational depth: A qualitative interview study. *Counselling and Psychotherapy Research*, 5(2), 87–95. DOI: 10.1080/17441690500211130

Cooper, M. (2005b, October). Working at relational depth. *Therapy Today*, 16(8), 16–20.

Cooper, M. (Ed.) (2006). Relational depth [Special issue] *Person-Centered & Experiential Psychotherapies*, 5(4).

Cooper, M. & Ikemi, A. (2012). Dialogue: A dialogue between focusing and relational perspectives. *Person-Centered & Experiential Psychotherapies*, 11(2), 124–136.

Cornell, W. F. (1988). Life script theory: A critical review from a developmental perspective. *Transactional Analysis Journal*, 18(4), 270–282.

Cornell, W. F. (2000). If Berne met Winnicott: Transactional analysis and relational analysis. *Transactional Analysis Journal*, 30(4), 270–275.

Cornell, W. F. & Eusden, S. (Eds.) (2011). Dialogues on ethics [Special issue]. *Transactional Analysis Journal*, 41(2).

Cornell, B., Heathcote, A., & Heiller, B. (2008). [Letter to John Parr]. *Transactional Analysis Journal*, 38(3), 263.

Coward, R. & Ellis, J. (1977). *Language and materialism*. London, UK: Routledge & Kegan Paul.

Cox, S. (2009). Relational depth: Its relevance to a contemporary understanding of person-centred therapy. *Person-Centered & Experiential Psychotherapies*, 8(3), 208–223. DOI: 10.1080/14779757.2009.9688489

Craib, I. (1987). The psychodynamics of theory. *Free Associations*, 10, 32–56.

Craig, E. (1978). *The heart of the teacher: A heuristic study of the inner world of teaching*. Unpublished doctoral dissertation, Boston University, Boston, Massachusetts, USA.

Crepet, P. & De Plato, G. (1983). Psychiatry without asylums: Origins and prospects in Italy. *International Journal of Health Services*, 13, 119–129.

Creswell, J. W. (2007). *Qualitative inquiry and research design: Choosing among five approaches* (2nd ed.). Thousand Oaks, CA: Sage.

Davies, D. & Neal, C. (Eds.) (1996). *Pink therapy*. Buckingham, UK: Open University Press.

Davies, D. & Neal, C. (Eds.) (2000). *Pink therapy. Vol. 2: Therapeutic perspectives on working with lesbian, gay and bisexual clients*. Buckingham, UK: Open University Press.

Davies, M. (1990, 21 June). When in Rome.... *The Health Service Journal*, 915.

Dawes, R. M. (1994). *House of cards: Psychology and psychotherapy built on myth*. New York, NY: Free Press.

Del Giudice, G., Evaristo, P., & Reali, M. (n.d.). *Can mental hospitals be phased out?* Unpublished paper, Trieste, Italy.

Dell'Acqua, G. & Mezzina, R. (n.d.). *La storia, il soggetto, la capacita de intendere e di volere*. [A person's history, self and the full possession of their faculties]. Unpublished manuscript, Trieste, Italy.

Dell'Acqua, G., Mezzina, R., & Cogliati, M.G. (1986, June). *Lesioni e minacce alla salute psichica nella "carrierra" del malato di mente*. [Injuries and threats to mental health of the psychiatric patient]. Paper presented at an international conference, Trieste, Italy.

Denman, J. & McDonald, P. (1996). Unemployment statistics from 1881 to the present day. *Labour Market Trends*, 5–18.

Department of Health (1989). *Caring for people*. London, UK: HMSO.

Department of Health (1990, May). *Specific grant for provision of social care for people with a mental illness*. Draft Health/Local Authority Circular. Not paginated.

Department of Health (1992). *The health of the nation*. London, UK: DoH.

Department of Health (1993). *The health of the nation: key area handbook mental illness*. London, UK: DoH.
Department of Health (1999a). *National service framework for mental health*. London, UK: DoH.
Department of Health (1999b). *Our healthier nation*. London, UK: DoH.
Department of Health (2001). *Making it happen*. London, UK: DoH.
Department of Health (2011). *Enabling excellence: Autonomy and accountability for healthcare workers, social workers and social care workers*. London, UK: DoH.
Department of Health and Social Security (1983, March). *Health Service Development Care in the Community and Joint Finance* DHSS HC(83)8 LAC (83)5. London, UK: HMSO.
Department of Health and Social Security (1983, April). *Treatment and rehabilitation: Report of the Advisory Council on the Misuse of Drugs (ACMD)*; Central Funding Initiative DHSS HN(83)13 LASSL (83)1. London, UK: HMSO.
Department of Health and Social Security (1986). *Health and personal social services statistics for England*. London, UK: HMSO.
Dillon, G. (2011). The road to registration: The New Zealand Association of Psychotherapists and its long search for identity and recognition through legislation. In K. Tudor (Ed.), *The turning tide: Pluralism and partnership in psychotherapy in Aotearoa New Zealand* (pp. 31–38). Auckland, Aotearoa New Zealand: LC Publications.
Director-General of Health (2009). *Review of the Health Practitioners Competence Assurance Act 2003. Wellington, Aotearoa New Zealand: Ministry of Health*. Retrieved from www.moh.govt.nz/moh.nsf/pagesmh/9103/$File/report-minister-hpca-jun09.pdf.
Donovan, A. & Oddy, M. (1982). Psychological aspects of unemployment: An investigation into the emotional and social adjustment of school leavers. *Journal of Adolescence*, *5*, 15–30.
Douglass, B. & Moustakas, C. (1985). Heuristic enquiry: The internal search to know. *Journal of Humanistic Psychology*, *25*(1), 39–55.
Downey, R. (1990, 12 July). Ready, steady – stop? *Social Work Today*.
Doyal, L. & Pennell, I. (1979). *The political economy of health*. London, UK: Pluto.
Doyle, R. (1989). A meeting of minds. *The Health Service Journal*, 1407.
Duff, K. (1993). *The alchemy of illness*. London, UK: Virago.
Durie, M. (1998). *Te mana, te kāwanatanga: The politics of Māori self-determination*. Auckland, Aotearoa New Zealand: Oxford University Press.
Durie, M. (2001). *Mauri ora: The dynamics of Māori health*. Auckland, Aotearoa New Zealand: Auckland University Press.
Durie, M. (2011, 24 August). *Ecoconnectedness and identity: Land, territory and psychotherapy*. Keynote speech at World Council for Psychotherapy 6th International Congress, Sydney, Australia.
Dylan, B. (1964). With God on our side. From B. Dylan, *The times they are a changin'* [Album]. New York, NY: Columbia Records.
Dylan, B. (1974). When you see her say hello. From B. Dylan, *Blood on the tracks* [Album]. New York, NY: Columbia Records.
Editorial (1980, 5 June). Parents warn of young glue sniffers [Editorial]. *Shepherds Bush Gazette & Hammersmith Post*, p. 3.
Edleson, M. (1970). *Sociotherapy and psychotherapy*. Chicago, MI: University of Chicago Press.
Eisner, E. W. (1991). *The enlightened eye*. New York, NY: Macmillan.
Ellingham, I. (2011). Carl Rogers' fateful wrong move in the direction of Rogerian relational therapy: Retitling "relational therapy" "non-directive therapy". *Person-Centered & Experiential Psychotherapies*, 10(3), 181–197. DOI: 10.1080/14779757.2011.599515
Embleton Tudor, L. (2011). The neuroscience and politics of regulation. In K. Tudor (Ed.), *The turning tide: Pluralism and partnership in psychotherapy in Aotearoa New Zealand* (pp. 167–176). Auckland, Aotearoa New Zealand: LC Publications.
Embleton Tudor, L. & Tudor, K. (1994). The personal and the political: Power, influence and authority in psychotherapy. In P. Clarkson & M. Pokorney (Eds.), *The handbook of psychotherapy* (pp. 384–402). London, UK: Routledge.

Embleton Tudor, L. & Tudor, K. (1997, September). *Sharing life therapy*. Presentation at Ten Years On International Conference on the Person-Centred Approach, University of Sheffield.
Embleton Tudor, L. & Tudor, K. (2009). Past present: Person-centred therapy with trauma and enactment. In D. Mann & V. Cunningham (Eds.), *The past in the present: Therapy enactments and the return of trauma* (pp. 136–154). London, UK: Routledge.
Embleton Tudor, L., Keemar, K., Tudor, K., Valentine, J., & Worrall, M. (2004). *The person-centred approach: A contemporary introduction*. Basingstoke, UK: Palgrave.
Engels, F. (1972). *The origin of the family, private property and the state*. London, UK: Lawrence & Wishart. (Original work published 1884)
Erikson, E. (1950). *Childhood and society*. New York, NY: Norton.
Erikson, E. (1956). The problem of ego identity. *Journal of American Psychoanalytic Association*, 4, 58–12.
Erikson, E. (1968). *Identity, youth and crisis*. New York, NY: Norton.
Ernst, F. Jr. (1971). The OK corral: The grid for Get-on-With. *Transactional Analysis Journal*, 1(4), 33–42. DOI: 10.1177/036215377100100409
Esterson, A. (1970). *Leaves of spring*. Harmondsworth: Penguin.
Etherington, K. (2004). *Becoming a reflexive researcher: Using our selves in research*. London, UK: Jessica Kingsley.
European Association for Transactional Analysis (2008). *Ethics and professional practice*. Retrieved from www.eatanews.org/pdf%20documents/June%2008%20final%20 ethics%20statement.pdf.
Fanon, F. (1963). *The wretched of the earth* (C. Farrington, Trans.). New York, NY: Grove Press (Original work published 1961)
Fay, J. (2008). Conservative, liberal and radical psychotherapy. *Forum* [The Journal of the New Zealand Association of Psychotherapists], 14, 103–110.
Fay, J. (2016). Decolonising mental health services one prejudice at a time: Psychological, sociological, ecological, and cultural considerations. *Settler Colonial Studies*. DOI: org/ 10.1080/2201473X.2016.1199828
Fernando, S. (1988). *Race and culture in psychiatry*. Beckenham, UK: Croom Helm.
Ferrera, M. (1980, 25–30 March). *The crisis of the Italian Welfare State*. A paper presented at the ECPR Joint Sessions of Workshops "A crisis of the European Welfare States?", Florence, Italy.
Feuerbach, L. (1854). *The essence of Christianity* (M. A. Evans, Trans.). London, UK: John Chapman. (Original work published 1841)
Fife, B. (1997). *The healing crisis*. Colorado Springs, CO: Piccadilly Books.
Finch, J. (1986, Summer). Community care and the invisible welfare state. *Radical Community Medicine*, 15–22.
Foreman, A. (1977). *Femininity as alienation*. London, UK: Pluto.
Foulkes, S. H. (1975). *Group analytic psychotherapy: Method and principles*. London, UK: Gordon & Breech, Science Publishers Ltd.
Fox, N. J. (1999). *Beyond health: Postmodernism and embodiment*. London, UK: Free Association Books.
Francis, E., David, J., Johnson, N., & Sashidharan, S.P. (1989). Black people and psychiatry in the UK. *Psychiatric Bulletin*, 13, 482–485.
Freire, P. (1972). *Pedagogy of the oppressed*. Harmondsworth, UK: Penguin.
French, J. & Adams, L. (1986). From analysis to synthesis. Theories of health education. *Health Education Journal*, 45, 71–74.
Freud, S. (1959). The question of lay analysis: Conversations with an impartial person. In *The standard edition of the complete psychological works of Sigmund Freud, Vol XX* (J. Strachey, Trans. & Ed.; pp. 177–250). London, UK: The Hogarth Press/The Institute of Psycho-Analysis. (Original work published 1926)
Freud, S. (1961). Civilization and its discontents. In *The standard edition of the complete psychological works of Sigmund Freud, Vol. XXI* (J. Strachey, Trans. & Ed.; pp. 59–148). London, UK: Hogarth Press and Institute of Psycho-Analysis. (Original work published 1930)
Freud, S. (1984). Formulations on the two principles of mental functioning. In A. Richards (Ed.), *Beyond the pleasure principle* (J. Strachey, Trans. & Ed.). Harmondsworth, UK: Penguin. (Original work published 1911)

Friedli, L. (2009). *Mental health, resilience and inequalities.* Copenhagen, Denmark: World Health Organization.
Friend, A. & Metcalf, A. (1981). *Slump city: The politics of mass unemployment.* London, UK: Pluto Press.
Fromm, E. (1971). *The crisis of psychoanalysis.* London, UK: Cape.
Gabbard, G. O. (1989). Two subtypes of narcissistic personality disorder. *Bulletin of the Menninger Clinic*, 53, 527–532.
Gabbard, G. O. (1990). *Psychodynamic psychiatry in clinical practice.* Washington, DC: American Psychiatric Press.
Gabriel, S. (1987). *The schizophrenic label and Afro-Caribbeans in Britain: Diagnosis or misdiagnosis?* Unpublished manuscript available from the Bristol Inner City Mental Health Project, The Manse, Conduit Place, St Werburgh's, Bristol, UK.
Gaglio, A. & Sarli, E. (1977). Bisogni e practica psichiatrica. [Needs and psychiatric practice]. *Aut-Aut*, 162, 61–74.
Gallio (1983). La memoria del manicome. Fasi della de-intitutionalizzazione: Alune parole-ciave. [The memory of illness. Phases of de-institutionalisation: A few key word]. In G. Gallio, M. G. Giannichedda, O. De Leonardis, & D. Mauri *La libertà é terapeutica. L'esperienza psichiatrica di Trieste* (pp. 17–60), Milano, Italia: Feltrinelli.
Gardner, H. (1993). *Frames of mind: the theory of multiple intelligences* (2nd ed.). London, UK: Fontana Press.
Gellert, S. D. (1975). Drivers. *Transactional Analysis Journal*, 5(4), 422–425. DOI: 10.1177/036215377500500425
Gelso, C. J. & Carter, J. A. (1985). The relationship in counseling and psychotherapy: Components, consequences and theoretical antecedents. *The Counseling Psychologist*, 13(2), 115–243. DOI: 10.1177/0011000085132001
Gendlin, E. (1961). Experiencing: A variable in the process of therapeutic change. *American Journal of Psychotherapy*, 15, 233–245.
Gendlin, E. (1978). *Focusing.* New York, NY: Bantam.
Giesekus, U. & Mente, A. (1986). Client empathic understanding in client-centered therapy. *Person-Centered Review*, 1(2), 163–171.
Gillon, E. (2007). *Person-centred counselling psychology.* London: Sage.
Goldberg, D. & Hillier, V. (1979). A scaled version of the General Health Questionnaire. *Psychological Medicine*, 9(1), 139–145.
Goldstein, K. (1995). *The organism.* New York, NY: Zone Books. (Original work published 1934)
Goleman, D. (1996). *Emotional intelligence: Why it can matter more than IQ.* London, UK: Bloomsbury.
Goulding, M. M. & Goulding, R. L. (1979). *Changing lives through redecision therapy.* New York, NY: Brunner/Mazel.
Goulding, R. (1974). Thinking and feeling in psychotherapy: Three impasses. *Voices*, 10(1), 11–13.
Goulding, R. L. & Goulding, M. M. (1976). Injunctions, decisions, and redecisions. *Transactional Analysis Journal*, 6(1), 41–48. DOI: 10.1177/036215377600600110
Graham, H. (1992). Imaginative assessment of personal health needs. In D.R. Trent (Ed.), *Promotion of mental health. Vol. 1* (pp. 53–62). Aldershot, UK: Avebury.
Green, S. & Tudor, K. (Eds.), Dillon, G., Duncan, A., Fay, J., Land, C., Morice, M. P., & Woodard, W. (2014). Ngā Ao e Rua | The two worlds: Psychotherapy, biculturalism, and professional development in Aotearoa New Zealand. *Psychotherapy & Politics International*, 12(2), 129–150.
Greenberg, J. & Mitchell, S. A. (1983). *Object relations in psychoanalytic theory.* Cambridge, MA: Harvard University Press.
Griffiths, R. (1988). *Community care: Agenda for action.* London, UK: HMSO.
Groder, M. (1977). Asklepieion: An integration of psychotherapies. In G. Barnes (Ed.), *TA after Eric Berne* (pp.134–137). New York, NY: Harper & Row.
Grof, C. (1993). *The thirst for wholeness: Attachment, addiction, and the spiritual path.* San Francisco, CA: Harper.

Gross, S. J. (1978). The myth of professional licensing. *American Psychologist*, 33, 1009–1016. DOI: 10.1037/0003-066X.33.11.1009

Gurney, R. M. (1980). Does unemployment affect the self-esteem of school leavers? *Australian Journal of Psychology*, 32(3), 175–182. DOI: 10.1080/00049538008254687

Hagehülsmann, H. (1984). The "Menschenbild" in transactional analysis: Conceptions of human nature. In E. Stern (Ed.), *TA: The state of the art. A European contribution* (pp. 39–59). Dordrecht, The Netherlands: Foris Publications.

Hall, A., Morice, M. P., & Wilson, C. (2011). Waka Oranga: The development of an indigenous professional organisation within a psychotherapeutic discourse in Aotearoa New Zealand. *Psychotherapy and Politics International*, 10(1), 7–16.

Hargaden, H. & Sills, C. (2002). *Transactional analysis: A relational perspective.* Hove, UK: BrunnerRoutledge.

Harré, R. (1983). *Personal being*. Oxford, UK: Blackwell.

Harris, T. (1990, 10 January). Time to change the record. *Insight*, p. 8.

Harrison, G., Owens, D., Holton, A., Neilson, D., & Boot, D. (1988). A prospective study of severe mental disorder in Afro-Caribbean patients. *Psychological Medicine*, 18, 3, 643–657. DOI: 10.1017/S0033291700008321

Hartley, J. (1980). Psychological approaches to unemployment. *Bulletin of the British Psychological Society*, 33, 412–414.

Hartmann, H. (1942). Psycho-analysis and the concept of health. *International Journal of Psycho-Analysis*, 20, 308–321.

Hartmann, H. (1958). *Ego psychology and the problem of adaptation*. London, UK: Imago. (Original work published 1939)

Hathaway, S. R. & McKinley, J. C. (1970). *The Minnesota multiphasic personality inventory manual.* New York, NY: Psychological Corporation. (Original work published 1940)

Hazell, J. W. (1989). Drivers as mediators of stress responses. *Transactional Analysis Journal*, 19(4), 212–223. DOI: 10.1177/036215378901900406

Health Professions Council (2009). *The statutory regulation of psychotherapists and counsellors. Consultation on the recommendations of the psychotherapists and counsellors professional liaison group. Appendix 2: Standards of proficiency for psychotherapists and counsellors – Draft for consultation.* Retrieved from www.hpc-uk.org/assets/documents/100029C2Draftstandardsofproficiencyforcounsellorsandpsychotherapists.pdf.

Heathcote, A. (2008). Letter from the Coeditor. *Transactional Analysis Journal*, 38(1), 2–4.

Heginbotham, C. (1984, 20 February). Lessons from the Italian school. *Social Work Today*, p. 18.

Heginbotham, C. (1990, 31 January). A classic example. *Insight*, p. 25.

Heron, J. (1997). A self-generating practitioner community. In. R. House & N. Totton (Eds.), *Implausible professions: Arguments for pluralism and autonomy in psychotherapy and counselling* (pp. 241–254). Ross-on-Wye, UK: PCCS Books.

Herrman, H., Saxena, S., & Moodie, R. (Eds.) (2005). *Promoting mental health: Concepts, emerging evidence, practice.* Geneva, Switzerland: World Health Organization.

Heyward, C. (1993). *When boundaries betray us: Beyond illusions of what is ethical in therapy and life.* San Francisco, CA: Harper.

Higgins, R. (1996). *Approaches to research.* London, UK: Jessica Kingsley.

Hillman, J. & Ventura, M. (1992). *We've had a hundred years of psychotherapy and the world's getting worse.* San Francisco, CA: Harper.

Hilton, J. & Canavan, S. (2008). *Embodied relating: Perspectives on the landscape of relational depth.* Unpublished manuscript.

Hogan, D. B. (1979). *The regulation of psychotherapists* (Vol. 1–4). Cambridge, MA: Ballinger.

Holland, R. (1981). From perspectives to reflexivity. In H. Bonarius, R. Holland & S. Rosenberg (Eds.), *Personal construct psychology: Recent advances in theory and practice* (pp. 23–29). London, UK: Macmillan.

Holland, R. (1987). *Experiments in perfectly reflexive teaching: The sociology of knowledge and science.* Unpublished manuscript, University of London, Kings College, Centre for Environmental Studies, London, UK.

Holland, R. (1988). *Sociopsychological studies: Course S3*. Document available from the Management Centre, King's College, University of London, London, UK.

Holland, R. (1990a). Scientificity and psychoanalysis: Insights from the controversial discussions. *The International Review of Psycho-Analysis*, 17, 133–158.

Holland, R. (1990b). The paradigm plague: prevention, cure and inoculation. *Human Relations*, 1, 23–48.

Holland, R. (1992). Sanity, necessary complexities and mental health promotion. *Changes*, 10, 136–145.

Holland, R. (1999). Reflexivity. *Human Relations*, 52(4), 463–484.

Holland, S. (1979). The development of an action and counselling service in a deprived urban area. In M. Meacher (Ed.), *New methods of mental health care* (pp. 95–106). London, UK: Pergamon.

Holland, S. (1985, June). *Loss, rage and oppression. Neighbourhood psychotherapy with working class, black and national minority women.* Paper presented at the Pam Smith Memorial Lecture, Polytechnic of North London.

Holland, S. (1988). Defining and experimenting with prevention. In S. Ramon & M.G. Giannichedda (Eds.), *Psychiatry in transition* (pp. 125–137). London, UK: Pluto Press.

Holland, S. (1990). Psychotherapy, oppression and social action: gender, race and class in black women's depression. In R. Perelberg & A. Miller (Eds.), *Gender and power in families* (pp. 256–269). London, UK: Routledge.

Holland, S. & Hoggett, P. (1977). People's aid and action centre. *Humpty Dumpty Radical Psychology Magazine*, 8, 18–23.

House, R. (2003). *Therapy beyond modernity: Deconstructing and transcending profession-centred therapy*. London, UK: Karnac.

House, R. (2009). The PLG's proposals for the statutory regulation of counselling & psychotherapy. In D. Postle & R. House (Eds.), *Compliance? Ambivalence? Rejection? Nine papers challenging the health professions council proposals for the state regulation of the psychological therapies* (pp. 93–123). London, UK: Wentworth Learning Resources/eIpnosis.

House, R. & Totton, N. (Eds.) (1997). *Implausible professions: Arguments for pluralism and autonomy in psychotherapy and counselling*. Ross-on-Wye, UK: PCCS Books.

House, R. & Totton, N. (Eds.) (2011). *Implausible professions: Arguments for pluralism and autonomy in psychotherapy and counselling* (extended 2nd ed.). Ross-on-Wye, UK: PCCS Books.

Howell, J. (1981). Big Flame: resituating socialist strategy and organisation. In R. Miliband & J. Saville (Eds.), *Socialist register, Vol. 18* (pp. 207–220). London, UK: Merlin Press.

Hunt, J., Leaman, R., Tudor, K., & White, J. (1988). *Disability in Cuba: Cuba Rehabilitation Study Tour 1985*. Report available from Britain–Cuba Resource Centre, c/o CARILA, 29 Islington Park Street, London N1 1QB, UK.

Illich, I. (1978). *The right to useful unemployment and its professional enemies*. London, UK: Marion Boyars.

Institute of Transactional Analysis (2013). *Code of practice for psychotherapy trainers and training establishments*. Cambridge, UK: ITA.

International Transactional Analysis Association (2010). *Transactional analysis*. Retrieved from www.itaa-net.org/ta/index.htm.

Ioane, J. & Tudor, K. (2016). *The Fa'ásamoa, person-centred theory, and cross-cultural practice*. Manuscript submitted for publication.

Jacobs, A. (1987). Autocratic power. *Transactional Analysis Journal*, 17(1), 59–71. DOI: 10.1177/036215378701700303

Jacobs, A. (1990). Nationalism. *Transactional Analysis Journal*, 20(4), 221–228. DOI: 10.1177/036215379002000403

Jacobs, A. (1991). Autocracy: Groups, organizations, nations, and players. *Transactional Analysis Journal*, 21(4), 199–206. DOI: 10.1177/036215379102100402

Jacobs, A. (1996). Strength without justice. *Transactional Analysis Journal*, 26(3), 206–213.

Jacobs, A. (1997). Eric Berne memorial award speech: Transactional analysis and social applications. *Transactional Analysis Journal*, 27(1), 11–14. DOI: 10.1177/036215379702700105

Jacoby, R. (1977). *Social amnesia*. Hassocks, UK: Harvester.

Jaggi, M. (1977). *Red Bologna*. Littlehampton, UK: Littlehampton Books Services.

Jahoda, M. (1958). *Current concepts of positive mental health*. New York, NY: Basic Books.

Jahoda, M. (1979). The impact of unemployment in the 1930s and the 1970s. *Bulletin of the British Psychological Society*, 32, 309–314.

James, N. (1989). Emotional labour: Skill and work in the social regulation of feelings. *Sociological Review*, 37(1), 15–42.

Janis, I. L. (1972). *Victims of groupthink*. New York, NY: Houghton Mifflin.

Jefferson, T. (2005). *Light and liberty: Reflections on the pursuit of happiness* (E. S. Petersen, Ed.). New York, NY: The Modern Library. (Original work published 1791)

Johns, C. (1995). Framing learning through reflection within Carper's fundamental ways of knowing in nursing. *Journal of Advanced Nursing*, 22(2), 226–234.

Johnson, S. M. (1994). *Character styles*. New York, NY: Norton.

Joines, V. & Stewart, I. (2002). *Personality adaptations: A new guide to understanding psychotherapy and counselling*. Nottingham, UK: Lifespace Publishing.

Jones, J. M. (1972). *Prejudice and racism*. Reading, MA: Addison-Wesley.

Jones, K. & Poletti, A. (1984, 4 October). The mirage of reform. *New Society*, 147(2), 10–12.

Jones, K. & Poletti, A. (1985). Understanding the Italian experience. *British Journal of Psychiatry*, 147, 341–347.

Jordan, J. V., Kaplan, A. G., Baker Miller, J., Stiver, I. P., & Surrey, J. (1991). *Women's growth in connection. Writings from the Stone Centre*. New York, NY: Guilford Press.

Jordan, J. V., Walker, M., & Harling, L. M. (Eds.) (2004). *The complexity of connection. Writings from the Stone Center's Jean Baker Miller Training Institute*. New York, NY: Guilford Press.

Joubert, N. & Raeburn, J. (1998). Mental health promotion: People, power and passion. *International Journal of Mental Health Promotion*, 1(1), 15–22.

Jourard, S. (1971). *Self-disclosure*. London, UK: John Wiley & Sons.

Jung, C. G. (1959). The concept of the collective unconscious. In *The collected works of C. G. Jung* (Vol. 9, pp. 42–53; R. F. C. Hull, Trans.). Princeton, NJ: Princeton University Press. (Original work published 1936)

Kahler, T. (1974). [Letter to the Editor]. *Transactional Analysis Journal*, 4(4), 64. DOI: 10.1177/036215377400400419

Kahler, T. (1975). In response. *Transactional Analysis Journal*. 5(4), 425–428. DOI: 10.1177/036215377500500426

Kahler, T. (1979). *Process therapy in brief*. Little Rock, AR: Human Development Publications.

Kahler, T. I. (2008). [Letter to the Editors]. *Transactional Analysis Journal*, 38(3), 258–259.

Kahler, T. & Capers, H. (1974). The miniscript. *Transactional Analysis Journal*, 4(1), 26–42. DOI: 10.1177/036215377400400110

Kareem, J. (1992). The Nafsiyat intercultural therapy centre: Ideas and experience in intercultural therapy. In J. Kareem & R. Littlewood (Eds.), *Intercultural therapy* (pp. 14–37). Oxford, UK: Blackwell Scientific Publications.

Karpman, S. (2008). [Letter to the Editors]. *Transactional Analysis Journal*, 38(3), 259.

Kearney, A. (1996). *Counselling, class and politics*. Manchester, UK: PCCS Books.

Kearney, A. (1997). Class, politics and the training of counsellors. *Person-Centred Practice*, 5(2), 11–15.

Keay, D. (1987, 31 October). AIDS, education and the year 2000 [Interview with Margaret Thatcher]. *Women's Own*, pp. 8–10.

Keyes, C. L. M. (2007). Promoting and protecting mental health as flourishing: A complementary strategy for improving national mental health. *American Psychologist*, 62(2), 95–108.

Kickbush, I. (1989). Healthy cities: A working project and a growing movement. *Health Promotion*, 4(1), 77–89.

King, L. & Moutsou, C. (2010). *Rethinking audit cultures: A critical look at evidence-based practice in psychotherapy and beyond*. Ross-on-Wye, UK: PCCS Books.
Kirsner, D. (2000). *Unfree associations: Inside psychoanalytic institutes*. London, UK: Process Press.
Klein, M. (1985). Ten personality types. *Transactional Analysis Journal*, 15(3), 224–231. DOI: 10.1177/036215378501500308
Knight, M. (1961). *Humanist anthology*. London, UK: Barrie & Rockliff.
Knox, R. (2008). Clients' experiences of relational depth in person-centred counselling. *Counselling and Psychotherapy Research*, 8(3), 182–188. DOI: 10.1080/14733140802035005
Knox, R. & Cooper, M. (2010). Relationship qualities that are associated with moments of relational depth. *Person-Centered & Experiential Psychotherapies*, 9(3), 236–256.
Kohut, H. (1971). *The analysis of the self: A systematic approach to the psychoanalytic treatment of narcissistic personality disorders*. New York, NY: International Universities Press.
Komiya, N. & Tudor, K. (2016). "Reading the air", finding common ground: Reconsidering Rogers' therapeutic conditions as a framework for understanding therapy in Japan. *Asia Pacific Journal of Counselling & Psychotherapy*, 17(1&2), 26–38.
Koocher, G. (1979). Credentialing in psychology: Close encounters with competence? *American Psychologist*, 34, 696–702. DOI: 10.1037/0003-066X.34.8.696
Kovel, J. (1981). *The age of desire: Case histories of a radical psychoanalyst*. New York, NY: Pantheon Books.
Kuhn, T. (1996). *The structure of scientific revolutions*. Chicago, IL: University of Chicago Press. (Original work published 1962)
Kunnes, R. (1971). How to be a radical therapist. In The Radical Therapist Collective. *The radical therapist* (J. Agel, Ed.; pp. 27–34). New York, NY: Ballantine Books.
Kupers, T. (1971). Radical therapy needs revolutionary theory. In The Radical Therapist Collective. *The radical therapist* (J. Agel, Ed.; pp. 35–46). New York, NY: Ballantine Books.
Lago, C. (1994). The need for connectedness and community: Therapy for a masturbatory society. *Counselling*, 5(2), 120–124.
Laing, R. (1967). *The politics of experience*. Harmondsworth, UK: Penguin.
Lalonde, M. (1975). *A new perspective on the health of Canadans*. Ottawa, Canada: Information Canada.
Lasch, C. (1979). *Culture of narcissism: American life in an age of diminishing expectations*. New York, NY: Warner Books.
Lather, P. (1993). Fertile obsession: Validity after poststructuralism. *Sociological Quarterly*, 34(4), 673–693.
Lees, J. (2009). *Revisions required by examination board following an oral examination*. [Form RD (E-Revs) 2003 to the candidate]. Middlesex University, London, UK.
Lees, J. (2010). *Further revisions required by examination board following an oral examination*. [E-mail to the candidate]. Middlesex University, London, UK.
Leonard, P. (1984). *Personality and ideology*. Basingstoke, UK: Macmillan.
LeVine, R. A. (1990). Infant environments in psychoanalysis: A cross-cultural view. In J. W. Stigler, R. A. Shweder & G. Herdt (Eds.), *Cultural psychology* (pp. 454–476). Cambridge, UK: Cambridge University Press.
Lewin, K. (1952). *Field theory in social science*. London, UK: Tavistock.
Lincoln, Y. S. & Guba, E. G. (1985). *Naturalistic inquiry*. Newbury Park, CA: Sage.
Lindner, R. (1953). *Prescription for rebellion*. London, UK: Gollancz.
Littlewood, R. & Cross, S. (1980). Ethnic minorities and psychiatric services. *Sociology of Health and Illness*, 2, 194–201.
Littlewood, R. & Lipsedge, M. (1982). *Aliens and alienists: Ethnic minorities and psychiatry*. Harmondsworth, UK: Penguin.
Lomas, P. (1987). *The limits of interpretation*. Harmondsworth, UK: Penguin.
Lotringer, S. & Marazzi, C. (1980). *Autonomia: Post-political politics*. New York, NY: Semiotext(e).

Luft, J. & Ingham, H. (1955). The Johari window, a graphic model of interpersonal awareness. In *Proceedings of the Western Training Laboratory in Group Development.* Los Angeles, CA: University of California Los Angeles.
Lukács, G. (1971). *History and class consciousness.* London, UK: Merlin.
Lukas, E. (1989, June). *From self-actualization to global responsibility.* Paper presented at the Seventh World Congress of Logotherapy, Kansas City, Kansas, USA.
McCarraher, L. & Daniels, L. (2000). *The work-life manual.* London, UK: The Industrial Society.
McCarraher, L. & Daniels, L. (2002). *The book of balanced living.* London, UK: The Work Foundation.
McCartney, P. (1970). Get back. On *Let it be* [Album]. London, UK: Apple.
McCulloch, G. (1999). Strategic approaches in Sheffield. Regeneration and mental health. *Briefing,* 1, 5.
McCulloch, G. F. & Boxer, J. (1997). *Mental health promotion: Policy, practice and partnerships.* London, UK: Baillière Tindall.
McDonald, G. & O'Hara, K. (1998). *Ten elements of mental health, its promotion and demotion: Implications for practice.* London, UK: Society of Health Promotion Specialists.
McMillan, M. & McLeod, J. (2006). Letting go: The client's experience of relational depth. *Person-Centered & Experiential Psychotherapies,* 5(4), 277–292. DOI: 10.1080/14779757.2006.9688419
McNulty, M. (1997). Promoting mental health. [Review of *Mental health promotion* by K. Tudor] *British Journal of Guidance & Counselling,* 25(1), 119–121.
Macleod, A. & McSherry, B. (2007). Regulating mental healthcare practitioners: Towards a standardised and workable framework. *Psychiatry, Psychology and Law,* 14(1), 45–55. DOI: 10.1375/pplt.14.1.45
Mahler, M. S., Pine, F., & Bergman, A. (1973). *The psychological birth of the human infant.* New York, NY: Basic Books.
Main, T. (1946). The hospital as a therapeutic institution. *Bulletin of the Menninger Clinic,* 10, 66–70.
Manning, N. (1979). *Therapeutic communities.* London, UK: Routledge & Kegan Paul.
Manning, S. (Ed.) (2006, August). *Registration* [Theme issue]. *NZAP Newsletter.*
Maranesi, T. & Piazza, A. (1986, September). Dossier: Dopo la 180 I dati della prima indagine sull'assistenza psichiatrica in Italia. [Dossier: After Law 180 The data from the first research on psychiatric welfare in Italy]. *Scienza Experienza,* 17–21.
Marcelloni, M. (1979). Urban movements and political struggle in Italy. *International Journal of Urban and Regional Research,* 3(2), 251–268.
Marcuse, H. (1968). *One dimensional man.* London, UK: Routledge & Kegan Paul.
Marcuse, H. (1969). *Eros and civilisation.* London, UK: Allen Lane.
Marks, D. F. (Ed.) (2002). *The health psychology reader.* London, UK: Sage.
Martin, P. (2011, 25 August). Indigenous population still falling through the gap. *Sydney Morning Herald.* Retrieved from http://www.smh.com.au/national/indigenous-population-still-falling-through-gap-20110824-1jadq.html.
Marx, K. (1962). *Capital: A critique of political economy.* Vol. III (F. Engels, Ed., S. Moore & E. Aveling, Trans.) Moscow, USSR: Progress. (Original work published 1894)
Marx, K. (1971). *Grundisse.* Harmondsworth, UK: Penguin (Original work published 1858)
Marx, K. (1975a). Economic and philosophical manuscripts. In L. Colletti (Ed.), *Karl Marx. Early writings* (G. Benton, Trans.; pp. 279–400). Harmondsworth, UK: Penguin. (Original work published 1832)
Marx, K. (1975b). Theses on Feuerbach. In L. Colletti (Ed.), *Karl Marx. Early writings* (G. Benton , Trans.; pp. 421–423). Harmondsworth, UK: Penguin. (Original work published 1888)
Marx, K. & Engels, F. (1964). *The German ideology.* London, UK: Lawrence & Wishart. (Original work published 1846)
Massey, R. (1996). Transactional analysis as a social psychology. *Transactional Analysis Journal.* 26(1), 91–99. DOI: 10.1177/036215379602600114

Masterson, L. F. (1988). *The search for the real self: Unmasking the personality disorders of our age*. New York, NY: The Free Press.

Matthews, F. (1991). *The ecological self*. London, UK: Routledge.

Maturana, H. (1995). *The nature of time*. Retrieved, 30 June, 2011, from www.inteco.cl/biology/nature.htm.

Mead, G. (1980). *The philosophy of the present* (A. E. Murphy, Ed.). Chicago, IL: University of Chicago Press. (Original work published 1932)

Mearns, D. (1996). Working at relational depth with clients in person-centred therapy. *Counselling*, 7(4), 306–311.

Mearns, D. (1998, 11 December). *Person-centred therapy with configurations of the self*. Public Lecture, Athens, Greece.

Mearns, D. (1999). Person-centred therapy with configurations of the self. *Counselling*, 10(2), 125–130.

Mearns, D. & Cooper, M. (2005). *Working at relational depth in counselling and psychotherapy*. London, UK: Sage.

Mearns, D. & Thorne, B. (2000). *Person-centred therapy today: New frontiers in theory and practice*. London, UK: Sage.

Mearns, D. & Thorne, B. (2007). *Person-centred counselling in action*. London, UK: Sage.

Mebane-Francescato, D. & Jones, S. (1973). Radical psychiatry in Italy: "Love is not enough". In The Radical Therapist Collective. *The radical therapist* (J. Agel, Ed.; pp. 43–49). New York, NY: Ballantine Books.

Medicina Democratica [Democratic Medicine] (1985, January/February and March/April). Handicap: Prevenzione, riabilitazione e lavoro [Handicap: Prevention, Rehabilitation and Work] [Special Issue]. *Medicina Democcratica*, 46/47.

Meredith, K. (2000). Control: The fourth psychological hunger. *Transactional Analysis Journal*, 30(4), 285–291. DOI: 10.1177/036215370003000405

Merry, T. (Ed.) (2000). *The BAPCA reader*. Ross-on-Wye, UK: PCCS Books.

Merry, T. (2004). Supervision as heuristic research inquiry. In K. Tudor & M. Worrall (Eds.), *Freedom to practise: Person-centred approaches to supervision* (pp. 189–199). Ross-on-Wye, UK: PCCS Books.

Mills, M. & Topolski, C. (1996). Shanti: A women's therapy centre. *Counselling*, 7, 108–112.

Minikin, K. & Tudor, K. (2016). Gender psychopolitics: Men being, becoming, and belonging. In R. Erskine (Ed.), *Transactional analysis in contemporary psychotherapy* (pp. 257–275). London, UK: Karnac.

Minister of National Health and Welfare (1988). *Mental health for Canadians*. Ottawa, Canada: MNHW.

Ministry of Health (2010a). *Health Practitioners Competence Assurance Act 2003. Guidelines for the operation of restricted activities under the Health Practitioners Competence Assurance Act 2003*. Retrieved from www.moh.govt.nz/moh.nsf/indexmh/hpca-restricted-guidelines#amends.

Ministry of Health (2010b). *How do we determine if statutory regulation is the most appropriate way to regulate health professions? Discussion document*. Wellington, New Zealand: Ministry of Health. Document also available online at: www.health.govt.nz/publication/how-do-we-determine-if-statutory-regulation-most-appropriate-way-regulate-health-professions.

Ministry of Health | Manatu Hauora (2002). *Building on strengths: A new approach to promoting mental health in New Zealand/Aotearoa*. Wellington, Aotearoa New Zealand: Ministry of Health | Manatu Hauora.

Mitchell, J. (1975). *Psychoanalysis and feminism*. Harmondsworth, UK: Penguin.

Moiso, C. (1995). The commitments. *Transactional Analysis Journal*, 25(1), 75–76.

Moiso, C. (1998). Being and belonging. An appreciation and application of Berne's social psychiatry. *The Script*, 28(9), 1, 7.

Money, M. (1993). *Health and community*. Dartington, UK: Green Books.

Montero, M. (1984). *Ideología, alienación e identidad nacional* [Ideology, alienation and national identity]. Caracas, Venezuela: Ediciones de la Biblioteca de la Universidad Central de Venezuela.

Montero, M. (2007). The political psychology of liberation: from politics to ethics and back. *Political Psychology*, 5, 517–533. DOI: 10.1111/j.1467-9221.2007.00588.x

Moore, J. (1997). Who is the "person" in the person-centred approach? *Person-Centred Practice*, 5(2), 11–15.

Moreno, J. L. (1964). *Psychodrama. Vol 1* (rev. ed.). Beacon, NY: Beacon House. (Original work published 1946)

Moreno, J. L. (1978). *Who shall survive? Foundations of sociometry, group psychotherapy and sociodrama* (2nd ed.). Beacon, NY: Beacon House.

Morrell, J., Ricketts, T., Tudor, K., & Williams, C. (2011). Training health visitors in cognitive behavioural and person centred approaches for depression in postnatal women as part of a cluster randomised trial and economic evaluation in primary care: The PoNDER trial. *Primary Health Care Research & Development*, 12(1), 1–10. DOI: 10.1017/S1463423610000344

Mosher, L. R. & Burti, L. (1989). *Community mental health*. New York, NY: W. W. Norton.

Moustakas, C. (1961). *Loneliness*. Englewood Cliffs, NJ: Prentice Hall.

Moustakas, C. (1990). *Heuristic research: Design, methodology and applications*. London, UK: Sage.

Mowbray, R. (1995). *The case against psychotherapy registration*. London, UK: Transmarginal Press.

Murray, H. A. (1938). *Explorations in personality*. Oxford, UK: Oxford University Press.

Nandy, A. (1983). *The intimate enemy: Loss and recovery of self under colonialism*. Oxford, UK: Oxford University Press.

National Health Service Scotland (2001). *Our national health: A plan for action, a plan for change*. Edinburgh, UK: Scottish Executive.

National Institute for Health and Clinical Excellence (2009). *Defining mental health*. Retrieved from www.library.nhs.uk/mentalhealth/viewresource.aspx?resid=105867.

Naughton, M. & Tudor, K. (2006). Being white. *Transactional Analysis Journal*, 36(2), 159–171.

Neal, C. & Davies, D. (Eds.) (2000). *Pink therapy. Vol. 3: Issues in therapy with lesbian, gay, bisexual and transgender clients*. Buckingham, UK: Open University Press.

Neumann, J., Schroeder, H., & Voss, P. (1989). Mental health and well-being in the context of the health promotion concept. In J. Neumann, H. Schroeder & P. Voss (Eds.), *Mental health within the health promotion concept* (pp.3–17). Dresden, Germany: German Hygiene Museum/Copenhagen: WHO.

New Zealand Association of Counsellors (2010). *Discussion paper on the possibility of self-regulation for the counselling profession*. Retrieved from www.nzac.org.nz/Self%20Regulation%20Discussion%20Paper.pdf.

New Zealand Association of Psychotherapists. (2008). *Code of ethics*. Wellington, Aotearoa New Zealand: NZAP.

Nobles, W. W. (1973). Psychological research and the black self-concept: A critical review. *Journal of Social Issues*, 29(1), 11–31. DOI: 10.1111/j.1540–4560.1973.tb00055.x

Nocon, A. (1990, 11 April). No role for collaboration in the market place. *Insight*, 27.

Nuttall, J. (2009). *Revisions required by examination board following an oral examination*. [Form RD (E-Revs) 2003 to the candidate]. Middlesex University, London, UK.

Nuttall, J. (2010). *Further revisions required by examination board following an oral examination*. [E-mail to the candidate]. Middlesex University, London, UK.

Ogden, C. L., Carroll, M. D., Curtin, L. R., McDowell, M. A., Tabak, C. J., & Flegal, K. M. (2006). Prevalence of overweight and obesity in the United States, 1994–2004. *Journal of the American Medical Association*, 295(13), 1549–1555. DOI: 10.1001/jama.295.13.1549

O'Hara, M. (1986). Heuristic inquiry as psychotherapy. *Person-Centered Review*, 1(2), 172–184.

Onnis, L. & Lo Rosso, G. (Eds.) (1980). *Dove va la Psichiatria?* [Where is psychiatry going?] Milano, Italy: Feltrinelli.

Orange, D. (2012). Clinical hospitality: Welcoming the face of the devastated other. *Ata: Journal of Psychotherapy Aotearoa New Zealand*, 16(2), 165–178.

Panksepp, J. (1998). *Affective neuroscience: The foundations of human and animal emotions*. Oxford, UK: Oxford University Press.
Papeschi, R. (1985). The denial of the institution: A critical review of Franco Basaglia's writings. *British Journal of Psychiatry*, 146, 247–254. DOI: 10.1192/bjp.146.3.247
Parker, I. & Revelli, S. (Eds.) (2008). *Psychoanalytic practice and state regulation*. London, UK: Karnac.
Parkinson, J. (2007). *Establishing a core set of national, sustainable mental health indicators for adults in Scotland: Rationale paper*. Glasgow, UK: NHS Health Scotland. Paper also available online at: www.healthscotland.com/uploads/documents/5289-Final%20rationale%20paper.pdf.
Parmar, P. (Producer) (2013). *Alice Walker: Beauty in Truth* [Film]. San Francisco, CA: Kali Films.
Parr, J. (2008). [Letter to the Editors]. *Transactional Analysis Journal*, 38(3), 259–260.
Penn, B. & Langton, J. (1980, 10 July). Special report on a habit that can kill. *Shepherds Bush Gazette & Hammersmith Post*, p. 5.
Perls, F. S., Hefferline, R. F., & Goodman, P. (1973). *Gestalt therapy: Excitement and growth in the human personality*. Harmondsworth, UK: Penguin. (Original work published 1951)
Petchkovsky, L., San Roque, C., & Beskow, M. (2003). Jung and the dreaming: analytical psychology's encounters with Aboriginal culture. *Transacultural Psychiatry*, 40(2), 208–238. DOI: 10.1177/1363461503402005
Phillips, A. (1995). *On flirtation*. London, UK: Faber & Faber.
Philpot, T. (1990, 26 July). Comment, April fooled. *Community Care*, p. 13.
Pihama, L. (1993). *Tungia te ururua, kia tupu whakaritorito te tupu o te harakeke: A critical analysis of parents as first teachers* (Master's thesis). University of Auckland: Auckland, Aotearoa New Zealand.
Pihama, L. (2001). *Tihei mauri ora, honouring our voices: Mana wahine as a kaupapa Māori theoretical framework*. Unpublished doctoral dissertation, University of Auckland, Auckland, Aotearoa New Zealand.
Pine, F. (1990). *Drive. ego. object and self: A synthesis for clinical work*. New York, NY: Basic Books.
Piro, S. & Oddati, A. (1983). *La riforma psichiatrica del 1978 e il Meridone d'Italia*. [The 1978 psychiatric reform and Southern Italy.] Roma, Italia: Il Pensiero Scientifico Editore.
Pohatu, T. W. (2005). *Āta: Growing respectful relationships*. Unpublished doctoral dissertation, University of Auckland: Auckland, Aotearoa New Zealand.
Polanyi, M. (1964). *Science, faith and society*. Chicago, IL: University of Chicago Press.
Polanyi, M. (1969). *Knowing and being* (M. Grene, Ed.). Chicago, IL: University of Chicago Press.
Polanyi, M. (1983). *The tacit dimension*. Gloucester, MA: Peter Smith.
Porter, R. (1990). *Mind-forg'd manacles*. London, UK: Penguin.
Postle, D. (2007). *Regulating the psychological therapies: From taxonomy to taxidermy*. Ross-on-Wye, UK: PCCS Books.
Postle, D. & House, R. (Eds.), (2009). *Compliance? Ambivalence? Rejection? Nine papers challenging the Health Professions Council proposals for the state regulation of the psychological therapies*. London, UK: Wentworth Learning Resources/Eipnosos.
Pressman, E. R. (Producer) & Stone, O. (Director) (1987). *Wallstreet* [Film]. Los Angeles, CA: 20th Century Fox.
Preston, G. H. (1943). *The substance of mental health*. New York, NY: Farrar & Rinehart.
Price, D. A. (1978). Social-psychological roots of transactional analysis: Exchange as symbolic interaction. *Transactional Analysis Journal*, 8(3), 212–215. DOI: 10.1177/036215377800800306
Prochaska, J. O. & DiClemente, C. C. (1992). *The transtheoretical approach: Crossing the traditional boundaries of therapy*. Homewood, IL: Dow Jones-Irwin.
Prouty, G. F. (1994). *Theoretical evolutions in person-centered/experiential therapy: Applications to schizophrenic and retarded psychoses*. Westport, CT: Praeger.
Prouty, G. F., Van Werde, D., & Pörtner, M. (2002). *Pre-therapy*. Ross-on-Wye, UK: PCCS Books.

Pullman, P. (2003–2007). *His dark materials trilogy*. New York, NY: Laurel Leaf.
Radical Therapist Collective (1971). *The radical therapist* (J. Agel, Ed.). New York, NY: Ballantine Books.
Raeburn, J. & Rootman, I. (1998). *People-centred health promotion*. Chichester, UK: Wiley.
Ramon, S. (1982). The logic of pragmatism in mental health policy: The implications of the government position on mental health in the 1959 debate for the 80s. *Critical Social Policy*, 2(2), 38–54.
Ramon, S. (1983). Psichiatrica democratica: A case study of an Italian community mental health service. *International Journal of Health Services*, 13, 307–324.
Red Notes and Conference of Socialist Economists (1979). *Working class autonomy and the crisis*. London, UK: Red Notes/CSE Books.
Reich, W. (1970). *The mass psychology of fascism* (V. R. Carfagno, Trans.). Harmondsworth, UK: Penguin. (Original work published 1933)
Reich, W. (1972a). *Character analysis* (V. R. Carfagno, Trans.; 3rd ed.). New York, NY: Farrar, Straus & Giroux. (Original work published 1933)
Reich, W. (1972b). What is class consciousness? In L. Baxandal (Ed.), *Sex-pol essays, 1929–1934* (A. Bostock, T. DuBose & L. Baxandal, Trans.; pp. 276–319). New York, NY: Vintage. (Original work published 1934)
Riebel, L. (1996). Self-sealing doctrines, the misuse of power, and recovered memory. *Transactional Analysis Journal*, 26(1), 40–45. DOI: 10.1177/036215379602600108
Rigney, M. (1981). *A critique of Maslow's self-actualization theory: The "highest good" for the aboriginal is relationship* [Videotape]. Aboriginal Open College, Adelaide, Australia.
Rogers, A. & Faulkner, A. (1987). *A place of safety*. London, UK: MIND Publications.
Rogers, C. R. (1942). *Counseling and psychotherapy: Newer concepts in practice*. Boston, MA: Houghton Mifflin.
Rogers, C. R. (1951). *Client-centered therapy*. London, UK: Constable.
Rogers, C. R. (1957). The necessary and sufficient conditions of therapeutic personality change. *Journal of Consulting Psychology*, 21(1), 95–103.
Rogers, C. R. (1959). A theory of therapy, personality, and interpersonal relationships as developed in the client-centered framework. In S. Koch (Ed.), *Psychology: The study of a science Vol. 3. Formulations of the person and the social context* (pp. 184–256). New York, NY: McGraw-Hill.
Rogers, C. R. (1963). The actualizing tendency in relation to "motive" and to consciousness. In M. Jones (Ed.), *Nebraska symposium on motivation 1963* (pp. 1–24). Lincoln, NE: University of Nebraska Press.
Rogers, C. R. (1967a). A process conception of psychotherapy. In *On becoming a person* (pp. 125–159). London, UK: Constable. (Original work published 1958)
Rogers, C. R. (1967b). Some of the directions evident in therapy. In *On becoming a person* (pp. 73–106). London, UK: Constable. (Original work published 1953)
Rogers, C. R. (1969). *Freedom to learn*. Columbus, OH: C. E. Merrill.
Rogers, C. R. (1973a). *Carl Rogers on encounter groups*. New York, NY: Harper and Row. (Original work published 1970)
Rogers, C. R. (1973b). Some new challenges to the helping professions. *American Psychologist*, 28(5), 379–387.
Rogers, C. R. (1978). *Carl Rogers on personal power: Inner strength and its revolutionary impact*. London, UK: Constable.
Rogers, C. R. (1980). *A way of being*. Boston, MA: Houghton Mifflin. (Original work published 1977)
Rogers, C. (1983). *Freedom to learn for the 80s*. New York, NY: Macmillan. (Original work published 1969)
Rogers, C. R. (1990a). Some new challenges to the helping professions. In H. Kirschenbaum & V. L. Henderson (Eds.), *The Carl Rogers reader* (pp. 357–375). London, UK: Constable. (Original work published 1973)
Rogers, C. R. (1990b). The necessary and sufficient conditions of therapeutic personality change. In H. Kirschenbaum & V. L. Henderson (Eds.), *The Carl Rogers reader* (pp. 219–235). London, UK: Constable. (Original work published 1957)

Rogers, C. R. & Freiberg, H. J. (1994). *Freedom to learn* (3rd ed.). Columbus, OH: Charles E. Merrill.

Rogers, N., Tudor, K., Embleton Tudor, L., & Keemar, K. (2012). Person-centred expressive arts therapy: A theoretical encounter. *Person-Centered & Experiential Psychotherapies*, 11(1), 31–47. DOI: 10.1080/14779757.2012.656407

Ronningstarn, E. (2005). *Identifying and understanding the narcissistic personality*. Oxford, UK: Oxford University Press.

Rough Times Staff (1973). *Rough times* (J. Agel, Producer). New York, NY: Ballantine Books.

Rowan, J. (1985). Listening as a four-level activity. *British Journal of Psychotherapy:* 1(4) 274–285.

Roy, B. (1988). Loss of power – Alienation. In B. Roy & C. Steiner (Eds.), *Radical psychiatry: The second decade* (pp. 3–13). Retrieved 8 December, 2007, from www.emotional-literacy.comlrpO.htm.

Roy, B. & Steiner, C. M. (Eds.) (1988). *Radical psychiatry: The second decade*. Unpublished manuscript available from Beth Roy, 270 Street, San Francisco, USA.

Royal College of Psychiatrists' Council (1988). The Royal College of Psychiatrists' comments on the Griffiths Report: "Community care: Agenda for action". *Bulletin of the Royal College of Psychiatrists*, 12(9), 385–388.

Rust, M.-J. (2004). Creating psychotherapy for a sustainable future. *Psychotherapy and Politics International*, 2(1), 50–63. DOI: 10.1002/ppi.69

Sacks, O. (1991). *Awakenings*. London, UK: Picador.

Sacks, O. (1995). *An anthroplogist on Mars: Seven paradoxical tales*. London, UK: Picador.

Samuels, A. (1993). *The political psyche*. London, UK: Routledge.

Samuels, A. (1997). Pluralism and the future of psychotherapy. In S. Palmer & V. Varma (Eds.), *The future of psychotherapy and counselling* (pp. 132–152). London, UK: Sage.

Sanders, P. & Tudor, K. (2001). This is therapy: A person-centred critique of the contemporary psychiatric system. In C. Newnes, G. Holmes & C. Dunn (Eds.), *This is madness too: Critical perspectives on mental health Services* (pp. 147–160). Ross-on-Wye, UK: PCCS Books.

Sandle, R. (2015). Viewing conflict through a reconstruction of the application of psychodynamic sexual theory in transactional analysis. *Transactional Analysis Journal*, 45(4), 289–300.

Sayce, L. (1989). Community mental health centres – Rhetoric and reality. In A. Brackx & C. Grimshaw (Eds.), *Mental health care in crisis* (pp. 158–174). London, UK: Pluto Press.

Sayce, L. (1990, August/September). Case reforms dislocated. *OpenMind*, 46, 5.

Schmid, P. (1998). On becoming a person-centred approach: A person-centred understanding of the person. In B. Thorne, & E. Lambers (Eds.), *Person-centred therapy: A European perspective* (pp. 38–52). London, UK: Sage.

Schmid, P. (2006a). [Review of *Working at relational depth in counselling and psychotherapy*, by D. Mearns & M. Cooper]. *Person-Centered & Experiential Psychotherapies*, 5(2), 149–151.

Schmid, P. (2006b). The challenge of the Other: Towards dialogical person-centered psychotherapy. *Person-Centered & Experiential Psychotherapies*, 5(4), 240–254. DOI: 10.1080/14779757.2006.9688416

Schmid, P. (2007). *Psychotherapy is political or it is not psychotherapy: The actualizing tendency as personalizing tendency*. Keynote speech, Annual Conference of the British Association for the Person-Centred Approach, Cirencester, UK.

Schmid, P. (2012). Psychotherapy is political or it is not psychotherapy: The person-centred approach as an essentially political venture. *Psychotherapy and Politics International*, 12(1), 4–17.

Schofield, M. (1971). *The strange case of pot*. Middlesex, UK: Penguin.

Schon, D. A. (1983). *The reflective practitioner*. New York, NY: Basic Books.

Schumacher, E. F. (1989). *Small is beautiful: Economics as if people mattered*. New York, NY: Harper & Row. (Original work published 1973)

Schutzman, M. (1994). Brechtian shamanism: The political therapy of Augusto Boal. In M. Schutzman & J. Cohen-Cruz (Eds.), *Playing Boal: Theatre, therapy and activism* (pp. 137–156). London, UK: Routledge.

Scottish Council Foundation (2001). *The possible human: America's approach*. Edinburgh: Scottish Council Foundation.

Sève, L. (1975). *Marxism and the theory of human personaliy*. London, UK: Lawrence & Wishart.

Seyle, H. (1956). *The stress of life*. New York, NY: McGraw-Hill.

Shakespeare, W. (1997). *Macbeth* (A. R. Braunmuller, Ed.). Cambridge, UK: Cambridge University Press. (Original work published 1623)

Shenker, B. (1986). *Intentional communities: Ideology and alienation in communal societies*. London, UK: Routledge & Kegan Paul.

Shweder, R. A. (1990). Cultural psychology – What is it? In J. W. Syigler, R. A. Schweder & G. Herdt (Eds.), *Cultural psychology*. Cambridge, UK: Cambridge University Press.

Sills, C. & Hargaden, H. (2003). An introduction, some reflections and a challenge. In C. Sills & H. Hargaden (Eds.), *Ego states* (Key concepts in transactional analysis: Contemporary views) (pp. ix–xxiii). London, UK: Worth Publishing.

Singh, J. & Tudor, K. (1997). Cultural conditions of therapy. *The Person-Centred Journal*, 4(2), 32–46.

Smith, B. & Tudor, K. (2003). Oppression and pedagogy: Anti-oppressive practice in the education of therapists. In. C. Lago & B. Smith (Eds.), *Anti-discriminatory counselling practice* (pp. 135–150). London, UK: Sage.

Smith, C. J. (1984). Geographical approaches to mental health. In H. L. Freeman (Ed.), *Mental health and the environment* (pp. 121–168). New York, NY: Churchill Livingstone.

Smith, G. (1997). *The development of kaupapa Māori theory and praxis*. Unpublished doctoral dissertation, University of Auckland: Auckland, Aotearoa New Zealand.

Smith, J. B. (2011). Licensing of psychotherapists in the United States: Evidence of societal regression? *Transactional Analysis Journal*, 41, 139–146. DOI: 10.1177/036215371104100209

Smith, K. & Tudor, K. (2015). To be or not to be registered: Is that the question? *Asia Pacific Journal of Counselling & Psychotherapy*, 1&2, 3–16. DOI: 10.1080/21507686.2015.1091020

Smith, L. (1999). *Decolonizing methodologies: Research and indigenous peoples*. Dunedin, Aotearoa New Zealand: Zed Books.

Smith-Merry, J. (2008). Improving mental health and wellbeing in Scotland: A model policy approach. *Australian e-Journal for the Advancement of Mental Health*, 7(3), 1–10, www.auseinet.com/journal/vol7iss3/smith-merry.pdf.

Smuts, J. (1987). *Holism and evolution*. New York, NY: Macmillan. (Original work published 1926)

Sontag, S. (1978). *Illness as metaphor*. New York, NY: Farrar, Straus & Giroux.

Stafford, E. M. (1982). The impact of the youth opportunities programme on young people's employment prospects and psychological well-being. *British Journal of Guidance and Counselling*, 10(1), 12–21. DOI: 10.1080/03069888200760021

Stafford, E, M., Jackson, P. R., & Banks, M. H. (1980). Employment, work involvement and mental health in less qualified young people. *Journal of Occupational Psychology*, 53, 291–304.

Standing Nursing and Midwifery Advisory Committee (1999). *Mental health nursing: Addressing acute concerns*. London, UK: DoH.

Stark, M. (1999). *Modes of therapeutic action: Enhancement of knowledge, provision of experience, engagement in relationship*. Northvale, NJ: Jason Aronson.

Steiner, C. M. (1966). Script and counterscript. *Transactional Analysis Bulletin*, 5(18), 133–135.

Steiner, C. M. (1971a). *Games alcoholics play: The analysis of life scripts*. New York, NY: Ballantine Books.

Steiner, C. M. (1971b). Radical psychiatry manifesto. In The Radical Therapist Collective. *The radical therapist* (J. Agel, Ed.; pp. 280–282). New York, NY: Ballantine Books.

Steiner, C. M. (1971c). Radical psychiatry: Principles. In The Radical Therapist Collective. *The radical therapist* (J. Agel, Ed.; pp. 3–7). New York, NY: Ballantine Books.

Steiner, C. M. (1971d). The stroke economy. *Transactional Analysis Journal*, 1(3), 9–15.

Steiner, C. M. (1981). *The other side of power*. New York, NY: Grove Press.

Steiner, C. M. (1984). Emotional literacy. *Transactional Analysis Journal*, 14, 162–173. DOI: 10.1177/036215379602600107

Steiner, C. M. (2000). Radical psychiatry. In R. J. Corsini (Ed.), *Handbook of innovative therapy* (pp. 578–586). Chichester, UK: Wiley.

Steiner, C. M. (2003). Core concepts of a stroke-centered transactional analysis. *Transactional Analysis Journal*, 33(2), 178–181. DOI: 10.1177/036215370303300209

Steiner, C. & Tudor, K (2014, 7 August). *Still radical after all these years: TA and politics*. Workshop presented at the International Transactional Analysis Association World Conference, San Francisco, California, USA.

Steiner, C. & Wyckoff, H. (1975). Alienation. In C. Steiner, H. Wyckoff, O. Goldstine, P. Lariviere, R. Schwebel, J. Marcus & Members of The Radical Psychiatry Center (Eds.), *Readings in radical psychiatry* (pp. 17–27). New York, NY: Grove Press.

Steiner, C., Wyckoff, H., Goldstine, O., Lariviere, P., Schwebel, R., Marcus, J., & Members of The Radical Psychiatry Center (Eds.) (1975). *Readings in radical psychiatry*. New York, NY: Grove Press.

Stephens, T. (1998). *Population health in Canada*. Toronto, Canada: Health Canada Mental Health Promotion Unit.

Stephens, T., Dulberg, C., & Joubert, N. (1999). Mental health of the Canadian population: A comprehensive analysis. *Chronic Diseases in Canada*, 20(3), 18–126.

Stern, D. (1985). *The interpersonal world of the infant: A view from psychoanalysis and developmental psychology*. New York, NY: Basic Books

Stern, D. N. (2004). *The present moment: In psychotherapy and everyday life*. New York, NY: W. W. Norton.

Stewart, I. (1996). *Developing transactional analysis counselling*. London, UK: Sage.

Stewart, I. & Joines, V. (2002). *Personality adaptations: A new guide to human understanding in psychotherapy and counselling*. Nottingham, UK: Lifespace Publishing.

Stewart, I. & Joines, V. (2012). *Personality adaptations: A new guide to human understanding in psychotherapy and counselling* (2nd ed.). Nottingham, UK: Lifespace Publishing.

Stewart, S. (Ed.) (1998). *The possible Scot: Making healthy public policy*. Edinburgh, UK: Scottish Council Foundation.

Stewart-Harawira, M. (2005). *The imperial order: Indigenous responses to globalization*. Wellington, Aotearoa New Zealand: Huia.

Stone, O. (Director) (1987). *Wall Street*. Los Angeles, CA: 20th Century Fox.

Summers, G. & Tudor, K. (2000). Cocreative transactional analysis. *Transactional Analysis Journal*, 30,(1), 23–40. DOI: 10.1177/036215370003000104

Suzuki, S. (1999). *Zen mind, beginner's mind* (rev, ed.). New York, NY: Weatherhill.

Symor, N. K. (1977). The dependency cycle: Implications for theory, therapy and social action. *Transactional Analysis Journal*, 7(1), 37–43.

Taft, J. (1933). *The dynamics of therapy in a controlled relationship*. New York, NY: Macmillan.

Thomlison, B. (1999). [Review of *Mental health promotion* by K. Tudor]. *Community Mental Health*, 35(5), 478–479.

Thorne, B. (1995). The accountable therapist: Standards, experts and poisoning the well. *Self & Society*, 23(4), 31–38.

Tosi, M. T., Cassoni, E., Cavallero, G., Moiso, C., Novellino, M., Quagliotti, L. ... Scilligo, P. (2008). Perspectives on theories of the unconscious in transactional analysis. *Transactional Analysis Journal*, 38(3), 247–257.

Totton, N. (1997). The Independent Practitioners Network: A new model of accountability. In R. House & N. Totton (Eds.), *Implausible professions: Arguments for pluralism and autonomy in psychotherapy and counselling* (pp. 287–293/41). Ross-on-Wye, UK: PCCS Books.

Totton, N. (1999). The baby and the bathwater: "Professionalisation" in psychotherapy and counselling. *British Journal of Guidance and Counselling*, 27(3), 313–324.

Totton, N. (2000). *Psychotherapy and politics*. London, UK: Sage.

Travis, A. & Brindle, D. (1990, 11 July). Howe signals delay in care programme. *The Guardian*, p. 20.

Trevillian, S. (1988/1989). Griffiths and Wagner: Which future for community care? *Critical Social Policy*, 24, 65–73.

Truax, C. B. & Carkhuff, R. R. (1967). *Toward effective counseling and psychotherapy. Training and practice*. Chicago, IL: Aldine.

Tudor, K. (1979). *The wrongs of women: Feminism and theory, women and crime*. Unpublished master's dissertation, Department of Social Work, University of Kent at Canterbury, UK.

Tudor, K. (1988). *"Truth is sweet": A critical overview of Italian mental health reform*. Unpublished manuscript.

Tudor, K. (1989, 2 May). People in glass houses. *The Voice*, p. 2.

Tudor, K. (1990a, 28 June). *Conceptualising mental health promotion*. Paper presented at Health in Mind conference organised by South East Thames Regional Health Authority, Canterbury, Kent, UK.

Tudor, K. (1990b). One step back, two steps forward: Community care and mental health. *Critical Social Policy*, 10(30), 5–22.

Tudor, K. (1992). Community mental health promotion – A paradigm approach. In D. R. Trent (Ed.), *Promotion of mental health*. Vol. 1 (pp. 127–138). Aldershot, UK: Avebury.

Tudor, K. (1993). *Masculinity and violence*. Unpublished research monograph. Management Centre, King's College, University of London, UK.

Tudor, K. (1996a). Mental health promotion at work. In D. R. Trent & C. A. Reed (Eds.), *Promotion of mental health*. Vol. 5 (pp. 127–143). Aldershot, UK: Avebury.

Tudor, K. (1996b). *Mental health promotion: Paradigms and practice*. London, UK: Routledge.

Tudor, K. (1996c). Transactional analysis *intra*gration: A metatheoretical analysis for practice. *Transactional Analysis Journal*, 26(4) 329–340.

Tudor, K. (1997a). Being at dis-ease with ourselves: Alienation and psychotherapy. *Changes*, 22(2), 143–150.

Tudor, K. (1997b). Mental health promotion: The contribution of psychotherapy. In M. Money & L. Buckley (Eds.), *Positive mental health and its promotion* (pp. 21–24). Liverpool, UK: John Moores University Institute for Health.

Tudor, K. (1997c). Social contracts: Contracting for social change. In C. Sills (Ed.), *Contracts in counselling* (pp. 207–215). London, UK: Sage.

Tudor, K. (1997d). The personal is political – and political is personal: A person-centred approach to the political sphere. *Person-Centred Practice*, 5(2), 4–10.

Tudor, K. (Ed). (1997e). The person-centred approach and the political sphere [Special issue]. *Person-Centred Practice*, 5(2).

Tudor, K. (1998). Value for money: Issues of fees in counselling and psychotherapy. *British Journal of Guidance and Counselling*, 26(4), 477–493. DOI: 10.1080/03069889808253858

Tudor, K. (1999a). *Group counselling*. London, UK: Sage.

Tudor, K. (1999b). Promoting mental health at work. In *Organisational, legal and political issues in occupational health care*. Distance learning paper. Aberdeen, UK: University of Aberdeen Faculty of Nursing, Midwifery and Community Studies.

Tudor, K. (1999c, 8 April). *The case against the state regulation of psychotherapy*. Talk to the Trainers' Meeting, Institute of Transactional Analysis Annual Conference, Edinburgh, UK.

Tudor, K. (1999d). What is mental health promotion? In *Organisational, legal and political issues in occupational health care*. Distance learning paper. Aberdeen, UK: University of Aberdeen Faculty of Nursing, Midwifery and Community Studies.

Tudor, K. (2000). The case of the lost conditions. *Counselling*, 11(1), 33–37.

Tudor, K. (2001). Change, time, place and community. In P. Lapworth, C. Sills & S. Fish *Integration in counselling and psychotherapy* (pp. 142–151). London, UK: Sage.

Tudor, K. (2003). The neopsyche: The integrating adult ego state. In C. Sills & H. Hargaden (Eds.), *Ego states* (pp. 201–231). London, UK: Worth Reading.
Tudor, K. (2006, 6 April). *All the "...onomies": Autonomy and homonomy in the face of heteronomy*. Pre Conference Institute, Institute of Transactional Analysis Annual Conference, Exeter, UK.
Tudor, K. (2007a, February). Exam exegesis. *EATA Newsletter*, 88, 16–20.
Tudor, K. (2007b). Geestelijk gezond; Autonoom én homonoom [Psychological health: Autonomy and homonomy]. *Tijdshrift Cliëntgerichte Psychotherapie*, 45(1), 5–18.
Tudor, K. (2007c, 4 July). *Independence day: Life, liberty and the pursuit of happiness, or, Interdependence* days: *Organismic life, freedom and the pursuit of homonomy*. Lecture to the Counselling Diploma Course, Faculty of Health and Applied Social Sciences, Liverpool John Moores University, Liverpool, UK.
Tudor, K. (2007d, 27 September). *In/out, this/that, we/them: Balancing polarities*. Keynote Speech to the First Conference of South Asian Association of Transactional Analysts, Coimbatore, Tamil Nadu, India.
Tudor, K. (2007e, 13 April). *On dogma*. Paper presented at the Institute of Transactional Analysis Annual Conference, York, UK.
Tudor, K. (2007f, 26 January). *Person-centred therapy: Foundations, fundamentals and fundamentalism*. Keynote speech at the Annual Congress of the Vereniging voor Cliëntgerichte Psychotherapie (VCgP) [Dutch Society of Client-Centered Therapy], Amersfoort, Holland.
Tudor, K. (2007g). Training in the person-centred approach. In M. Cooper, M. O'Hara, P. Schmid & G. Wyatt (Eds.), *The handbook of person-centred therapy* (pp. 379–389). Basingstoke, UK: Palgrave.
Tudor, K. (Ed.) (2008a). *Brief person-centred therapies*. London, UK: Sage.
Tudor, K. (2008b). L'analisi transazionale o è radicale o non è analisi transazionale [Transactional analysis is radical or it is not transactional analysis]. *Neopsiche*, 6, 8–20.
Tudor, K. (2008c). [Letter to the Editors]. *Transactional Analysis Journal*, 38(3), 260–262.
Tudor, K. (2008d). Person-centred therapy, a cognitive behavioural therapy. In R. House & D. Loewenthal (Eds.), *Against and for CBT: Towards a constructive dialogue?* (pp. 118–136). Ross-on-Wye, UK: PCCS Books.
Tudor, K. (2008e). Psychological health: Autonomy and homonomy. In B. Levitt (Ed.), *Reflections on human potential: Bridging the person-centered approach and positive psychology* (pp. 161–174). Ross-on-Wye, UK: PCCS Books.
Tudor, K. (2008f). "Take it": A sixth driver. *Transactional Analysis Journal*, 38(1), 43–57.
Tudor, K. (2008g). Therapy is a verb. *Therapy Today*, 19(1), 35–37.
Tudor, K. (2008h). Verbal being: From being human to human being. In B. Levitt (Ed.), *Reflections on human potential: Bridging the person-centered approach and positive psychology* (pp. 68–83). Ross-on-Wye, UK: PCCS Books.
Tudor, K. (2009a, 1 July). *Building bridges across troubled waters: Regarding humanistic and psychodynamic psychotherapies*. Talk given to the Hallam Institute, Sheffield, UK.
Tudor, K. (2009b, 24 September). *Building bridges across troubled waters: Regarding humanistic and psychodynamic psychotherapies*. Lecture given at the AUT Psychotherapy Forum, Auckland University of Technology, Auckland, Aotearoa New Zealand.
Tudor, K. (2009c). "In the manner of": Transactional analysis teaching of transactional analysts. *Transactional Analysis Journal*, 39(4), 276–292.
Tudor, K. (2009d, 7 November). *Psyche and society: The contribution of psychotherapy to community wellbeing*. Keynote speech at International Public Mental Health Symposium: Toward Global Wellbeing, Auckland University of Technology, Auckland, Aotearoa New Zealand.
Tudor, K. (2010a). Being in process, being in context: A person-centred perspective on happiness. In D. Loewenthal & R. House (Eds.), *Critically engaging CBT* (pp. 84–97). Buckingham, UK: Open University Press.
Tudor, K. (2010b). Building bridges across troubled waters: Regarding humanistic and psychodynamic psychotherapies. *Forum* [The Journal of the New Zealand Association of Psychotherapists], 15, 8–25.

Tudor, K. (2010c). Regulation and registration: Protection or protectionism? A plea for pluralism. *The TAttler* [Newsletter of the New Zealand Transactional Analysis Association], 14(2), 4–10.

Tudor, K. (2010d, 15 March). *Relational transactional analyses*. A talk given at the Auckland Transactional Analysis Training Institute, St Luke's Church Centre, Auckland, Aotearoa New Zealand.

Tudor, K. (2010e). *The fight for health: A heuristic enquiry into psychological well-being*. Unpublished context statement for PhD in Mental Health Promotion by Public (Published) Works, School of Health and Social Sciences, Middlesex University, London, UK.

Tudor, K. (2010f). The state of the ego: Then and now. *Transactional Analysis Journal*, 40(3&4), 261–277.

Tudor, K. (2011a). Empathy: A co-creative perspective. *Transactional Analysis Journal*, 41(4), 322–335.

Tudor, K. (2011b, 10 March). *Regulation and registration*. A talk at the New Zealand Association of Psychotherapists' Northern Branch Meeting, Parnell Community Centre, Auckland, Aotearoa New Zealand.

Tudor, K. (2011c). Rogers' therapeutic conditions: A relational conceptualization. *Person-Centered & Experiential Psychotherapies*, 10(3), 165–180. DOI: 10.1080/14779757.2011.599513

Tudor, K. (2011d). The law is an Act: The Health Practitioners Competence Assurance Act 2003. In K. Tudor (Ed.), *The turning tide: Pluralism and partnership in psychotherapy in Aotearoa New Zealand* (pp. 39–68). Auckland, Aotearoa New Zealand: LC Publications.

Tudor, K. (Ed.) (2011e). *The turning tide: Pluralism and partnership in psychotherapy in Aotearoa New Zealand*. Auckland, Aotearoa New Zealand: LC Publications.

Tudor, K. (2011f). Understanding empathy. *Transactional Analysis Journal*, 41(1), 39–57. DOI: 10.1177/036215371104100107

Tudor, K. (2011g, 1 July). *Transactional analysis, radical psychiatry, and politics*. A talk given to PerFormat [TA Training Institute], Pisa, Italy.

Tudor, K. (2012a). Ebb and flow: One year on from *The Turning Tide: Pluralism and Partnership in Psychotherapy in Aotearoa New Zealand*. *Psychotherapy and Politics International*, 10(2), 170–177. DOI: 10.1002/ppi.1271

Tudor, K. (Ed.) (2012b). Political Papers from the World Congress of Psychotherapy, Sydney 2011 [Special Issue]. *Psychotherapy and Politics International*, 10(2).

Tudor, K. (2012c). Southern psychotherapies. *Psychotherapy and Politics International*, 10(2), 116–129.

Tudor, K. (2013a). Back to the future: Carl Rogers' "new challenge" reviewed and renewed. *Self & Society: An International Journal for Humanistic Psychology*, 40(2), 17–24.

Tudor, K. (2013b). "Be careful what you wish for": Professional recognition, the statutory regulation of counselling, and the state registration of counsellors. *New Zealand Journal of Counselling*, 33(2), 46–69.

Tudor, K. (2013c). Person-centred psychology and therapy, ecopsychology and ecotherapy. *Person-Centred and Experiential Psychotherapies*, 12(4), 324–338. DOI: 10.1080/14779757.2013.855137

Tudor, K. (2013d, 4 July). *Politics, practice and the changing world*. Keynote speech to the New Zealand Tertiary Counsellors' Hui, AUT University, Auckland, Aotearoa New Zealand.

Tudor, K. (2014a). Introduction. In *Co-creative transactional analysis: Papers, dialogues, responses, and developments* (pp. xix–xxix). London, UK: Karnac Books.

Tudor, K. (2014b, 25 August). 疎外,異なる立場の専門家、精神科医 精神病理学への批判的かつ異文化的視点 [Alienation, aliens, and alienists: A critical and cross-cultural perspective on psychopathology]. Keynote speech to the Association of Japanese Clinical Psychology, Yokohama, Japan. Available at: http://www.ajcp.info/archive/33/000jikko0/data/20140825a_02.pdf.

Tudor, K. (2016a). Some critiques of person-centred theory from within and without the person centred "nation". In C. Lago & D. Charura (Eds.), *Person-centred counselling and psychotherapy: Origins, developments and contemporary applications*. Buckingham, UK: Open University/McGraw Hill.

Tudor, K. (2016b). "We are": The fundamental life position. *Transactional Analysis Journal*, 46(2), 164–176.

Tudor, K. & Begbie, F. (2005). *"Fit like?" Being, belonging and becoming in Grampian. A mental health promotion framework for Grampian 2005–2010*. Aberdeen, UK: NHS Grampian. Unpublished draft document. (A revised version published by NHS Grampian as *A Mental Health Improvement Framework for Grampian 2006–2008*)

Tudor, K. & Begg, K. (2016). Radical therapy: A critical review. *The Journal of Critical Psychology, Counselling and Psychotherapy*, 16(2), 81–92.

Tudor, K. & Grinter, C. (2014). Informing consent: Principles, process and practice. *Ata: Journal of Psychotherapy Aotearoa New Zealand*, 18(1), 51–65.

Tudor, K. & Hargaden, H. (2002). The couch and the ballot box: The contribution and potential of psychotherapy in enhancing citizenship. In C. Feltham (Ed.), *What's the good of counselling and psychotherapy: The benefits explained* (pp. 156–178). London, UK: Sage.

Tudor, K. & Hobbes, R. (2007). Transactional analysis. In W. Dryden (Ed.), *The handbook of individual therapy* (5th ed.; pp. 256–286). London, UK: Sage.

Tudor, K. & Merry, T. (2002). *Dictionary of person-centred psychology*. London, UK: Whurr.

Tudor, K. & Shaw, S. (2016). Health regulation and the prescription – and proscription – of educational practice. *Policy Futures in Education*, 14(2), 211–224.

Tudor, K. & Summers, G. (2014). *Co-creative transactional analysis: Papers, dialogues, responses, and developments*. London, UK: Karnac Books.

Tudor, K. & Widdowson, M. (2008). From client process to therapeutic relating: a critique of the process model and personality adaptations. *Transactional Analysis Journal*, 38(3), 218–232. DOI: 10.1177/036215370803800304

Tudor, K. & Worrall, M. (1994). Congruence reconsidered. *British Journal of Guidance and Counselling*, 22(4), 197–206.

Tudor, K. & Worrall, M. (Eds.) (2004). *Freedom to practise: Person-centred approaches to supervision*. Ross-on-Wye, UK: PCCS Books.

Tudor, K. & Worrall, M. (2006). *Person-centred therapy: A clinical philosophy*. London, UK: Routledge.

Tudor, K. & Worrall, M. (Eds.) (2007). *Freedom to practise II: Developing person-centred approaches to supervision*. Ross-on-Wye, UK: PCCS Books.

Union of Physically Impaired Against Segregation and The Disability Alliance (1976). *Fundamental principles of disability*. London, UK: Union of Physically Impaired Against Segregation and The Disability Alliance.

Union of Physically Impaired Against Segregation (1981, May). Aims and policy statement. *Disability Challenge*. http://disability-studies.leeds.ac.uk/files/library/UPIAS-fundamental-principles.pdf.

United Nations (1975). *Charter of rights for disabled people*. New York, NY: United Nations.

United Nations. (1979). *Convention on the elimination of all forms of discrimination against women*. New York, NY: Author.

United Nations. (1997). *Kyoto protocol to the United Nations framework convention on climate change*. New York, NY: Author.

United Nations. (1998). *Convention on the rights of the child*. New York, NY: Author.

Upstairs Project (1982). *The service and propoals for its evaluation*. Document available from The Upstairs Project (Hammersmith Crisi Centre Ltd.), 182 Hammersmith Road, Hammersmith, London W6 7DJ, UK.

van der Ploeg, J. (1993). Potatoes and knowledge. In M. Hobart (Ed.), *An anthropological critique* (pp. 209–226). London, UK: Routledge.

van Deurzen-Smith, E. (1996). Existential therapy. In W. Dryden (Ed.), *Handbook of individual therapy* (pp. 166–193). London, UK: Sage.

Viney, T. (1990). *Community care: Who's to benefit?* Unpublished manuscript. Available from Greenwich Welfare Rights Unit, Riverside House, Beresford St., London, UK.

Vitz, P. (1997). *Psychology as religion: The cult of self worship*. Grand Rapids, MI: William B. Eerdmans.

Waitangi Tribunal (2011). *The Treaty of Waitangi*. Retrieved 21 March, 2012, from www.waitangitribunal.govt.nz/treaty/

Wampold, B. (2001). *The great psychotherapy debate: Models, methods, and findings*. London, UK: Routledge.

Ware, P. (1983). Personality adaptations (Doors to therapy). *Transactional Analysis Journal*, 13(1), 11–19. DOI: 10.1177/036215378301300104

Ware, P. (1987). *Personality adaptations*. Workshop presented by the Southeast Institute for Group and Family Therapy, Chapel Hill, North Carolina, USA.

Warr, P. (1982). Psychological aspects of employment and unemployment. *Psychological Medicine*, 12, 7–11.

Warr, P. B., Cook, J. P., & Wall, T. D. (1979). Scales for the measurement of some work attitudes and aspects of psychological well-being. *Journal of Occupational Psychology*, 52, 129–148.

Watts, A. (1971). *Psychotherapy east and west*. London, UK: Vintage Books. (Original work published 1961)

Weare, K. (1996). Mental health in the school system: "The health promoting school" idea. In D. R. Trent & C. A. Reed (Eds.), *Promotion of mental health*. Vol. 5 (pp. 161–170). Aldershot, UK: Avebury.

Weare, K. (2000). *Promoting mental, emotional and social health: A whole school approach*. London, UK: Routledge.

West, M. (1990). *Lazarus*. London, UK: Methuen.

Westergren, R. M. (2011, 24 January). You say Australia, I say invasion. *The Economist*. Retrieved from www.economist.com.ezproxy.aut.ac.nz/blogs/banyan/2012/01/australias-aborigines.

Whitney, N. J. (1982). A critique of individual autonomy as the key to personhood. *Transactional Analysis Journal*, 12, 210–212.

Whittington, C. & Holland, R. (1985). A framework for theory in social work. *Issues in Social Work Education*, 5(1), 25–50.

Widiger, T. A. & Simonsen, E. (2006). Alternative dimensional models of personality disorder: Finding a common ground. In T. A. Widiger, E. Simonsen, P. J. Sirovatka & D. A. Regier (Eds.), *Dimensional models of personality disorders: Refining the research agenda for DSM–V* (pp. 1–21). Washington, DC: American Psychiatric Association.

Wiggins, S., Elliott, R., & Cooper, M. (2012). The prevalence and characteristics of relational depth events in psychotherapy. *Psychotherapy Research*, 22(2), 139–158. DOI: 10.1080/10503307.2011.629635

Wilde, O. (1997). The ballad of Reading gaol. In O. Wilde, *Collected works of Oscar Wilde* (pp. 891–909). London, UK: Wordsworth. (Original work published 1898)

Wilders, S. (2007, February). Relational depth and the person-centred approach. *Person-Centred Quarterly*, 1–4.

Windes, K. (1977). The three "C's" of corrections: Cops–Cons–Counselors. In G. Barnes (Ed.), *Transactional analysis after Eric Berne* (pp. 351–379). New York, NY: Harper's College Press.

Winnicott, D. W. (1986). Living creatively. In *Home is where we start from: Essays by a psychoanalyst* (C. Winnicott, R. Shepherd, & M. Davies, Comp. & Ed.) (pp. 35–55). New York: W. W. Norton. (Original work published 1970)

Winnicott, D. W. (1988). Introduction. In *Human nature* (pp. 1–3). London: Free Association Books.

Wood, J. K. (2008). *The person-centered approach of Carl Rogers: Toward an understanding of its implications*. Ross-on-Wye, UK: PCCS Books.

Woodard, W. (2008). *Entering the void: Exploring the relationship between the experience of colonisation and the experience of self for indigenous peoples of Aotearoa and the implications for clinical practice* (Unpublished master's dissertation). AUT University, Auckland, Aotearoa New Zealand.

Woollams, M. & Brown, M. (1978). *Transactional analysis*. Dexter, IL: Huron Valley Press.

World Health Organization (1978). *Mental disorders: Glossary and guide to their classification in accordance with the ninth revision of the International Classification of Diseases*. Geneva, Switzerland: WHO.

World Health Organization (1986). *Ottawa charter for health promotion*. Retrieved from http://www.who.int/healthpromotion/conferences/previous/ottawa/en/.

Wyckoff, H. (Ed.) (1976). *Love, therapy and politics*. New York, NY: Grove Press.

Wyss, D. (1966). *Depth psychology: A critical history*. London, UK: Allen & Unwin.

Yalom, I. D. (1985). *The theory and practice of group psychotherapy* (3rd ed.). New York, NY: Basic Books.

Zalcman, M. (1990). Game analysis and racket analysis: Overview, critique, and future developments. *Transactional Analysis Journal*, 20(1), 4–19. DOI: 10.1177/036215379002000102

Zimring, F. M. (1988). Attaining mastery. The shift from the "me" to the "I". *Person-Centered Review*, 3(2), 165–175.

Zuboff, S. & Maxmin, J. (2004). *The support economy: Why corporations are failing individuals and the next episode of capitalism*. London, UK: Penguin.

AUTHOR INDEX

Given the nature of the book, I have not indexed my own work, except where it is co-authored.

For Product Safety Concerns and Information please contact our EU
representative GPSR@taylorandfrancis.com
Taylor & Francis Verlag GmbH, Kaufingerstraße 24, 80331 München, Germany

www.ingramcontent.com/pod-product-compliance
Ingram Content Group UK Ltd.
Pitfield, Milton Keynes, MK11 3LW, UK
UKHW011002180926
475701UK00004B/519

9781138207851